The use of embryonic and fetal tissues in the treatment and repair of diseased organs is a rapidly advancing field of scientific medicine. Sophisticated techniques offer the potential for powerful new forms of treatment. Our understanding of the processes involved in organ development and gene expression have considerable clinical implications and also lead to questions of ethical concern.

Professor Edwards is a pioneer of much of the research in applied human embryology and he has made a significant and invaluable contribution to knowledge in this field. In this book, he has brought together the research experience of many prominent scientists and clinicians whose work is at the forefront of current knowledge. The most recent scientific and clinical developments and techniques are presented, including both the transplantation of fetal tissue into mature recipients and the grafting of donor cells into fetuses which are known to be carrying genetic disease. The successes and failures of these techniques as a clinical treatment and therapeutic tool are discussed. The book begins with an overview of embryologic development: from fertilization to differentiation of cell lines and organogenesis. The transplantation of specific cell lines and tissue types is then considered. Transplantation techniques, donor–host interactions and immunology, cell and tissue storage are all discussed, as are the ethical issues and the legal implications.

This book will be of the greatest interest to clinicians and scientists concerned with human embryology as well as to neurologists, endocrinologists and others in fields where fetal tissue transplantation has clinical potential.

Fetal tissue transplants in medicine

Fetal tissue transplants
in medicine

Edited by

Robert G. Edwards

Professor Emeritus, Cambridge University
Extraordinary Fellow, Churchill College, Cambridge, UK

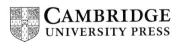
CAMBRIDGE
UNIVERSITY PRESS

Published by the Press Syndicate of the University of Cambridge
The Pitt Building, Trumpington Street, Cambridge CB2 1RP
40 West 20th Street, New York, NY 10011-4211, USA
10 Stamford Road, Oakleigh, Victoria 3166, Australia

First published 1992

Printed in Great Britain at the University Press, Cambridge

A catalogue record for this book is available from the British Library

Library of Congress cataloguing in publication data

Fetal tissue transplants in medicine / edited by Robert G. Edwards.
p.   cm.
Includes index.
ISBN 0-521-41075-4 (hardback)
1. Fetal tissues – Transplants. I. Edwards, R. G. (Robert Geoffrey), 1925–
[DNLM: 1. Fetal Tissue Transplants. WO 665 F419]
RD120.9.F48   1992
617.9'5 – dc20 91-37656 CIP
DNLM/DLC
for Library of Congress

ISBN 0 521 41075 4 hardback

SE

Contents

Contributors

M. ADINOLFI
Division of Medical and Molecular Genetics, Paediatric Research Unit, Prince Philip Research Laboratories, 7th and 8th Floors, Guy's Tower, Guy's Hospital, London SE1 9RT, UK.

M. J. ASHWOOD-SMITH
Department of Biology, University of Victoria, PO Box 1700, Victoria, British Columbia, Canada.

P. BRUNDIN
Department of Medical Cell Research, University of Lund, Biskopsgatan 5, S-223 62 Lund, Sweden.

M. J. COWAN
Department of Pediatrics, University of California, San Francisco, CA 94143-0105, USA.

S. B. DUNNETT
Department of Experimental Psychology, Downing Street, Cambridge CB2 3EB, UK.

R. G. EDWARDS
Churchill College, Storey's Way, Cambridge CB3 0DS, UK.

M. ELDER
Department of Pediatrics, University of California, San Francisco, CA 94143-0105, USA.

M. S. GOLBUS
Department of Obstetrics, Gynecology and Reproductive Sciences, Reproductive Genetics Unit, Room U-262, University of California, San Francisco, California 9413-0720, USA.

R. G. GOSDEN
Department of Physiology, University Medical School, Teviot Place, Edinburgh EH8 9AG, UK.

J. M. McCUNE
SyStemix Inc, 3400 W. Bayshore Road, Palo Alto, California 94303, USA.

J. KROWKA
SyStemix Inc, 3400 W. Bayshore Road, Palo Alto, California 94303, USA.

R. NAMIKAWA
SyStemix Inc, 3400 W. Bayshore Road, Palo Alto, California 94303, USA.

B. PÉAULT
SyStemix Inc, 3400 W. Bayshore Road, Palo Alto, California 94303, USA.

J. C. POLKINGHORNE
Queen's College, Silver Street, Cambridge CB3 9ET, UK.

T. W. SADLER
Department of Cell Biology and Anatomy, 108 Taylor Hall, CB 7090, University of North Carolina at Chapel Hill, Chapel Hill, NC 27599-7090, USA.

H. SAUER
Department of Medical Physiology, Pettenkoferstr. 12, D-8000 Munich 2, Germany.

J.-L. TOURAINE
Pavilion P, Département de Néphrologie, Médecine de Transplantation et Immunologique Clinique, Hôpitaux de Lyon, Lyon, France.

B. E. TUCH
Department of Medicine, University of Sydney, New South Wales 20066, Australia.

H. J. VÖLKER-DIEBEN
Diaconessenhuis, Houtlaan 55, 2334 CK Leiden, The Netherlands.

L. WONG
MRC Tissue Bank, Royal Marsden Hospital, Fulham Road, London SW3 6JJ, UK.

Preface

THE SUBJECT OF THIS BOOK has held my interest for many years. It was greatly stimulated in 1962, in John Paul's laboratory in Glasgow University, as we saw various types of tissue differentiate in outgrowths of stem cells from rabbit blastocysts. The implications of the work led me to the concept of using human blastocysts to obtain tissue cultures of stem cells for human grafting, and became one of the driving forces leading me to undertake human in vitro fertilization. Success has not come easily in obtaining these cell outgrowths from human embryos, although there are now promising leads in this direction. I trust that my dedication to the clinical application of this field is reflected in the pages of this book, and that it will stimulate more studies on grafting fetal tissue.

The book focusses on one of the many clinical uses of fetal tissue: for grafting into sick fetuses, children and adults of all ages. Fetal tissue has various known benefits. Tissues that are difficult to obtain from adults are more readily available from fetuses. Fetal tissue has already been widely applied in some forms of grafting, as in the reconstitution of the haemopoietic system in adults, even though tissue from adult donors who are closely related to the recipient is used more often. Large numbers of dynamic and adaptable fetal cells are available, capable of a sustained and widespread colonization of many tissues in both fetal and adult recipients. Fetal tissue might also offer advantages in avoiding graft rejection in a manner not matched by adult donor tissues. Finally, the astonishing ability of embryonic stem cells, sometimes modified genetically, to colonize preimplantation embryos may be of considerable value if it could be adapted for grafting into fetuses or adults.

The book is designed to progress through modern knowledge, beginning with chapters by Sadler and myself which provide the framework of embryonic differentiation and organogenesis in man. Successive contributions on the ontogeny of human immunity by Elder and co-authors, and on the value of experimental animals as experimental models by Péault and his colleagues provide data that is essential to investigate the value of fetal tissue in grafting. Most of the remaining chapters of the book describe specific clinical advantages of fetal tissue in the recolonization of particular recipient organs. These include its value for the restitution of haemopoietic tissue, brain, pancreas, cornea and reproductive tissues, in chapters written by Touraine, Sauer and co-authors, Tuch, Völker-Dieben and Gosden. The enormous clinical benefits now within sight in some of these fields are stressed, for some improvements recorded in some of the fetal or adult recipients are deeply impressive and promise to become widespread. Embryonic and fetal cells could also provide a permanent therapy for enzyme deficiencies in many recipients, and could be modified genetically before grafting, as discussed by Adinolfi. Ashwood-Smith deals with the low-temperature preservation of fetal cells, a necessity if they are to be of widespread use in grafting.

Despite these potential benefits, many people will object to the transplantation of fetal tissues, fearing that abortions will be done deliberately or indiscriminately, or fetuses will be conceived, to satisfy the need for donor tissues. Stringent ethical safeguards are therefore essential to guard against misconduct by professionals or patients. Two chapters deal with such ethical problems that are raised by the use of fetal tissue. Wong discusses how the procurement of fetal tissue has to be done with great care while maintaining a high ethical stance. Polkinghorne provides the background to guidelines issued on the complex and difficult ethical and legal issues raised by fetal tissue transplantation, and provides details of the new regulations which now control work on the collection and grafting of fetal tissues in the UK.

Editing this book has proved to be most stimulating and thought provoking. I thank the authors for their excellent contributions and my secretary Bev Watts for all her help.

R. G. Edwards
Churchill College
Cambridge

The front cover design includes a photograph by courtesy of T. W. Sadler (see p. 59); the back cover design includes a photograph by courtesy of R. G. Gosden (see p. 268).

CHAPTER 1

Differentiation and transplantation of embryonic cells in mammals

R. G. EDWARDS

CONTENTS

MANY INSIGHTS ON REGENERATION by grafting fetal and adult tissue into recipients can be gained by studying the differentiation and formation of the embryo. This chapter will relate work on grafting embryonic cells to knowledge on early mammalian embryology, and especially the regulatory factors involved in tissue formation. It is not intended to be a comprehensive analysis of early embryology, and cited references to books and review should be consulted for this purpose. References to work on amphibians and insects will be made where necessary. The differentiation of the human embryo to approximately day 20 will be considered to be the end of the embryonic phase when the primary organ systems have been established.

Embryonic differentiation to the blastocyst

Formation of the blastocyst

The initial stages of embryonic growth involve a cascade of regulatory events. After sperm entry into the oocyte, the sperm chromatin forms when disulphide bonds are cleaved and nuclear proteins degraded as

Table 1.1. *Approximate timing of some events during the first 14 days of human embryonic growth*

Day	Event	Carnegie Stage	Comment
0	Sperm entry	1	Maternal mRNA transcribed
1	2-cell	2	
2	4–8 cell		Embryonic mRNA transcribed
			Transcripts of HCGβ
			Polarization
3	Morula		Compaction
4–5	Formation of blastocyst	3	Blastocoel formed
			Transcripts for growth factors
6–7	Enlarging blastocyst	4–5	Hatching
			Secretion of HCG
			Epiblast forms
			Extraembryonic endoderm forms
8–9	Implantation	5	Syncytiotrophoblast forms
10	Amniotic cavity		Embryonic endoderm formed
13	Prechordal plate	6	Beginning of head process
14	Primitive streak		Colonization by embryonic mesoderm
			Axes of embryo established
16	Notochord	7	
18	Neural folds	8	

histones from the oocyte replace the protamines (Yanagimachi, 1988; Tesarik, 1992). Paternal and maternal pronuclei undergo DNA synthesis, the initiation of the S phase in the cell cycle being regulated by cytoplasmic factors in many species and probably in man (Laskey *et al.*, 1989); the pronuclei persist for approximately fifteen hours in human eggs (Edwards, 1980).

The first cleavage results in two equal-sized blastomeres and one of these divides before the other; the right-angled orientation of their cleavage planes being an indication of the tight regulation of embryonic growth. Early embryos might release trophic factors, e.g. platelet activating factor (PAF) (O'Neill *et al.*, 1989).

Blastomeres of approximately equal size formed in successive cleavages are associated by microvilli; their cytoplasmic organelles differentiate; and compaction in 8-cell embryos heralds the formation of outer trophectoderm cells associated by desmosomes and tight junctions which enclose one or more inner cells. The human blastocyst initially has 32–64 cells at 4–5 days (Table 1.1), a blastocoelic cavity, an inner cell mass and large secretory-like cells adjacent to it (Figures 1.1– 1.4) (Edwards, 1980). In mice, the inner cell mass regulates the overlying polar trophectoderm which colonizes the mural trophecto- derm lining the blastocoel. Inbuilt 'clocks' time embryonic growth, for

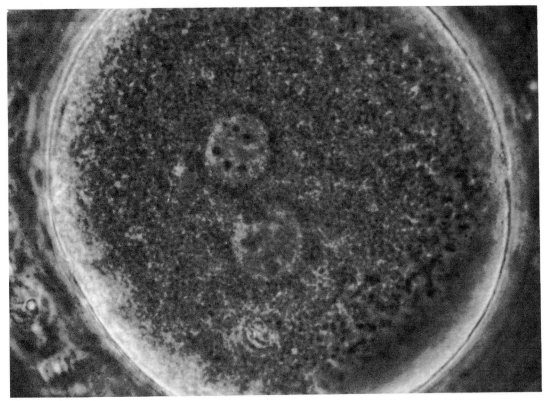

Figure 1.1. A fertilized human egg containing two pronuclei, with the surrounding zona pellucida.

blastulation occurs as expected when cell number in cleaving embryos is reduced (Edwards, 1980). Cell allocation to various tissues is organized, perhaps from the first cleavage division (Kelly *et al.*, 1978).

Compaction and cell migration involve β1,4-galactosyl transferase (GalTase), acting as a ligand on glycoproteins expressed on the cell surface (Shur, 1977; Bayna *et al.*, 1988); any distortions in its expression mimic morphological anomalies typical of t^{12}/t^{12} in mouse embryos. At least two families of adhesion molecules participate in 8-cell mouse embryos, including calcium-dependent fucosylated glycoproteins of approximately 120 kd (Damsky *et al.*, 1985) and complex glycoproteins (lactosaminoglycans) with repeating *N*-acetyllactosamine units (Muramatsu *et al.*, 1983). CAM and CAD molecules are also expressed in early mouse embryos. Cytokeratin and filamentous proteins form in intercellular junctions between trophectoderm cells in mice (Iwakura & Nozaki, 1989).

A human blastocyst flushed from the uterus had 69 mural and 30 polar trophectoderm cells, eight cells comprising ectoderm and flattened primitive endoderm, and a primordial germ cell (Hertig, 1968), i.e. stage 3–4 of the Carnegie classification. A single layer of

3

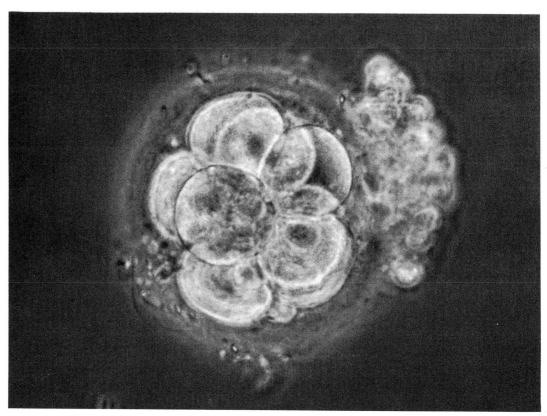

Figure 1.2. Human 8-cell embryo, the blastomeres being distinct and even-sized showing that compaction has not begun; the zona pellucida is distinct.

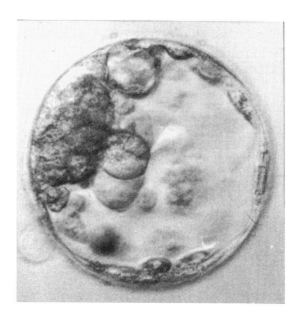

Figure 1.3. Human blastocyst grown *in vitro* with a distinct inner cell mass, a single layer of trophectoderm cells enclosing the blastocoelic cavity, secretory-like cells adjacent to the inner cell mass, and an enclosing zona pellucida.

4

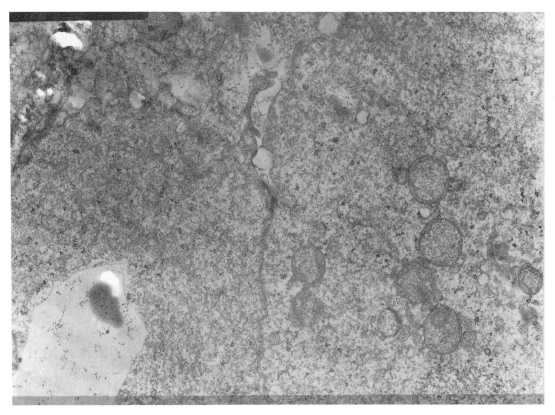

Figure 1.4. Electron micrograph of two blastomeres in a human 16 to 32-cell embryo, showing junctional complexes, mitochondria, endoplasmic reticulum and a few microvilli (Edwards, 1980).

primitive (extraembryonic) endoderm differentiates after day 5 from inner cell mass, which becomes epiblast; the embryonic disc forms and includes epiblast and underlying, small vesiculated cells of embryonic endoderm. Endoderm near the epiblast forms proximal (visceral) endoderm, and that lining the blastocoel forms distal (parietal) endoderm associated with trophoblast, i.e. Heuser's membrane or the exocoelomic membrane. Embryos now implant in the uterus.

The ratio of inner cell mass to trophectoderm cells in blastocysts is achieved between 8-cells and 32-cells in mice (Fleming, 1987), and component cells of blastocysts increasingly resemble normal somatic cells. The absence of a basal lamina between inner cell mass and trophectoderm might assist repair mechanisms in embryos (Enders, 1989). Human blastocysts expand 5 to 7 days after fertilization (Table 1.1), as the zona pellucida thins and the embryo 'hatches' from it perhaps by means of 'strypsin' produced in mural trophectoderm in mice, although there is some debate on this point (Figure 1.5) (Perona & Wassarman, 1986; Chan, 1987; Cohen *et al.*, 1989; Yamazaki & Kato, 1989). Abnormal hatching might cause the death of human

5

Figure 1.5. A hatched human blastocyst grown to day 9 *in vitro*, showing its slightly flattened appearance, distinct epiblast and trophectoderm; the zona pellucida contains a few cells or remnants (Edwards & Surani, 1978).

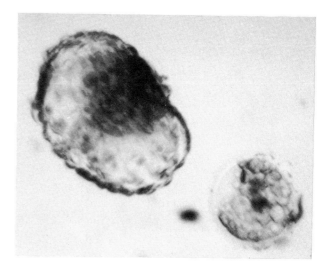

blastocysts, and partial hatching could cause identical twinning (Edwards *et al.*, 1986).

Transcription in oocytes, cleaving embryos and blastocysts

Two sources of genetic information exist in early embryos. 'Maternal' mRNA in oocytes encodes for proteins active in maturation, fertilization and cleavage, and embryonic mRNA is synthesized after fertilization. Maternal poly (A^+) RNA encodes glycoproteins of the zona pellucida and other enzymes (Wassarman, 1990), and for connexon, a precursor of junctional complexes (Kidder & McLachlin, 1985). Much of it and its encoded proteins are degraded after fertilization in mouse eggs and presumably in human eggs (Paynton *et al.*, 1988). Some specific transcripts are destroyed at this time, including c-*mos* protein which is involved in oocyte maturation (Sagata *et al.*, 1988; Watanabe *et al.*, 1990). Some maternal transcripts seem to persist into blastocysts including those encoded by c-*mos*.

Regulatory genes in amphibians and *Drosophila* code for factors enhancing or repressing transcription, e.g. graded doses of XTC–MIF, a homologue of activin A, invoke stepwise transitions in *Xenopus* embryos (Green & Smith, 1990). Regulation is imposed at the molecular level too, e.g. through RNA splicing or other post-transcriptional modifications. Mammalian regulatory genes are active in embryo cell lineages and cells derived from embryos, known as embryonic or teratocarcinoma cell lines (ES and EC respectively) as described below. Enhancers isolated from EC cells contain endogenous retrotransposon elements expressed in early embryos (Brûlet *et al.*, 1983), which remain active only until the cells begin to differentiate (Okamoto *et al.*, 1990). Two enhancers contain an octamer motif (ATTTGCAT) and an AT-rich sequence TTAAAATTCA, as in recognition sequences in *Drosophila* En protein, and a factor corresponding to *oct*-3 binds to these sequences, and is also inactivated as cells differentiate. *Oct*-3 probably confers totipotency or multipotency on embryonic cells (Okamoto *et al.*, 1990).

Oct-3 is synthesized in maturing oocytes with two protective RNA species of 442 and 380 base pairs respectively. It has homeodomains but is unlike other homeodomain-encoding genes in being active in totipotent and pluripotential stem cells and being down-regulated as endoderm and mesoderm differentiate (Lenardo *et al.*, 1989; Okamoto *et al.*, 1990; Rosner *et al.*, 1990; Schöler *et al.*, 1990).

Embryonic genes encode for various proteins in early cleavage, including heat-shock proteins and paternal gene variants of β_2-microglobulin (β_{2M}) in 2 to 4-cell mouse embryos (Sawicki *et al.*, 1982; Bolton *et al.*, 1984). Uridine incorporation increases fifty-fold per embryo by the blastocyst stage (Clegg & Piko, 1983). Translational efficiency rises after the 2-cell stage in mice.

Embryonic transcription begins in 4 to 8-cell human embryos (Tesarik *et al.*, 1987; Braude *et al.*, 1988), although some data imply that it might begin in pronucleate eggs (Tesarik, 1992). Transcripts for human chorionic gonadotrophin β subunit (hCGß) presumably embryonic, are present in 8-cell human embryos (Bonduelle *et al.*, 1988). Maternal transcripts apparently persist into blastocysts, and may be responsible for the constant levels of many enzymes including glucose phosphate isomerase, hexosaminidase, β-galactosidase and of hypoxanthine guanine phosphoribosyl transferase (HGPRT) in human preimplantation embryos (Leese *et al.*, 1991); the sharp increase in levels of other enzymes signals the onset of embryonic gene activity.

mRNA forms approximately 6–8% of total RNA in mouse embryos, and heterogeneous RNA in rabbit blastocysts corresponds with approximately 2% of unique sequence DNA; cytoplasmic RNA can evidently specify for 6000 polypeptides (Manes *et al.*, 1981; Piko & Clegg, 1982). Much of the mRNA codes for the three histones and for actin present in large amounts in early embryos (Schultz, 1986). A differentiated cell usually contains thousands of copies of ten or fewer mRNA species, and a few copies of the other species (Lewin, 1980).

Embryos must inherit paternal and maternal genomes to grow normally, for gynogenetic and androgenetic embryos lacking a genetic contribution from one parent develop abnormally; this phenomenon is

Table 1.2. *Maternal and paternal gene expression in human syndromes*

Syndrome	Cause
Hydatidiform mole	Paternal genome duplicated, no maternal genome
Wilm's tumour	Paternal 11p chromosome duplicated
Neurofibromatosis I	Severity increases with maternal transmission
Huntington's chorea	Early onset with paternal inheritance
Myotonic dystrophy	Congenital form associated with maternal transmission

Source: Surani *et al.*, 1990.

an example of genomic imprinting evidently caused by variable degrees of methylation of certain genes in the ovary or testis (Surani *et al.*, 1990) (Table 1.2). An imprinted gene might remain inactive over long periods in embryos and adults – even permanently. This explains why some human genetic diseases can be inherited from one parent, for example the Prader–Willi syndrome from the father, for the maternal allele is not expressed in fetus or adult. In contrast, the mother transmits the active gene for Angelman syndrome and the paternal gene remains inert. The receptor for insulin-like growth factor type 2 (IGF2r) is another example of imprinting, for only the gene which is carried on the maternal chromosome is expressed (Barlow *et al.*, 1991). Genomic imprinting is also involved when a maternal chromosome replaces the paternal chromosome in some patients (i.e. maternal heterodisomy), as in the non-deletion Prader–Willi syndrome (Nicholls *et al.*, 1989). Some chromosomal sites are demethylated in preimplantation embryos (Manes & Menzel, 1981).

Some genes impair embryonic growth, e.g. T-alleles and homozygotes for Tail short, oligosyndactyly and Yellow in mice (Magnuson, 1986; Magnuson & Epstein, 1987). Transcripts in blastocysts encode for growth factors (Rappolee *et al.*, 1988). *Oct*-3 transcripts are produced in inner cell mass, epiblast and primitive ectoderm, with little or none in trophectoderm, trophoblast, primitive endoderm and mesoderm. After day 8, the gene is expressed in primordial germ cells only (Rosner *et al.*, 1990).

Both paternal and maternal X chromosomes are active during cleavage. In female embryos, genes on the two X chromosomes are active until late cleavage or the morula, but one of them is then largely inactivated in the blastocyst. Inactivation occurs at different times in various tissues of the mouse embryo, for example in trophectoderm first and then in inner cell mass, and reactivation is rare except in oogonia (Chapman, 1986). Cytosine methylation in gene promotor sites and regulatory regions might be responsible for this large-scale inactivation (Wolf & Migeon, 1985). Many genes on the 'inactivated' X chromosome remain functional, especially those on or adjacent to the pairing region with the Y chromosome or on the long arm of the human X chromosome, and the gene XIST (X_i-specific transcripts) might control X inactivation; it is located near the X-inactivation centre and is functional in the 'inactive' X, but the allele located on the 'active' X in female embryos and the gene present on the X chromosome in male embryos remain inert (Brown *et al.*, 1991).

An inactive X chromosome replicates slowly and forms sex chromatin in blastocysts. The two X chromosomes may not be inactivated at random in different cells of the embryo, for the maternal X might remain active in mouse trophectoderm, and possibily in human proximal endoderm and extraembryonic ectoderm (Takagi *et al.*, 1982). The maternal X also remains active in yolk sac and extraembryonic lineages; the paternal X being inert (Chapman, 1986).

Genes which are inserted into mouse eggs ('transgenes') may be expressed in many cell types in the resulting fetus, and transgenes include transferrin, growth hormone, elastase, myosin light chains, α-fetoprotein, globins, immunoglobulins, and fusion genes composed of promoter and structural gene (Gordon *et al.*, 1980; Brinster *et al.*, 1981; Gordon & Ruddle, 1981; Palmiter *et al.*, 1982; Hammer *et al.*, 1985; Wagner & Stewart, 1986; Wagner 1990). The c-fos oncogene with 5′ regulating elements, e.g. human metallothionein promoter, is expressed in many cell types of the resulting embryo. The gene Sry, which is the primary sex determinant in mammals, will switch female to male differentiation when incorporated as a functional transgene in pronucleate mouse eggs. A transgene activating adenylyl cyclase produces gigantism in mice (Burton *et al.*, 1991).

The foreign DNA is usually injected into the male pronucleus, the larger of the two pronuclei, and can become selectively incorporated into paternal gene sites. Viruses, especially cloned retroviruses, can be vectors with genes up to 6–8 kb. The integrated DNA might invoke chromosomal rearrangements or deletions; it can also serve to tag, isolate and extract nearby host DNA to characterize the afflicted gene. Transgenic animals can also be established by transfection embryonic cell lines growing *in vitro*, as described below, where further examples of gene modification will be described.

Disorders in DNA synthesis occur in human embryos with multinucleated blastomeres, and RNA transcription is impaired in abnormal or retarded human embryos with a retarded ultrastructural pattern; many of these degenerate cells are expelled into the space between the zona pellucida and the trophectoderm (Tesarik, 1992).

Factors regulating embryonic differentiation

An understanding of the factors regulating primary embryonic differentiation could help to establish lines of cells from early embryos. Primary differentiation provides the cells needed to form inner cell mass and trophectoderm, and further tissues can then differentiate through the processes of induction, e.g. between inner cell mass and trophectoderm (Gurdon *et al.*, 1990; Hartshorne & Edwards, 1991).

In invertebrates and amphibians, an animal–vegetal axis in ovarian oocytes establishes the polarity needed for primary differentiation (Gerhart, 1980; Schroeder, 1986), but mammalian oocytes do not seem to be polarized. Some evidence suggested that mouse oocytes are polarized, because membranal microvilli are absent from the membrane overlying the second meiotic spindle. Microvilli are present in this site in human oocytes, indicating that polarity is not a general feature of the mammalian oocyte (Maro *et al.*, 1984; Johnson *et al.*, 1990).

Cell membranes and cytoplasm become polarized in 2 and 4-cell mouse embryos. This is seen in the distribution of membranal carbohydrates, alkaline phosphatase and 5′-nucleotidase in regions of cell contact (Ziomek, 1982; Richa & Solter, 1986), and the presence of permanent microvilli on outward-facing poles of blastomeres of 8-cell embryos as compared with the distribution of labile microvilli in areas of cell contact. It is also detected by exclusion of actin and myosin from regions of cell contact, the distribution of lectins, proteins and antigens on membranes of 16-cell and later embryos and of membrane proteins and of β_{2M} on the apical surface of trophectoderm (Calarco-Gillam, 1986).

Polarization could be initiated by transcellular ion currents (Nuccitelli & Wiley, 1985), microfilaments and microtubules (Johnson & Maro, 1984), and components of the extracellular matrix including laminin, fibronectin and some forms of collagen (Calarco-Gillam, 1986). Polarized cells produce either two polarized descendants which form trophectoderm or one polar and one non-polar descendant, the latter becoming inner cells in 16-cell embryos and forming the inner cell mass (Fleming, 1987; Johnson, 1989). Similar forms of cell allocation could arise in other types of cell aggregates, as in cells on the free border of isolated cell masses or of aggregates of embryonal carcinoma cells (Wiley, 1984). Trophectoderm formation resembles the differentiation of an epithelium, and transepithelial movements of ions and water could establish the blastocoelic cavity. Alternatively, the cavity may be formed in response to the synthesis of ATP and water in association with mitochondria, lipid droplets and Na^+/K^+ ATPase on basal membranes of outer blastomeres, the ATP enabling Na^+ to be pumped into intracellular spaces, with water following (Overstrom et al., 1989).

Growth factors enable embryonic tissues to communicate with each other or with the uterus (Brigstock et al., 1989; Heyner et al., 1989), but there is no clear consensus on their functions and inter-relationships. Receptor profiles might be related to cell density (Rizzino, 1988). Growth factors exist in multiple related forms, some latent, and have varying affinities for different factors, e.g. TGF-α binds to EGF receptors. Blastocysts synthesize transcripts for platelet derived growth factor (PDGF), transforming growth factors (TGF-α and TGF-β_1) including TGF-β_1, IGF-II, receptors for all three, and possibly FGF; EGF, basic FGF, nerve growth factor (NGF-β) and granulocyte colony-stimulating factor are not produced by cleaving mouse embryos (Massague, 1983; Smith et al., 1987; Mercola & Stiles, 1988; Rappolee et al., 1988, 1989; Graham et al., 1990).

Mouse morulae and blastocysts do not produce insulin but incorporate maternal insulin which passes through trophectoderm to the inner cell mass; it might promote DNA, RNA and protein synthesis and support cell division (Heyner et al., 1989). EGF receptors formed in morula and blastocysts in mice become restricted to trophectoderm. EGF stimulates protein synthesis, possibly via Na^+/K^+ ATPase (Wood & Kaye, 1989), enhances the growth of 8-cell mouse embryos (Paria & Dey, 1990) and promotes the production of human chorionic gonadotrophin by syncytiotrophoblast (Maruo & Mochizuki, 1987).

Grafting cells from preimplantation embryos

The changing properties of embryonic cells during differentiation is reflected in their properties of regeneration and colonization. Disaggregated embryos reform in culture, and cells from several cleaving embryos will aggregate into a single embryo which forms a complex chimaera. Disaggregated blastocysts can also reform, their constituent cells reoccupying their original place (Johnson, 1989).

Each blastomere in 2-cell and perhaps in 4-cell embryos can produce an entire fetus, a property known as totipotency (Nicholas & Hall, 1940; Seidel, 1952). By the 8-cell stage, single blastomeres are losing their capacity to form blastocysts (Tarkowski & Wroblewska, 1967), but 8-cell embryos of animals and man can recover when most of the blastomeres are destroyed during cryopreservation, and such a human embryo has grown into a normal child (Veiga et al., 1987).

Restraints are imposed on the developmental potential of blasto-meres by the third cleavage division in mice, when compaction and cell allocation to trophectoderm are well advanced (Johnson & Maro,

11

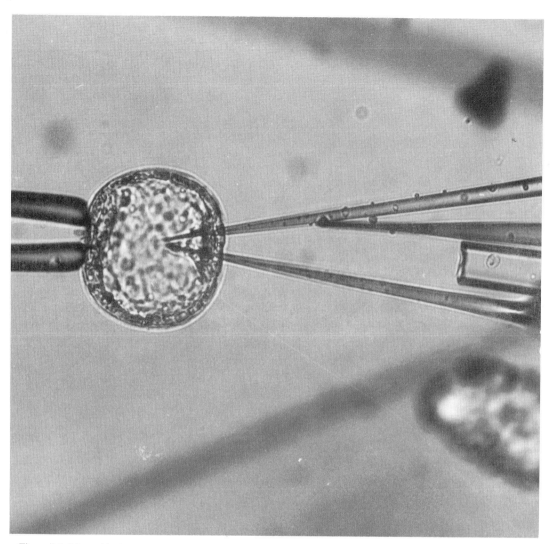

Figure 1.6. Mouse blastocyst held on a large suction pipette as fine needles perforate the trophectoderm to permit the passage of a transfer pipette into the blastocoelic cavity and so inject a donor cell or inner cell mass. Courtesy of Professor R. L. Gardner.

1986). Some blastocyst cells are 'multipotent' with a restricted capacity to differentiate into various tissues, although isolated inner cell masses can reconstitute a complete blastocyst and identical twins arise when cow blastocysts are cut in half (Ozil, 1983). Trophectoderm might be able to reconstitute parts of the blastocyst (Dyce *et al.*, 1987; Winkel & Pedersen, 1988).

The considerable degree of totipotency or multipotency in the cells of early embyros is revealed by their facility to colonize many tissues when injected into a recipient embryo. Cleaving embryos will fuse

12

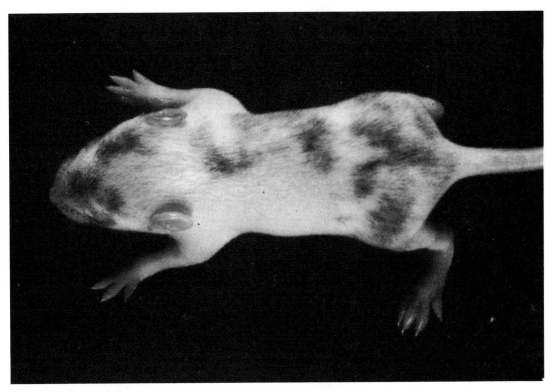

Figure 1.7. A mouse chimaera resulting from the injection of cells carrying a pigmented gene into the blastocoelic cavity of a blastocyst carrying albinism. The pigmented areas reveal the extent of chimaerism in the coat and hair. Courtesy of Professor R. L. Gardner.

together when placed in close proximity to each other, to form aggregation chimaeras, and individual or groups of disaggregated blastomeres can be combined with oocytes, cleaving embryos and blastocysts, but not with older embryos. Isolated mouse blastomeres are able to colonize many different organs when used to form chimaeras by injecting them into 8-cell embryos (Gardner, 1968). Single inner cell mass cells placed in the blastocoelic cavity retain the property of colonizing all the tissues of fetuses and offspring including the germ line (Figures 1.3, 1.6 and 1.7). As a result, spermatozoa originating from the donor cell are formed, and are able to fertilize eggs and develop into offspring; in effect, an animal is created from a donated cell, a most unusual form of animal breeding! Cells transferred from $4\frac{1}{2}$-day old mouse embryos into $3\frac{1}{2}$-day blastocysts also colonize all tissues of the resulting chimaeras, but similar grafts of extraembryonic ectoderm yield only ectoplacental cone and trophoblast giant cells, and epiblast has lost the capacity for widespread colonization.

Donor cells from rat blastocysts will colonize extensive areas of the resulting mouse–rat chimaeric fetus when placed in mouse blastocysts (Gardner & Johnson, 1973). Even more extraordinary, adult sheep–

goat chimaeras have been produced by blastomere aggregation or the injection of inner cell mass and trophectoderm of one species into blastocysts of the other (Fehilly *et al.*, 1984).

These are extreme examples showing how graft and host cells survive together in aggregation chimaeras. There does not seem to be much evidence of the rejection of these grafts. Perhaps they do not express the major histocompatibility antigens, although the zona pellucida is believed to protect embryos against the mother's immune response, and becomes coated with maternal proteins, IgA-secreting plasma cells, T cells and peritoneal macrophages (Bernard *et al.*, 1977). Breaches in it apparently permit maternal scavenging cells to destroy the embryos (Willadsen, 1979). Early pregnancy factor released from cleaving embryos under the influence of platelet activating factors might be an immunosuppressant (Bose *et al.*, 1989).

Chimaeras produced by grafting embryonic cells into recipient embryos display wide variations in mosaicism, from barely any to almost total colonization by descendants of donor cells. Donor cells cannot be directed to a particular organ. Perhaps the scarcity of donor cells from cleaving embryos and blastocysts has precluded the grafting of embryonic cells into fetuses or adult recipients, since there are only twenty or so in a human blastocyst. Fortunately, the astonishing properties of embryonic cells to differentiate and colonize all the organs of a recipient embryo can be mimicked by using cell lines formed from cell outgrowths of blastocysts, and these cells can be obtained in very large numbers.

Teratocarcinoma and embryonic cell lines

Studies on embryonic differentiation have been enormously simplified by the introduction of embryonic stem cell lines (ES cells) and embryonal carcinoma cell lines (EC cells). They offer ready sources of cells for investigation or grafting; can be modified genetically; and, when replaced in recipient embryos, are able to differentiate into all tissues of the body.

Two types of ES cell lines exist, differentiated and undifferentiated. The latter are subdivided into 'determined' stem cells which self-replicate but have a limited capacity for development (e.g. similar to haemopoietic stem cells) and 'undetermined' stem cells (or pluripotential stem cells, which have the capacity for differentiation into many, but not all, organs) with self-renewal, a wider potency and the ability to produce determined cells (Robertson & Bradley, 1986). Differentiation can be achieved *in vitro* by adding substrates to the medium, e.g.

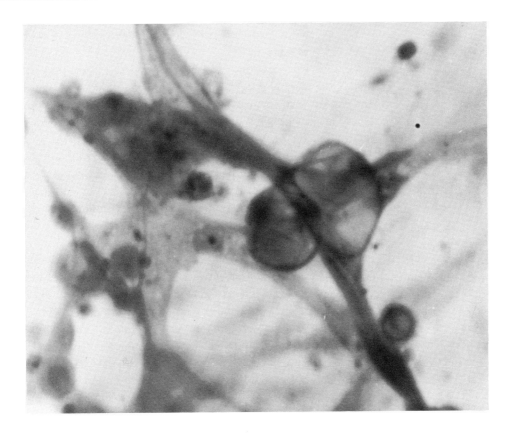

Figure 1.8. Detail of a cell outgrowth from a rabbit blastocyst *in vitro*. (Cole *et al.*, 1967).

retinoic acid, or by changing the culture conditions. The gene *oct*-3 is expressed in undifferentiated ES cells, but not when they are induced to differentiate (Rosner *et al.*, 1990).

Embryonic stem cells were initially grown as outgrowths from rabbit blastocysts on trophoblast monolayers, and they differentiated into various tissues especially when exposed to 'mesodermal inducers' which were extracted from bone marrow (Cole *et al.*, 1967) (Figure 1.8). Cell lines were established from embryonic cells but their potential for colonizing blastocysts could not be tested, since the methods had not been introduced.

Embryonic cell outgrowths from mouse blastocysts formed embryoid bodies *in vitro*, which could be grown as cell lines (Evans & Kaufman, 1981); they were also produced from cell colonies established by embryo transfers to ectopic sites in recipient animals. ES cells arise from the inner cell mass or epiblast, contain many pluripotential stem cells and can be propagated by serial transfers into recipients or by repeated passage *in vitro*. So far, similar cell lines have not been

15

obtained from human blastocysts, because cells of the inner cell mass cells and trophoblast do not persist in monolayer cultures (Fishel *et al.*, 1984; Lopata & Hay, 1989).

EC cells were developed from several sources. They arose spontaneously in testis tumours in strain 129 mice (Stevens & Little, 1954), and were formed when grafts of genital ridges of mouse embryos were placed into the testes of recipient animals, although their origin from spermatogonia or spermatocytes may be an inadequate model of embryonic cells. EC cells have also been derived from spontaneous teratocarcinomas in the ovaries of LT strain mice, where they are derived from parthenogenetically-activated oocytes or from stem cells, which might provide a better model (Stevens & Varnum, 1974). Human teratocarcinoma cell lines display varying properties *in vitro*, although similar overall to mouse EC cells (Pera *et al.*, 1990).

EC and ES progenitor cells probably resemble definitive embryonic ectoderm at $5\frac{1}{2}$ days, or perhaps epiblast, rather than cells of the inner cell mass. Accordingly, many of these cell lines differentiate into parietal and visceral endoderm. These cell lines are invaluable for the study of lethal mutants: to characterize molecules involved in growth and differentiation; to analyse the protein composition or other aspects of stem cells and differentiating cells; and to test the effects of changing environments on cell differentiation.

ES cells remain undifferentiated in the presence of leukaemia inhibitory factor (LIF), which is related to interleukin, and in the absence of heterologous feeder layers; this evidence indicates that LIF might regulate the formation of pluripotential embryonic ectoderm (Smith *et al.*, 1988; Williams *et al.*, 1988). ES cells differentiate into endoderm-like cells in suspension cultures, when exposed to retinoic acid, or after their transfection with the f-*mos* proto-oncogene (Wagner, 1990), and the resulting changes resemble the initial stages of embryogenesis.

Retinoic acid (RA) is a morphogen which induces cell differentiation and morphogenesis. It binds to a nuclear receptor called retinoic acid receptor (RAR), and the RA/RAR complex presumably recognises control regions for particular genes and activates or represses them. The *oct*-3 gene is evidently regulated by retinoic acid, for the amount of *oct*-3 mRNA declines by 90% soon after cells are exposed to it and this action precedes the commitment of stem cells to various tissues. Therefore, it is essential to repress *oct*-3 in order to invoke the differentiation of ES cells into stem cells for various lineages. Retinoic acid can induce neuroglia and astroglia or fibroblasts, according to the nature of the treatment of the cells.

16

Multipotent EC cell lines may differentiate into endoderm-like cells in serum-free medium containing fibronectin, insulin, transferrin and HDL (Rizzino, 1988). Others release TGF-like factors enhancing the growth of NRK cells on agar, but not after they have differentiated into endoderm. The TGF is not TGFα or TGFβ, and appears to be an embryonic form also released from human placenta, implying it has a role in growth and differentiation (Adamson, 1986). Endoderm cells form on the outside of EC cell aggregates within forty eight hours, and other cell types appear later, especially if promoters are used (Martin *et al.*, 1977). EC cells in long-term propagation become restricted in their properties of differentiation.

EC lines have varied chromosome complements, although many are diploid. Some lines have two functioning X chromosomes, others have an active and an inactive X chromosome (Chapman, 1986). The induction of endodermal differentiation by retinoic acid or the removal of feeder layers inactivates one X chromosome in those lines with two active chromosomes (Takagi & Martin, 1984). X inactivation is induced in some somatic cells by 5-azacytidine.

Grafting embryonal cell lines

A single cell or a group of cells isolated from the inner cell mass have been injected into recipient blastocysts, and they can colonize extensive areas of the resulting chimaeric mouse, including the gonads and gametes as described above (Gardner, 1968). This powerful embryonic method is also effective with ES and to some extent with EC cells, which vary in their capacity to colonize recipient embryos. EC cells can be incorporated into blastocysts (Brinster, 1974) or cleaving embryos (Stewart, 1982), but might colonize only extraembryonic tissues; few EC cell lines are as effective at colonization as cells from the inner cell mass. Many chimaeric fetuses resulting from grafts of EC cells into blastocysts are abnormal and die *in utero*, and one-fifth of the offspring display tumours, colonization is patchy, and few offspring display germ-line chimaerism.

In contrast, most ES cell lines colonize large areas of recipient embryos, and proliferate and integrate into many organ systems (Evans *et al.*, 1985); they closely resemble inner cell mass cells in this respect. One-third of the offspring are chimaeric, there are few fetal losses, colonization of the chimaera is extensive and reaches 50% in many of them, and ES cells from parthenogenetic animals are as effective as any others. ES cells colonize the germ line routinely and, although many males fail to breed, others transmit only spermatozoa

17

derived from the ES cells. Some of these difficulties with breeding presumably arise through the transfer of XY stem cells to XX hosts or vice versa.

Genes can be inserted or ablated from ES and EC cells to study differentiation or to introduce new genetic variants, e.g. the c-*fos* proto-oncogene, to promote differentiation as described above. The insert usually contains dominant gene markers in order to select the transfected cells. Transgenic offspring are obtained when the trans-fected cells are injected into blastocysts to form chimaeras (Wagner, 1990), and this approach offers an alternative to the injection of DNA into fertilized eggs to produce transgenic animals. These methods are being extended to rabbits and farm animals.

Genes can be ablated from ES cells by introducing an artificial gene construct into targetted gene sites to disrupt the reading frame (Doetschman *et al.*, 1987; Thomas & Capecchi, 1987, 1990; Kim & Smithers, 1988; Mansour *et al.*, 1988; McMahon & Bradley, 1990). The procedure involves using a cloned fragment of a gene which has known intron–exon boundaries and contains an insert such as *neoSOr*. It is incorporated into ES cells using electroporation, i.e. passing a high voltage current for a few minutes through a mixture containing ES cells and the insert. Many cells are killed, but the gene is incorporated into the target site in some survivors and into random sites in others.

Cells with the incorporated gene are selected by 'positive–negative' selection. A substrate including neomycin is added to the medium to select cells which have been transformed, since only they can metabolize it. Cells with the insert correctly targetted are then identified and sorted using a vital dye binding to the target site, or by use of the polymerase chain reaction with primers flanking the insertion site (Joyner *et al.*, 1988).

Some examples will reveal the scope of the method. The *int*-1 proto-oncogene encodes for a protein found in a group of cells in the neural plate, and it might be a patterning gene involved in cell–cell signals in the extracellular matrix. It was ablated from ES cells using the methods just described, and these cells were used to make and breed chimaeric mice and obtain fetuses homozygous for the ablated gene; these fetuses displayed major abnormalities of the dorsal midbrain and hindbrain (McMahon & Bradley, 1990; Thomas & Capecchi, 1990). The homeobox gene *hox* 1.5 was disrupted by targetting in mouse ES cells, and offspring carrying the ablated gene were athymic, aparathyroid, had defects of the heart and arteries and died at birth; they had resemblances to the human DiGeorge syndrome (Chisaka & Capecchi, 1991). Lastly, the disruption of an exon of the gene encoding the immunoglobulin μ-chain resulted in the birth of mice with no B cells (Kitamura *et al.*, 1991).

ES and perhaps EC cells should also offer enormous scope for grafting into fetal or adult recipients in animals and man. The easy ability to grow them *in vitro*; to induce some forms of differentiation along chosen pathways, e.g. by the use of retinoic acid; their immense properties of colonization; and the availability of methods to insert or ablate genes could make them invaluable in all forms of grafting for every body tissue. The increasing ability to insert or ablate genes in specific targetted sites makes them excellent carriers of genetic information of all kinds, to repair an enzyme deficiency or metabolize an excess substrate. They might escape rejection in the recipient, and it might be possible to tailor their histocompatibility system by inserting inactive genes such as HLA-G, which apparently protects trophoblast from rejection as described below. They can be frozen-stored for transfer, after being modified.

Surprisingly, their potential for this purpose has apparently not been assessed in animals, yet there could be fascinating prospects for clinical and agricultural work as described on earlier occasions (Edwards, 1982, 1989). This omission is all the more surprising because human EC lines are now available. It may be necessary to induce specific forms of differentiation in ES cells before they are grafted, in order to direct them to their target organ in the recipient, and simple methods might be effective for this purpose such as coculturing them with samples of the tissue to be colonized. The clinical opportunities are even greater when the work on inserting or ablating genes is taken into account, for there could be enormous prospects for the alleviation of deficiency diseases in the recipients. (See note, p. 37.)

Gastrulation

Two major types of tissue form the basis of embryonic organs. These are: epithelia, i.e. sheets of cells with junctional complexes and polarized as illustrated by the formation of trophectoderm; and mesenchyme with its three-dimensional network, punctate junctions and production of an extracellular matrix (Hay, 1968). Primary mesenchyme cells in the sea urchin elongate and form apical cell processes which contact neighbouring cells (Solursh, 1986). Gastrulation in amphibians involves the involution of mesoderm through the inner blastoporal lip, to establish regional patterns in gastrula (Keller, 1986). Extracellular matrices, including the hyaline layer, mesodermal fibronectin and laminin are involved in differentiation, as advancing

19

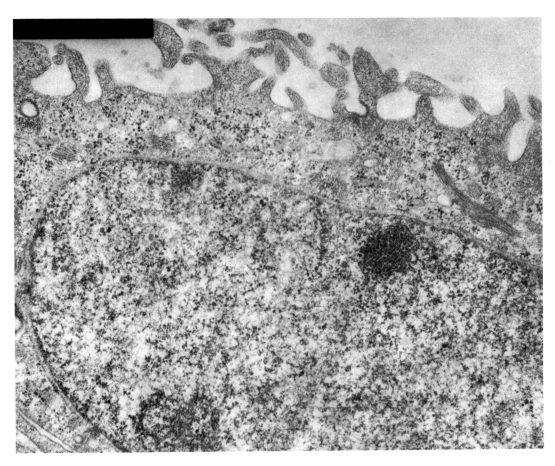

Figure 1.9. Electron micrograph of the mural trophoblast of the hatched human blastocyst growing *in vitro* at day 9; the living blastocyst is shown in Figure 1.5. There are extensive microvilli, desmosomes, tono filaments, glycogen and membrane-bound vesicles (Edwards, 1980).

mesodermal cells 'sample' adjacent cells by filopodia, forming contacts with some and rejecting others.

Fibronectin, glycosaminoglycans and other substrates may be involved in mesoderm migration and differentiation in mice, being found in blastocysts, trophoblast and visceral endoderm, while laminin is present from fertilization and type III collagen soon afterwards. Other types of collagen are produced later in mesenchyme, somites, embryonic membranes and parietal endoderm. Some EC cell lines differentiate into endoderm-like cells in medium containing fibronectin, insulin, transferrin and HDL as described above (Rizzino, 1988). Differentiation is regulated by internal clocks, e.g. the 'micromere clock' in sea urchins times the reaggregation of disaggregated embryonic cells (Spiegel & Spiegel, 1986), and blastocyst formation is timed in mouse embryos with normal or reduced cell numbers, as described above.

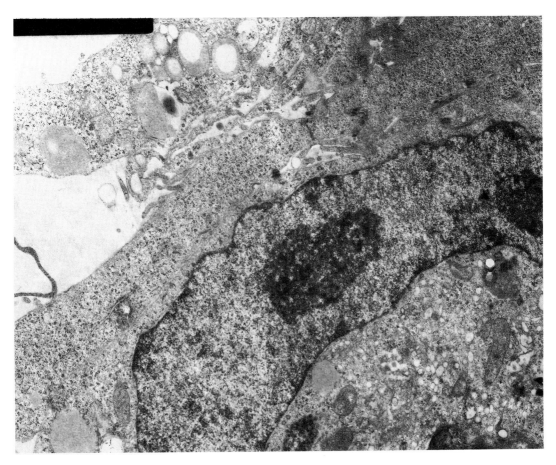

Figure 1.10. Electron micrograph of the hatched human blastocyst shown in Figure 1.5. It shows a large cytotrophoblast nucleus, filamentous structures and various inclusion bodies; there appears to be a portion of an embryonic cell in the upper part of the illustration. Normal and vacuolated mitochondria, rough endoplasmic reticulum, desmosomes and intercellular spaces can be seen (Edwards, 1980).

Morphogenesis of the human embryo to day 20

Gastrulation results in the formation of the three germ layers and in tissue differentiation in animals and man. Details of morphogenesis in human embryos have been described elsewhere (e.g. O'Rahilly & Muller, 1987; see Chapter 2, this volume); difficulties in gaining access to implanting embryos limit detailed studies on mammals, although rat fetuses can be cultured from blastocysts to the end of organ differentiation (New, 1991). Human embryos grow to day 9 *in vitro* (Figures 1.5, 1.9 and 1.10; Table 1.1) (Edwards & Surani, 1978; Edwards & Hollands, 1988; Lopata & Hay, 1989); and a human fetus implanted in a uterus maintained *in vitro* (Bulletti *et al.*, 1988), reaching day 11 with the formation of an amniotic cavity.

Tissue movements in blastocysts lead to the formation of ectoderm, mesoderm and endoderm. The epiblast is the precursor of embryonic

Figure 1.11. Human embryo at day 9 surrounded by predecidual tissue with leucocytes. Bilaminar germ disc, small amniotic cavity, lacunae within peripheral syncytiotrophoblast communicating with dilated endometrial sinusoids (upper right); cytotrophoblast around chorionic cavity thin at embryonic pole, thick and irregular at opposite pole and masses project into syncytiotrophoblast as villi primordia. Exocoelomic membrane (Heuser's) continuous with primitive endoderm. Reprinted by courtesy of Dr A. Hertig (Hertig & Rock, 1949).

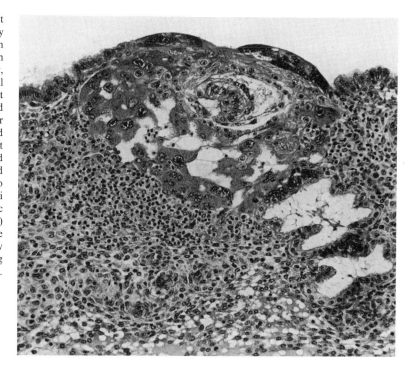

ectoderm, embryonic endoderm and embryonic and extraembryonic mesoderm; extraembryonic and chorionic ectoderm evidently arise from trophectoderm (Luckett, 1978; Gardner, 1982). The fate map of these tissues is consistent in mice and primates (Gardner, 1982, 1985). The form of differentiation could depend on cell position in the embryo, e.g. cells exposed to blastocoelic fluid might differentiate into extraembryonic endoderm in a manner resembling the inside–outside formation of the blastocyst.

The amniotic cavity appears in Stage 5a at about 7–8 days within the embryonic disc or between it and overlying trophoblast (O'Rahilly & Muller, 1987); its roof and walls are lined by amniotic cells which may develop from trophectoderm, and its floor by epiblast (Hertig, 1968). The primary yolk sac forms as endoderm colonizes the blastocoelic cavity from day 9 (Figures 1.11 and 1.12).

The axis of the bilaminar embryonic disc might be established by the condensation of extraembryonic mesoblast at its caudal end (also called mesenchyme or primitive mesoderm), in a 'precocious primitive streak' giving rise to extraembryonic mesoderm. Mesoblast derivatives during stage 5c, i.e. at 11–12 days, include angioblast, the precursor of blood vessels, and the coelomic cavity formed from isolated spaces in extraembryonic mesoderm, demarcating primary endoderm from the

Figure 1.12. Detail of an implanted human embryo at day 14. The embryonic disc and the amniotic cavity, large secondary yolk sac adjacent to the embryo, and the enclosing chorion lined with extraembryonic mesoderm can be seen (Hertig, 1975). Reprinted by courtesy of Dr A. Hertig.

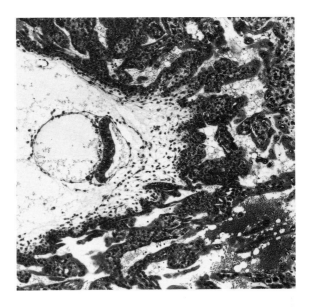

exocoelomic membrane of the yolk sac. The prechordal plate might form at this stage, as a thickening of endoderm at the rostral end of the embryonic disc.

Gastrulation is characterized in mammals by the appearance of the primitive streak, which is formed in stage 6 in human embryos, as embryonic mesoderm derived from epiblast invaginates and migrates between ectoderm and endoderm. The head process is formed at the anterior end of the streak from invaginated epiblast. Increasing cell specialization is reflected in the activity of *oct*-3 in mouse fetuses, its transcripts being restricted successively to primitive ectoderm, undifferentiated ectoderm, and finally to primordial germ cells (Rosner *et al.*, 1990).

By stage 6, 13 days after ovulation, extraembryonic mesoblast extends into chorionic villi, angiogenesis has begun in the chorionic mesoblast and blood islands have formed in the yolk sac (sometimes called the umbilical vesicle) at the margin of the embryonic disc (O'Rahilly & Muller, 1987). The amnion is well formed, and the long axis of the embryonic disc is coincident with the primitive streak. Some epiblast cells enter the streak, those remaining on the dorsal aspect of the embryo becoming embryonic ectoderm. The primitive streak contains many migratory differentiating cells passing from outer layers of the embryo to form mesoderm and endoderm by 'ingression' as the underlying basal lamina is lost (Bellairs, 1986).

The prechordal plate, the rostrocaudal axis of the embryo and its left and right sides are now established. A secondary yolk sac is 'pinched

23

off' (see O'Rahilly & Muller, 1987) and primordial germ cells and haemopoietic cells which are present in the yolk sac endoderm may have originated earlier in the embryonic disc. Cells producing fetal haemoglobin appear at 2 weeks in the yolk sac, and they might have a different origin from the fetal haemopoietic system which differentiates later. The cloacal membrane, allantoic diverticulum and connecting stalk appear in stage 6.

By stage 6, therefore, major positional decisions have been taken, and the appearance of the prechordal plate as a thickened area of endoderm on day 13 is perhaps the first indication of axis formation. Stages 7–9, lasting until day 20 approximately, are the final stages of what many embryologists consider to be the embryonic period, as organ rudiments are formed (for details, see O'Rahilly & Muller, 1987). The neural plate, neural folds and neural groove form by day 18 and are prominent by day 20, with the three major divisions of the brain appearing before the neural tube is formed. The otic disc is formed by day 20. Mitotic cells in the mesencephalic and rhombencephalic areas may represent the origin of the neural crest.

Embryonic mesoblast spreads laterally and rostrally from the primitive streak, and the notochord may be involved in the later formation of somites. The prechordal plate, destined to form the rostral region of the head, becomes continuous with the notochord and rotates in association with the head fold. Somites are visible in stage 9, around day 20. Isolated spaces appear in the mesoblast, to form the pericardial cavities in the rostral half of the embryo, and the endocardial plexus and cardiogenic plate are forerunners of myocardium and endocardium. Nephric structures appear after stage 9 is completed. Extraembryonic mesoblast continues to invade the yolk sac, where modified mesenchymal cells, haemocytoblasts and primitive erythroblasts accumulate in blood islands. The regions of the gut develop from recesses in the yolk sac.

Cell lineages

The developmental fate of every cell can be traced in embryos of some invertebrates, cell lineages being fixed from fertilization, and being virtually invariant (Rossant, 1986). The pattern in *Drosophila* is different, since individual cells are not committed to single types of development, and groups of cells are allocated to specific patterns or compartments. This form of allocation occurs in early mammalian development, with extensive cell mixing during differentiation, so that a coherent and clonal form of differentiation is unlikely.

Trophectoderm and primitive endoderm are committed to their fate

Table 1.3. *Some derivatives of the tissues of the mouse blastocyst*

Inner cell mass		Trophectoderm
Primitive ectoderm	Primitive endoderm	Mural and polar trophectoderm
	Visceral endoderm	Extraembryonic and chorionic ectoderm
Fetal soma and germ line	Parietal endoderm	
Amniotic ectoderm		
Extraembryonic mesoderm		

Note:
The fate map of the rhesus monkey and perhaps the human embryo appears to be similar in most respects to that of the mouse (Luckett, 1978).
Source: Gardner, 1985.

by day $4\frac{1}{2}$ in mice; the former is restricted to extraembryonic derivatives, and the latter to extraembryonic derivatives including endoderm of the visceral yolk sac and parietal endoderm. Their characteristics are precocious differentiation, limited potential, preferential inactivation of the paternal X chromosome, and undermethylation of repetitive and structural DNA sequences. Their undermethylation might be inherited from embryonic cells, and not imposed during development (Rossant, 1986). Extraembryonic ectoderm is a stem cell pool for various types of trophoblast cell. Embryonic endoderm in the distal embryonic cylinder in mice contributes to gut and notochord. There is conflicting evidence about the contribution of the head process endoderm to the formation of the foregut (Beddington, 1986). Forward embryonic endoderm colonizes the visceral yolk sac.

Epiblast in the primitive streak in mice has an enormous potential for differentiation, being the sole founder of the tissues of the fetus (Table 1.3). Its lability is curtailed as the head process appears when it can still produce mesoderm but not gut epithelium (Beddington, 1986) or teratocarcinoma cells in ectopic sites (Damanjov *et al.*, 1971). Anterior epiblast differentiates into neuroectoderm and surface ectoderm; the posterior part differentiates into embryonic and extraembryonic mesoderm, but will produce ectodermal derivatives if placed in the anterior region.

Gene regulation of stem cell migration and protein synthesis

The routes of stem cell migration are controlled by growth factors which are themselves regulated genetically, as clarified in *Steel* (*Sl*) and *W* mice. The *Sl* product is a growth factor binding specifically as a ligand to the c-*kit* proto-oncogene receptor, which is encoded by *W*. *Sl* factor is identical to SCF (stem cell factor), MGF (mast cell growth

25

factor), and KL (kit ligand); c-*kit* is a member of the transmembrane tyrosine kinase receptor class of oncogenes. Both genes have numerous alleles, each exerting varying effects.

This widespread genetic system functions in early myeloid and lymphoid cells, synergizing with interleukin 7 and granulocyte macrophage colony stimulating factor (GM-CSF), in bone, erythroid lineages, anaemia and mast cell deficiency, in bone marrow transplantation and the development of multipotential stem cells (Witte, 1990). The *W* gene is expressed autonomously in cells, whereas *Sl* affects the microenvironment for cell migration and the 'homing' sites of melanoblasts, germ cells and haemopoietic stem cells. In mouse embryos, Sl factor (SCF) is expressed in endoderm and mesoderm of yolk sac, hind gut and ventral wall of the dorsal aorta, and in embryonic liver (presumably related to the migratory routes of primordial germ cells and haemopoietic cells). It is present in stromal cells of the fetal genital ridges but not in germ cells, and its expression in bone is perhaps related to haemopoiesis. It also forms along some routes of neural crest migration. These include the routes of melanoblast precursors, as they migrate between ectoderm and the dorsal surface of somites, and also their 'homing' sites such as the ectoderm of whisker follicles, otic vesicle and dermis, and in spinal cord and brain (Matsui *et al.*, 1990). Transcripts of c-*kit* mRNA encoding for Sl (SCF) are produced in primordial cells in the genital ridge and in presumptive melanoblasts at $10\frac{1}{2}$ days.

Sets of genes coding for similar proteins are activated together in several differentiating tissues. Genes for albumin, α-fetoprotein, transferrin, α_1-antitrypsin and apolipoproteins are expressed in endoderm of the visceral yolk and fetal liver, and anti-α-chymotrypsin and some urinary proteins are produced in liver of older fetuses. α-Fetoprotein is also present in kidney (mesoderm), although it may be absorbed and not synthesized by this tissue. Epithelia are characterized by the formation of basement membranes, desmosomal plaques and tight junctions to interact with the cytoskeleton (Adamson, 1986). In mice, a product of the T gene is essential for mesoderm formation (Herrmann *et al.*, 1990).

Knowledge of the compounds produced by specific types of fetal cell could help in choosing the correct tissue for grafting into adult recipients. An example is the ontogeny of the human plasma proteins (Adinolfi & Adinolfi, 1976) where several opportunities are given including the value of fetal spleen cells in correcting the synthesis of complement 5. The ontogeny of fetal tissues is described in Chapter 2, this volume.

Growth factors and the differentiation of germ layers

TGF might stimulate the growth and differentiation of embryonic cells and ES cells in a timed and spatial sequence, and possibly in combinations with other growth factors. It might be the 'mesoderm inducer' recognized many years ago, for TGF-β, perhaps in combination with FGF, induces the formation of mesoderm in *Xenopus* (Kimelman and Kirschner, 1987). TGF-β_1 is produced by many cells, has distinct temporal and spatial distributions in mouse embryonic tissues during morphogenesis, and could invoke inhibitory and stimulatory effects depending on cell type (Rizzino, 1988). TGFs may stimulate angiogenesis locally, e.g. at the implantation site (Folkman & Klagsbrun, 1987).

Genes encoding TGF-β_1, TGF-β_2 and TGF-β_3 are transcribed in human embryos between 32 and 57 days gestation. The distribution of TGF-β_1, TGF-β_2 and TGF-β_3 is broadly similar to that in mice (Gatherer *et al.*, 1990): TGF-β_1 is expressed in haemopoietic, endothelial and osteogenic cells; TGF-β_2 is expressed in epithelium and nervous system; and TGF-β_2 and TGF-β_3 are expressed in many mesenchymal cells. These factors have homologies with Mullerian inhibitory substance.

EGF stimulates keratinocytes to produce keratin and influences the synthesis of fibronectin, hyaluronic acid and glycoaminoglycans produced by fibroblasts, and of HCG by choriocarcinoma cells (Benveniste *et al.*, 1988). Receptors for EGF are expressed in mouse embryos, e.g. in amnion, liver, myoblasts, epidermal cells, and also as teratocarcinoma stem cells differentiate into endoderm. They are not present on several types of stem cells.

PDGF produced by the inner cell mass may be an embryonic form influencing the growth of extraembryonic endoderm (Rizzino, 1988), and human cytotrophoblast produces and responds to it by cell division (Goustin *et al.*, 1985); the ability to produce and respond to PDGF also arises in some endoderm derivatives. PDGF may influence cell migration (Seppä *et al.*, 1982), and parietal endoderm might migrate from the egg cylinder to the inner surface of trophoblast in response to trophoblastic PDGF. Mesodermal derivatives such as vascular smooth muscle, megakaryocytes, glial cells, chondrocytes and endothelial cells, and several EC cell lines produce a factor like PDGF (Adamson, 1986).

EC cells, fetal liver, human embryonic fibroblast cells, placenta, kidney, allantois and amnion produce IGFs (Adamson, 1986). IGFs stimulate mouse fibroblasts and are involved in establishing pluripotential

27

cell lines from mouse embryos. IGF receptors that are present on endoderm derivatives of teratocarcinoma cells, and in human placentae might bind insulin as well as IGF (Heath *et al.*, 1981).

FGF affects myogenesis, stimulates cell growth and slows differentiation (Rizzino, 1988). bFGF is freely diffusible in extracellular matrices and basement membranes. It binds with heparin or heparan sulphate and then resists proteolysis and becomes more diffusible, affecting morphogenesis at greater distances (Haumenhaft *et al.*, 1990).

Grafting differentiating embryos and their outgrowths

There is an enormous richness of differentiating cell types in human fetuses between the blastocyst and day 20. Most organ primordia are laid down, stem cells have high rates of mitosis, and cells in early stages of differentiation are available in large numbers. Tissues can be collected from early abortuses, especially since the introduction of RU486 for elective abortion. Embryonic cell lines offer an alternative source of primary and differentiating cells.

Purified samples of specific types of cells might be obtained by adapting a technique pioneered in *Drosophila*. A transgene, *lacZ*, produces β-galactosidase in different cell types, which is detected using fluorigenic β-galactosidase substrates and fluorescent activated cell sorting. The transgene has many variants, each expressed in different tissues, and the desired cells can be isolated by choosing the appropriate variant (Krasnow *et al.*, 1991).

Virtually all studies on grafting these tissues are restricted to animals, but their clinical potential is becoming evident. Tissues isolated from differentiating embryos have been injected into embryos a day or so younger, e.g. extraembryonic or embryonic visceral endoderm from 6-day-old mouse embryos colonize the yolk sac and parietal endoderm (Gardner, 1982). Epiblast from the early primitive streak colonizes all the germ layers, and produces teratocarcinomas in recipients, but its capacity for wide differentiation is regionalized by the headfold stages (Grobstein, 1951; Skreb & Svajger, 1975; Svajger *et al.*, 1981; Beddington, 1986).

The success of these grafts in adult recipients will presumably depend on their antigenic properties (see Chapter 4, this volume). Most immunological studies have concerned the role of trophoblast in averting the mother's immune response, a topic outside the scope of this chapter. It is doubtful if forms of protection which are perhaps peculiar to pregnancy will protect embryonic grafts placed in fetal or adult recipients. Some tissue products might be effective, e.g. TGF-β may inhibit the immune system (Rizzino, 1988), and α-fetoprotein (AFP) is reported to suppress primary and secondary IgM, IgG and IgA responses *in vitro* and to inhibit lymphocyte proliferation but this effect might be due to a contaminant (Murgita and Tomasi, 1975; Yachnin & Lester, 1976). This property is also characteristic of pregnancy-associated α_2-glycoprotein (Stimson, 1972). Natural killer cells are less active during pregnancy, and retroplacental serum blocks the production of interleukin-2 by T cells (Nicholas & Panagi, 1985).

Transplants of embryonic haemopoietic tissue

Embryonic haemopoietic cells have been grafted into recipient fetuses or adults, mostly in mice, where blood islands form in the yolk sac by 7.5 days after fertilization (Metcalf & Moore, 1971). These tissues produce mostly large, nucleated erythrocytes containing embryonic haemoglobin to sustain the fetus for three days of growth (Russell & Bernstein, 1966). Erythropoiesis is then mainly achieved in fetal liver, the non-nucleated erythrocytes being slightly larger in size than those in adult animals at the onset of haemopoiesis and being capable of producing adult haemoglobins (Burgess & Nicola, 1983). The liver is seeded apparently by multipotential stem cells.

The proliferative ability of multipotential haemopoietic stem cells, sometimes called HSC, is highest in embryos and declines in fetuses and adults, although still considerable at all stages of growth and at all ages (Burgess & Nicola, 1983; Lord, 1983; Harrison *et al.*, 1988). In adults, these multipotential cells represent one cell among 100 000 marrow cells (Harrison *et al.*, 1988), and their bone marrow environment or 'niche' is tightly organized and regulated, although open to intercellular reactions and environmental influences.

Early studies showed how embryonic cells could colonize the haemopoietic system of lethally X-irradiated adult mouse recipients; the yield of cell colonies being estimated by the number of spleen colony-forming units (CFUs), which originate from a single stem cell (Till & McCulloch, 1961; Becker *et al.*, 1963). Cells from the yolk sac were reported to be less successful than liver cells for grafting into irradiated recipients (Moore & Metcalf, 1970), and this evidence, together with the high numbers of fetal cells reportedly needed for successful grafting as compared with adult bone marrow, led to a belief that early embryonic cells were not efficient in grafting although their efficiency was improved by culturing them for a short term (Perah & Feldman, 1976). However, it appears that CFUs are not formed from

29

primitive haemopoietic stem cells, and actually arise from myeloid precursor cells which differentiate into erythrocytes, granulocytes and platelets (Harrison *et al.*, 1988).

Embryonic grafts might avoid rejection by the recipient, unlike grafts from adults. Initially, grafts from younger fetuses were believed to be less efficient than those from older fetuses (Jacobson, 1956; Russell *et al.*, 1956). Nevertheless fetal liver grafts were not rejected, and the haemopoietic system of adult mice with inherited anaemia was colonized by grafts of syngeneic fetal liver, reversing the recipients' anaemia, without any need for irradiation (Uphoff, 1958; Bernstein & Russell, 1959). The local environment of the haemopoietic tissue influenced grafting; grafts of fetal liver are more successful in recipients with severe forms of anaemia (Seller, 1968), perhaps due to the 'empty space' of anaemic bone marrow and the higher proliferative potential of the donated cells.

The efficiency of haemopoietic stem cells from older embryos to colonize recipient fetuses and adult animals attracted increasing attention. Mononuclear blood islands transplanted from the visceral yolk sac of 9 to 11-day-old mouse fetuses into the yolk sac cavity of 9 to 12-day-old embryos colonized bone marrow, thymus and lymphoid tissue by birth (Weissman *et al.*, 1978). Approximately 100 000 fetal liver cells from 13-day-old mouse fetuses, and containing many haemopoietic stem cells, colonized erythroid and lymphoid tissues when injected into placental blood vessels of 11 to 12-day-old mouse fetuses and persisted for two years or more to repair the inherited macrocytic anaemia of the recipients (Fleischman & Mintz, 1979; Fleischman *et al.*, 1982; Farah *et al.*, 1986). The numbers of stem cells in some inocula were very low yet they achieved partial or whole colonization. Intraperitoneal injections of fetal liver cells into sheep fetuses colonized the recipients' haemopoietic tissues (Flake *et al.*, 1986).

Early-forming haemopoietic stem calls were then grafted into adults to utilize their wide and multipotential developmental capacity to colonize the recipients' haemopoietic system (Burgess & Nicola, 1983). These cells have considerable powers of self-renewal and differentiation, as the precursors of various types of secondary stem cells each committed to the development of a specific type of haemopoietic tissue or cell (Lord, 1983).

The most ambitious studies were carried out by Hollands (1987, 1988*a*, *b*, *c*, 1991). Mouse embryos aged 6–7 days, i.e. before the overt onset of haemopoiesis, were disaggregated and the resulting cell suspensions colonized the haemopoietic tissues of lethally irradiated adult recipients, untreated adult athymic nude mice and others with

Table 1.4. *Colonization of mouse liver and bone marrow on various days after grafting CBA-T6T6 embryonic cells into adult X-irradiated Balb/C recipients*

| | Number of recipients colonized[a] | | | |
| | Liver | | Bone marrow | |
Days after grafting	Low[b]	High	Low[b]	High
1	4	0	0	0
2	7	4	0	0
4	4	14	6	0
8	9	11	9	8
16	0	0	4	16
32	0	0	2	18
64	0	0	0	20

Notes:
[a] Twenty recipients examined on each day; those without colonization not shown.
[b] Classification: low, between 1 and 10 donor mitoses per slide; high $\geqslant 11$ mitoses per slide.
Source: Hollands, 1987.

genetic anaemia (Table 1.4). A day or so after grafting, the injected cells were found in the recipients' liver and they colonized bone marrow a day or two later, literally following the fetal pathway of migration in the adult recipient. Tissues from rat embryos also colonized adult mouse recipients, migrating via the recipients' liver, and persisting throughout their lifespan without any sign of rejection. Cell outgrowths from large groups of blastocysts formed embryoid bodies and blood islands, and also colonized irradiated adult mice. Chromosome and biochemical markers were used to measure the onset and degree of colonization, and show how grafted cells persisted for the full lifetime of recipients. Low rates of colonization were also achieved in intact untreated mice, the degree of success perhaps being restricted by the few niches available in the recipient bone marrow. Fewer than 50 000 cells, many of them not haemopoietic precursors, were grafted into some irradiated recipients, and conferred a survival rate of 80% on them.

Unfortunately, these observations were not confirmed. In one study, disaggregated tissues from 7-day embryos did not colonize adult recipients, whereas those from the yolk sac at day 11 which were used as controls did colonize some of them (Tomlinson, 1989). In another, embryonic mouse cells did not colonize immunocompetent recipients

(Brent *et al.*, 1990). Yet Hollands' work is likely to be correct because a minute proportion of stem cells with similar astonishing powers of colonization have been obtained from bone marrow of adult mice, and very few are needed to colonize adult recipients (Williams *et al.*, 1984; Keller, 1986; Spangrude *et al.*, 1988). The different types of bone marrow cells were identified and separated using monoclonal antibodies against the membrane markers Thy-1 and Sca-1, which characterized stem cells without membranal differentiation markers (Spangrude *et al.*, 1988).

These stem cells formed fewer than 0.05% of the bone marrow population; they were remarkably efficient in splenic assays, only forty being needed to colonize recipient thymus glands and as few as thirty to restore haematopoiesis in lethally X-irradiated adults. They were slow to form functional grafts, but gave permanent colonization, whereas committed precursor cells gave faster but less permanent grafting (Spangrude *et al.*, 1988; Jones *et al.*, 1989). Such techniques enriched primary haemopoietic stem cells and CFUs, and day 12 CFUs were supposed to be primitive multipotential haemopoietic progenitors, but it seems that neither they nor day 8 cells are (Bertoncello *et al.*, 1988; Jones *et al.*, 1989; Ploemacker & Brons, 1989). It is notable that the yolk sac cells used by Hollands did not form CFUs. Similar conclusions about the need for a few stem cells to colonize bone marrow in mouse fetuses were reached when transfected ES cells were injected into mouse blastocysts (Wagner, 1990).

Studies on the grafting of human fetal cells into fetuses and adults will be presented in Chapter 6, this volume.

Grafting neural crest cells

The neural crest is the source of an extraordinarily wide variety of tissues. It differentiates from the epidermis and then from neural epithelium, propagating rostro-caudally at about day 7–8 in the mouse. Cells emigrate from the caudal region before the neural folds fuse in this region although the neural tube and epidermal ectoderm have already formed in the trunk (Nichols, 1981). Cell migration begins as the basal lamina of the neural tube breaks down, or through changes in cell surface adhesiveness or mobility (Erickson, 1986). Neural crest cells arise from the neural plate and epidermis in axolotl, showing that the induction of neural crest is partly governed by local reciprocal interactions between epidermis and the neural plate (Moury & Jacobson, 1990).

Crest cells migrate along defined pathways in chick embryos. Cells in the mesencephalon are the first to migrate, colonizing tissues such as the ectoderm, the first visceral arch and ciliary ganglion. Crest cells from the prosencephalon move rostrally towards the optic stalks, while those migrating from the rhombencephalon move to the visceral and mandibular arches to form mesenchyme, and also form neurons and glia of several ganglia (Erickson, 1986). Crest cells from the trunk migrate to the dermis and epidermis to form pigment cells, and to the anterior dermatome-myotome. Basal laminae are barriers to migration, and fibronectin, collagen and glycosaminoglycans apparently guide their routes of migration. Crest cells do not produce fibronectin and are transported both actively and passively along specific pathways.

Embryonic neural crest cells have considerable abilities to colonize fetuses *in utero*. Cells resembling neural crest migrate from explanted neural tubes of mid-gestation mouse fetuses when cultured *in vitro*. They synthesize catecholamines and become dopa positive after several days' growth, indicating that they have differentiated into adrenergic and prepigment cells (Ito & Takeuchi, 1984).

Cell outgrowths from neural tubes of fetuses aged $8\frac{1}{2}$ days were grafted into recipient mouse fetuses aged $8\frac{1}{4}$, $8\frac{3}{4}$–$9\frac{1}{4}$ or $9\frac{3}{4}$ days; the cells on the outer edges of the outgrowth resembled neural crest cells whereas those in the centre had epithelial or neuronal morphology (Jaenisch, 1985). Sixty per cent of the fetuses survived and 15% were colonized and had pigmented areas in skin, trunk and iris typical of the donor tissue; the percentage rose to 30% with younger cultures indicating that predifferentiated cells had colonized the recipients. Only recipient fetuses aged between $9\frac{1}{4}$ and $9\frac{3}{4}$ days were colonized because donor cells were probably injected into the amniotic cavity of the recipient embryo and gained access to the fetus when the anterior and posterior neurophores were open (Jaenisch, 1985). Once again, a remarkable aspect of the study was the capacity of a few cells to colonize large areas of the recipient, for between 50 and 300 cells only were injected into each fetus.

Grafting primordial germ cells

Primordial germ cells reportedly originate from several tissue precursors. In mouse fetuses, eight of these cells were found at the end of gastrulation, 50–80 cells in mesoderm of the primitive streak and then in endoderm, and about 125 cells by day 8 in hindgut endoderm and the base of the allantois (Ginsburg *et al.*, 1990). Primordial germ cells display active locomotion *in vitro* (Wylie *et al.*, 1986), and possess membrane extensions and processes resembling pseudopodia (Makabe *et al.*, 1989). They move towards the allantois, become incorporated in the developing gut, then migrate through the dorsal mesentery to the genital ridge, evidently by elongation (Fujimoto *et al.*, 1977). Their migration might be mediated as fibronectin promotes cell-to-substrate adhesion, although other evidence implies that they do not adhere to fibronectin, laminin or collagen (Wylie *et al.*, 1986).

Primordial germ cells and those in early gametogenesis in female fetuses might be useful for various forms of grafting. Studies on animals, and possible clinical applications will be presented in Chapter 3, this volume.

Grafting donor ES cells into fetuses and adults

Embryonic or ES cells have mostly if not entirely been used for grafting into recipient blastocysts. They could well have considerable potential for grafting into fetuses, newborn children or adults. Like other grafts, they can be injected into the peripheral circulation of newborn babies and adults, or into specific tissues, and it will be a matter of great interest to find out if they are capable of colonizing tissues in the recipient. Such routes might not be feasible with fetuses, especially with those in early stages of differentiation and questions inevitably arise about the routes of grafting at various fetal ages. This is an important question, especially in view of the fact that the enormous potential of embryonic stem cells might enable them to colonize organs from early in embryonic growth and they might achieve extensive repairs in recipient fetuses.

The fetus is largely inaccessible from the late blastocyst, through the stages of implantation, until it becomes visible on ultrasound at day 25 or thereabouts. Grafts could be of great value at this time and later, as embryogenesis is in full flow in the fetus and grafted cells could well join in these large-scale cell movements and processes of differentiation. Transvaginal ultrasound using a 6.5 MHz vaginal probe now enables the gestational sac to be identified at four weeks and one day after the last menstrual period, i.e. at 20 days postfertilization (Timor-Tritsch & Rottem, 1988). The yolk sac and embryonic pole are visible at five weeks and at five weeks three days respectively, after the last menstrual period. Nevertheless, there seems to be no chance of using ultrasound to visualize the need for fetal organs to be repaired during these stages of growth, or indeed of using any other marker of organ deficiency. It also seems unlikely that such grafts could be carried out with any degree of control or success, short of randomly injecting them into the gestational sac.

Even by day 35 postfertilization, it is not possible to visualize fetal parts clearly, except for the distinct secondary yolk sac. This is seen by

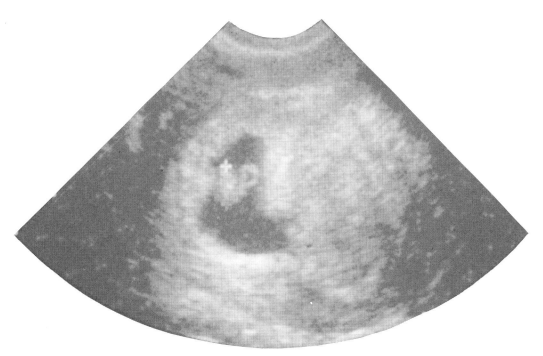

Figure 1.13. An implanted
human fetus seen by
ultrasound 35 days after IVF,
its crown–rump length being
marked. The secondary yolk
sac is seen as a clear ring to the
right of the fetus. Published by
courtesy of Dr Chris Steer.

day 30–35 and its remarkable reflections on ultrasound could serve as a
clear guide or site for the donation of cells. It is, indeed, a source of
various stem cells for the fetus at this stage of gestation. It is probably
too small to be considered as a site for the injection of donor cells, since
it apparently reaches a diameter of only 5 mm before it regresses
(Hamilton *et al.*, 1966; Moore, 1988). Later in development, it might be
possible to insert a fine-gauge needle into the chorionic cavity, or
especially the amniotic cavity, although such methods will require
considerable sophistication in view of the risks of damaging the
embryo which has a crown–rump length of 4–5 mm at 4 weeks and 18
mm at week 7 (Moore, 1988; Figure 1.13).

There is still no possibility of visualizing anomalies in the fetal
organs at these stages of growth, but some grafts might be valuable in
cases of genetic disease in the embryo. Recently, inherited disease has
been diagnosed in fetuses by an early form of placental aspiration from
6 weeks of amenorrhoea, i.e. at 30 days postfertilization or slightly
earlier, when the fetus has a crown–rump length of 4 mm (Brambati *et
al.*, 1988; Brambati, 1990). This represents another avenue of entry into
the embryo and fetus, and could be of great potential value, since the
donation of fetal cells at these ages could help in the colonization of
deficient organs of afflicted fetuses.

It is possible that donor cells injected into the gestational sac or into the peritoneal cavity will colonize the tissues of the growing fetus. Such operations can certainly be achieved at 12 weeks postfertilization, as shown by the successful intraperitoneal injection of three hundred million fetal liver cells into a human fetus described by Touraine (see Chapter 6, this volume). The placental veins also offer a route of access to the fetus in animals and man at these stages of growth, again as outlined in Chapter 6 (this volume), further details being available in a review by Harrison (1991).

Grafting cells from embryos of different ages into embryonic and fetal recipients at different stages of pregnancy has various implications. The extremely broad range of differentiation of embryo and ES cells when used for injection into blastocysts enables them to colonize all the organs of the recipient, so that virtually all tissues become chimaeric; this also occurs with injections of DNA into the male pronucleus of fertilized eggs. The intention of grafting is not to achieve such a widespread colonization: just the opposite is needed for a specific form of repair to a single organ, so that the fetus retains as much of its original identity as possible. In particular, the germ line should not be colonized for this could lead to genetic transmissions from the transplanted tissues.

The use of embryonic or ES cells after they have begun to differentiate should restrict their capacity for widespread colonization. This would obviously be desirable, and the injection of haemopoietic stem cells or primordial germ cells, or their immediate precursors, into the fetal spaces might enable these cells to join in the normal migratory pathways of native stem cells from the yolk sac and elsewhere. Whether these donated cells will be able to migrate and colonize a corresponding fetal organ remains a matter to be decided.

Conclusions

Analyses of early embryonic growth in mammalian cells open new concepts on grafting cells into recipients. Most work has involved their transfer to other embryos to study differentiation or to establish chimaeric animals, and has revealed their enormous capacity for colonizing virtually all organs of the body. The analysis of the actions of genes influencing stem cell formation, growth and differentiation, the roles of growth factors and substrates and the nature of interactions between tissues have been clarified.

Differentiating embryonic cells and tissues can be obtained from embryos or from ES and EC stem cells. Many of these cell lines can remain totipotent or can be induced to differentiate and they are evidently equivalent to ectoderm of the embryonic disc. Their use in grafting has so far been almost entirely restricted to embryos; they might colonize fetuses or adults especially if induced to differentiate along specific pathways before transfer. Genes can be inserted into fertilized eggs and ES and EC cells, or ablated from fertilized eggs. They can then be used: to study differentiation; to construct novel genotypes in offspring; to select various types of differentiating cells; or to inactivate specific genes.

Very small numbers of embryonic and possibly embryonic stem cells are needed to colonize the haemopoietic system and neural crest derivatives when grafted into fetuses or adult animals. Colonization of the haemopoietic system is slow but long lasting.

Acknowledgments

I am grateful to Drs Matteo Adinolfi and Geraldine Hartshorne for their helpful comments on this manuscript.

Note added in proof. A recent example has illustrated the considerable potential of grafting ES cells or other genetically-modified cell lines isolated from tissue outgrowths. Lines of mouse neural cells were established from the cerebellar external germinal layer which coats the developing cerebellar cortex. Clones of these cells were immortalized by incorporating the retrovirus-mediated gene v-*myc*, and single cells were multipotential since they developed *in vitro* into different morphological types expressing various antigens and markers. Clones were then marked by a second retrovirus encoding the *lacZ* reporter gene which helped to identify these cells after their grafting into the brain of recipient mice. These multipotential cells integrated and colonized specific sites in the developing cerebellum. They produced an exact cytoarchitecture, with neurons or glia differentiating according to the nature of the engraftment site. The grafted cells persisted for twenty two months, forming and receiving synapses, and caused no tumours (Snyder *et al.* (1992) *Cell*, **68**, 33–51).

References

ADAMSON, E. D. (1986) Cell-lineage-specific gene expression in development. In: *Experimental Approaches to Mammalian Embryonic Development*, p. 321–64. Eds. J. Rossant & R. A. Pedersen. Cambridge University Press, Cambridge.

ADINOLFI, M. & ADINOLFI, A. (1976) Ontogeny of human plasma proteins: Detection of the onset and site of synthesis using genetic markers and *in vitro* cultures. In: *Structure and Function of Plasma Proteins*, pp. 1–52. Ed. A. C. Allison. Plenum Press, New York.

BARLOW, D. P., STÖGER, R., HEREMANN, B. G., SAITO, K. & SCHWEITZER, N. (1991) The mouse insulin-like growth factor type 2 receptor is imprinted and closely linked to the *Tme* locus. *Nature*, **349**, 84–6.

BAYNA, E. M., SHAPER, J. H. & SHUR, B. D. (1988) Temporally specific involvement of cell surface galactosyl transferase during mouse embryos morula compaction. *Cell*, **53**, 145–7.

BECKER, A. J., McCULLOCH, E. A. & TILL, J. E. (1963) Cytological demonstration of the clonal nature of spleen colonies derived from transplanted mouse marrow cells. *Nature*, **197**, 452–4.

BEDDINGTON, R. (1986) Analysis of tissue fate and prospective potency in the egg cylinder. In: *Experimental Approaches to Mammalian Embryonic Development*, pp. 121–47. Eds. J. Rossant & R. A. Pedersen. Cambridge University Press, Cambridge.

BELLAIRS, R. (1986) The primitive streak. *Anatomy and Embryology*, **174**, 1–140.

BENVENISTE, R., CONWAY, M. C., PUETT, D. & RABINOWITZ, D. (1988) Heterogeneity of the human chorionic gonadotrophin α-subunit secreted by cultured choriocarcinoma (JEG) cells. *Journal of Clinical Endocrinology & Metabolism*, **48**, 85–91.

BERNARD, O., BENNETT, D. & RIPOCHE, M. (1977) Distribution of maternal immunoglobulins in the mouse uterus and embryo in the days after implantation. *Journal of Experimental Medicine*, **145**, 58–75.

BERNSTEIN, S. E. & RUSSELL, E. R. (1959) Implantation of normal blood-forming tissue in genetically anaemic mice, without X-irradiation of the host. *Proceedings of the Society for Experimental Biology and Medicine*, **101**, 769–73.

BERTONCELLO, I., HODGSON, G. S. & BRADLEY, T. R. (1988) Multiparameter analysis of transplantable haemopoietic stem cells. II Stem cells of long-term bone marrow – reconstituted recipients, *Experimental Haematology*, **16**, 245–9.

BOLTON, V. N., OADES, P. J. & JOHNSON, M. H. (1984) The relationship between cleavage, DNA replication, and gene expression in the mouse 2-cell embryo. *Journal of Embryology & Experimental Morphology*, **79**, 139–63.

BONDUELLE, M. L., DODD, R., LIEBAERS, I., VAN STEIRTEGHEM,

A., WILLIAMSON, R. & AKHURST, R. (1988) Chorionic gonadotrophin-β mRNA, a trophoblast marker, is expressed in human 8-cell embryos derived from tripronucleate zygotes. *Human Reproduction*, **3**, 909–14.

BOSE, R., CHENG, H., SABBADINI, E., McCOSHEN, J., MAHADEVAN, M. M. & FLEETHAM, J. (1989) Purified human early pregnancy factor possesses immunosuppressive properties. *American Journal of Obstetrics & Gynecology*, **160**, 954–60.

BRAMBATI, B. (1990) Fate of human pregnancies. In: *Establishing a Successful Human Pregnancy*, Serono Symposium no 66; pp. 269–81. Ed. R. G. Edwards. Raven Press, New York.

BRAMBATI, B., TULUI, L., SIMONI, G. & TRAVI, M. (1988) Prenatal diagnosis at 6 weeks. *Lancet*, **ii**, 397.

BRAUDE, P., BOLTON, V. & MOORE, S. (1988) Human gene expression first occurs between the four- and eight-cell stages of preimplantation development. *Nature*, **332**, 459–62.

BRENT, L., SHERWOOD, R. A., LINCH, D. C. & GALE, R. E. (1990) Failure of embryonic mouse cells to engraft in immunocompetent allogeneic recipients. *British Journal of Haematology*, **72**, 549–50.

BRIGSTOCK, D. R., HEAP, R. B. & BROWN, K. D. (1989) Polypeptide growth factors in uterine tissues and secretions. *Journal of Reproduction & Fertility*, **55**, 267–75.

BRINSTER, R. L. (1974) The effects of cells transferred into the blastocyst on subsequent development. *Journal of Experimental Medicine*, **140**, 1049–56.

BRINSTER, R. L., CHEN, H. Y. & TRUMBAUER, M. (1981) Somatic expression of herpes thymidine kinase in mice following injection of a fusion gene into eggs. *Cell*, **27**, 223–31.

BROWN, C. J., BALLABIO, A., RUPERT, J. L., LAFRENIERE, R. G., GROMPE, M., TONLORENZI, R. & WILLARD, H. F. (1991) A gene from the region of the human X inactivation centre is expressed exclusively from the inactive X chromosome. *Nature*, **349**, 38–44

BRÛLET, P., KAGHAD, M., XU, Y-S., CROISSANT, O. & JACOB, F. (1983) Early differential expression of transposon-like repetitive DNA sequences in the mouse. *Proceedings of the National Academy of Sciences, USA*, **80**, 5641–5.

BULLETTI, C., JASONNI, V. M., TABANELLI, S., GIANAROLI, L., CIOTTI, P. M., FERRARETTI, A. P. & FLAMIGNI, C. (1988) Early human pregnancy *in vitro* utilizing an artificially perfused uterus. *Fertility & Sterility*, **49**, 991–6.

BURGESS, A. & NICOLA, N. (1983) *Growth Factors and Stem Cells*. Academic Press, New York.

BURTON, F. H., HASEL, K. W., BLOOM, F. E. & SUTCLIFFE, J. G. (1991) Pituitary hyperplasia and gigantism in mice caused by a cholera toxin transgene. *Nature*, **350**, 74–77.

CALARCO-GILLAM, P. (1986) Cell–cell interactions in mammalian preimplantation development. In: *Developmental Biology, A Comprehensive Synthesis*, pp. 329–71. Ed. L. W. Browder. Plenum Press, New York.

CHAN, P. J. (1987) Developmental potential of human oocytes according to zona pellucida thickness. *Journal of In Vitro Fertilization and Embryo Transfer*, **4**, 237–41.

CHAPMAN, V. M. (1986) X-chromosome regulation in oogenesis and early mammalian development. In: *Experimental Approaches to Mammalian*

Embryonic Development, pp. 365–98. Ed. J. Rossant & R. A. Pedersen. Cambridge University Press, Cambridge.

CHISAKA, O. & CAPECCHI, M. R. (1991) Regionally restricted developmental defects resulting from targeted disruption of the mouse homeobox gene *hox-1.5*. *Nature*, **350**, 473–9.

CLEGG, K. B. & PIKO, L. (1983) Quantitative aspects of RNA synthesis and polyadenylation in 1-cell and 2-cell mouse embryos. *Journal of Embryology & Experimental Morphology*, **74**, 169–82.

COHEN, J., ELSNER, C., KORT, H., MALTER, H., MASSEY, J., MAYER, M. P. & WEIMER, K. (1989) Impairment of the hatching process following IVF in the human and improvement of implantation by assisting hatching using micromanipulation. *Human Reproduction*, **5**, 7–13.

COLE, R. J., EDWARDS, R. G. & PAUL, J. (1967) Cytodifferentiation and embryogenesis in cell colonies and tissue cultures derived from ova and blastocysts of the rabbit. *Developmental Biology*, **13**, 385–407.

DAMANJOV, I., SOLTER, D. & SKREB, N. (1971) Teratocarcinogenesis as related to the age of embryos grafted under the kidney capsule. *Wilhelm Roux's Arch. Entwickl. Org.*, **173**, 228–4.

DAMSKY, C. H., RICHA, J., WHEELOCK, M., DAMJANOV, I. & BUCK, C. (1985) Characteristics of cell-CAM 120/80 and the role of surface membrane adhesion glycoproteins in early events in mouse embryo morphogenesis. In: *The Cell in Contact: Adhesions and Junctions as Morphogenetic Determinants*, pp. 235–55. Eds. G. M. Edelman & J.-P. Thiery, Wiley & Sons, New York.

DOETSCHMAN, T., GREGG, R. G., MAEDA, N., HOOPER, M. L., MELTON, D. W., THOMPSON, S. & SMITHIES, O. (1987) Targetted correction of a mutant HPRT gene in mouse embryonic stem cells. *Nature*, **330**, 576–8.

DYCE, J., GEORGE, M. A., GOODALL, H. & FLEMING, T. P. (1987) Do cells belonging to trophectoderm and inner cell mass in the mouse blastocyst maintain discrete lineages? *Development*, **100**, 685–98.

EDWARDS, R. G. (1980) *Conception in the Human Female*. Academic Press, London.

EDWARDS, R. G. (1982) The case for studying human embryos and their constituent tissues *in vitro*. In: *Human Conception in Vitro*, pp. 371–88. Eds. R. G. Edwards & J. M. Purdy. Academic Press, London.

EDWARDS, R. G. (1989) *Life Before Birth*, Century Hutchinson, London.

EDWARDS, R. G. & HOLLANDS, P. (1988) New advances in human embryology: implications of the preimplantation diagnosis of genetic disease. *Human Reproduction*, **3**, 549–56.

EDWARDS, R. G., METTLER, L. & WALTERS, D. E. (1986) Identical twins and in vitro fertilization. *Journal of In Vitro Fertilization & Embryo Transfer*, **3**, 114–17.

EDWARDS, R. G. & SURANI, M. A. H. (1978) The primate blastocyst and its environment. *Uppsala Journal of Medical Science*, Supplement, **22**, 39–50.

ENDERS, A. C. (1989) Morphological manifestations of maturation of the blastocyst. *Progress in Clinical & Biological Research*, **294**, 151–70.

ERICKSON, C. A. (1986) Morphogenesis of the neural crest. In: *Developmental Biology, A Comprehensive Synthesis*, pp. 481–543. Ed. L. W. Browder. Plenum Press, New York.

EVANS, M., BRADLEY, A. & ROBERTSON, E. J. (1985) EK contribution to chimaeric mice: from tissue culture to sperm. In: *Genetic Manipulations of the Mammalian Ovum and Early Embryos*. Banbury Report. Cold Spring Harbor New York: Cold Spring Harbor Laboratory.

EVANS, M. J. & KAUFMAN, M. H. (1981) Establishment in culture of pluripotential stem cells from mouse embryos. *Nature*, **292**, 154–5.

FARAH, S. B., SIMPSON, T. J. & GOLBUS, M. S. (1986) Haemopoietic stem cells for the treatment of genetic disease. *Clinical Obstetrics & Gynecology*, **29**, 543–50.

FEHILLY, C. B., WILLADSEN, S. M. & TUCKER, E. M. (1984) Interspecific chimaerism between sheep and goat. *Nature*, **307**, 634–6.

FISHEL, S. B., EDWARDS, R. G. & EVANS, C. J. (1984) Human chorionic gonadotropin secreted by preimplantation embryos cultured *in vitro*. *Science*, **223**, 816–18.

FLAKE, A. W., HARRISON, M. R., ADZICK, N. S. & ZANJANI, E. D. (1986) Transplantation of foetal haemopoietic stem cells *in utero*: the creation of haemopoietic chimaeras. *Science*, **233**, 776–8.

FLEISCHMAN, R. A., CUSTER, R. P. & MINTZ, B. (1982) Totipotent hemopoietic stem cells: Normal self renewal and differentiation after transplantation between mouse fetuses. *Cell*, **30**, 351–9.

FLEISCHMAN, R. A. & MINTZ, B. (1979) Prevention of genetic anaemias in mice by microinjection of normal haemopoietic stem cells into the fetal placenta. *Proceedings of the National Academy of Sciences, USA*, **76**, 5736–40.

FLEMING, T. P. (1987) A quantitative analysis of cell allocation to trophectoderm and inner cells mass in the mouse blastocyst. *Developmental Biology*, **119**, 520–31.

FOLKMAN, J. & KLAGSBRUN, M. (1987) Angiogenic factors. *Science*, **235**, 442–7.

FUJIMOTO, T., MIYAYAMA, T. & FUYUTA, M. (1977) The origin, migration and fine morphology of human primodial germ cells. *Anatomical Record*, **188**, 315–67.

GARDNER, R. L. (1968) Mouse chimaeras obtained by the injection of cells into the blastocyst. *Nature*, **220**, 596–7.

GARDNER, R. L. (1982) Investigation of cell lineage and differentiation in the extraembryonic endoderm of the mouse embryo. *Journal of Embryology & Experimental Morphology*, **68**, 175–98.

GARDNER, R. L. (1985) Origin and development of the trophectoderm and inner cell mass. In: *Implantation of the Human Embryo*, p. 155. Eds. R. G. Edwards, J. M. Purdy & P. C. Steptoe. Academic Press, London.

GARDNER, R. L. & JOHNSON, M. H. (1973) Investigation of early mammalian development using interspecific chimaeras between rat and mouse, *Nature, New Biology*, **246**, 86–9.

GATHERER, D., TEN DIJKE, P., BAIRD, D. T. & AKHURST, R. J. (1990) Expression of TGF-β isoforms during first trimester human embryogenesis. *Development*, **110**, 445–60.

GERHART, J. (1980) Mechanisms regulating pattern formation in the amphibian egg and early embryo. In: *Biological Regulation and Development*, vol 2, pp. 133–6. Ed. R. Goldberger. Plenum Press, New York.

GINSBURG, M., SNOW, M. M. L. & McLAREN, A. (1990) Primordial germ cells in the mouse embryo during gastrulation. *Development*, **110**, 521–28.

GORDON, J. W. & RUDDLE, F. H. (1981) Integration and stable germ line transmission of genes injected into mouse pronuclei. *Science*, **214**, 1244–6.

GORDON, J. W., SCANGOS, G. A., PLOTKIN, D. J., BARBOSA, J. A. & RUDDLE, F. H. (1980) Genetic transformation of mouse embryos by microinjection of purified DNA. *Proceedings of the National Academy of Sciences, USA*, **77**, 7380–4.

GOUSTIN, A. S., BETSCHOLTZ, C., PFEIFFER-OHLSSON, S., PERSSON, H., RYDNERT, J., BYWATER, M. HOLMGREN, G., HELDIN, C. M., WESTERMARK, B. & OHLSSON, R. (1985) Coexpression of sis and myc protooncogenes in developing human placenta suggests autocrine control of trophoblastic growth. *Cell*, **41**, 301–12.

GRAHAM, C. F., ELLISS, C. J., BRICE, A. L., RICHARDSON, L. J., MARSHAL, H. & SCHOFIELD, P. N. (1990) Growth factors and early mammalian development. In: *Establishing a Successful Human Pregnancy*, pp. 239–54. Ed. R. G. Edwards. Serono Symposia Publications 66, Raven Press, Rome.

GREEN, J. B. A. & SMITH, J. C. (1990) Graded changes in dose of a *Xenopus* activin A homologue elicit stepwise transitions in embryonic cell fate. *Nature*, **347**, 391–4.

GROBSTEIN, C. (1951) Intraocular growth and differentiation of the mouse embryonic shield implanted directly and following in vitro cultivation. *Journal of Experimental Zoology*, **116**, 501–25.

GURDON, J. B., MOHUN, T. J., SHARPE, C. R. & TAYLOR, M. V. (1990) Induction, gene activation and embryonic differentiation. In: *Establishing a Successful Human Pregnancy*, pp. 155–69. Ed. R. G. Edwards. Serono Symposia Publications 66, Raven Press, Rome.

HAMILTON, W. J., BOYD, J. D. & MOSSMAN, H. W. (1966) *Human Embryology*. Heffer, Cambridge.

HAMMER, R. E., PURSEL, V. G., REXROAD, C. E. Jr, WALL, R. J., BOLT, D. J., EBERT, K. M., PALMITER, R. D. & BRINSTER, R. L. (1985) Production of transgenic rabbits, sheep and pigs by microinjection. *Nature*, **315**, 680–3.

HARRISON, D. E., ASTLE, C. M. & LERNER, C. (1988) Number and continuous proliferation pattern of transplanted primitive immunohaemopoietic stem cells. *Proceedings of the National Academy of Sciences, USA*, **85**, 222–6.

HARRISON, M. R. (1991) Selection for treatment: Which defects are correctable? In: *The Unborn Patient*, pp. 159–65. Eds. M. R. Harrison, M. S. Golbus & R. A. Filly. W. B. Saunders, Philadelphia.

HARTSHORNE, G. M. & EDWARDS, R. G. (1991) The role of embryonic factors in implantation: recent developments In: *Factors of Importance for Implantation*, pp. 133–58. Ed. M. Seppala. Baillière Tindall, London.

HAUMENHAFT, R., MOSCATELLI, D. & RIFKIN, D. B. (1990) Heparin and heparan sulfate increase the radius of diffusion and action of basic fibroblast growth factor. *Journal of Cell Biology*, **111**, 1651–9.

HAY, L. J. (1968) Organization and fine structure of epithelium and mesenchyme in the developing chick embryo. In: *Epithelial-Mesenchyme Interactions*, pp. 31–55. Eds. R. Fleischmajor & R. E. Billingham. Williams & Wilkins, Baltimore.

HEATH, J. K., BELL, S. & REES, R. (1981) Appearance of functional insulin-receptor during the differentiation of embryonal carcinoma cells. *Journal of Cell Biology*, **91**, 293–7.

HERRMANN, B. G., LABEIT, S., POUSTKA, A., KING, T. R. & LEHRACH, H. (1990) Cloning of the T gene required in mesoderm formation in the mouse. *Nature*, **343**, 617–22.

HERTIG, A. T. (1968) *Human Trophoblast*. C. C. Thomas, Springfield.

HERTIG, A. T. (1975) Implantation of the human ovum: the histogenesis of some aspects of spontaneous abortion. In: *Progress in Infertility*, p. 411. Eds. S. J. Behrman & R. W. Kistner. Little Brown & Co., Boston.

HERTIG, A. T. & ROCK, J. (1949) Two human ova at the pre-villous stage, having a developmental age of about eight and nine days respectively. *Carnegie Institute Contributions to Embryology*, No 221, **33**, 169–86.

HEYNER, S., RAO, L. V., JARETT, L. & SMITH, R. M. (1989) Preimplantation mouse embryos internalise maternal insulin via receptor-mediated endocytosis: Patterns of uptake and functional correlations. *Developmental Biology*, **134**, 48–58.

HOLLANDS, P. (1987) Differentiation and grafting of haemopoietic stem cells from early postimplantation mouse embryos. *Development*, **99**, 69–76.

HOLLANDS, P. (1988*a*) Embryonic haemopoietic stem cell grafts in the treatment of murine genetic anaemia. *British Journal of Haematology*, **70**, 157–63.

HOLLANDS, P. (1988*b*) Differentiation of embryonic haemopoietic stem cells from mouse blastocysts grown *in vitro*. *Development*, **102**, 135–41.

HOLLANDS, P. (1988*c*) Transplantation of embryonic haemopoietic stem cells without prior recipient X-irradiation. *British Journal of Haematology*, **69**, 437–40.

HOLLANDS, P. (1991) Embryonic stem cell grafting: the therapy of the future? *Human Reproduction*, **6**, 79–84.

ITO, K. & TAKEUCHI, T. (1984) The differentiation *in vitro* of the neural crest cells of the mouse embryo. *Journal of Embryology & Experimental Morphology*, **84**, 46–62.

IWAKURA, Y. & NOZAKI, M. (1989) Role of cell surface glycoproteins in the early development of the mouse embryo. *Progress in Clinical Biology & Research*, **294**, 199–210.

JACOBSON, L. O. (1956) Modification of radiation injury in the rabbit. *Proceedings of the Society for Experimental Biology and Medicine*, **91**, 135–9.

JAENISCH, R. (1985) Mammalian neural crest cells participate in normal development when microinjected into preimplantation mouse embryos. *Nature*, **318**, 181–3.

JOHNSON, M. H. (1989) How are two lineages established in early mouse development? *Progress in Clinical Biology & Research*, **294**, 189–98.

JOHNSON, M. H. & MARO, B. (1984) The distribution of cytoplasmic actin in mouse 8-cell blastomeres. *Journal of Embryology & Experimental Morphology*, **82**, 97–117.

JOHNSON, M. H. & MARO, B. (1986) Time and space in the early mouse embryo. In: *Experimental Approaches to Mammalian Embryonic Development*, pp. 35–65. Eds. J. Rossant & R. A. Pedersen. Cambridge University Press, Cambridge.

JOHNSON, M. H., VINCENT, C., BRAUDE, P. R. & PICKERING, S. J. (1990) The cytoskeleton of the oocyte: Its role in the generation of normal and aberrant pre-embryos. In: *Establishing a Successful Human Pregnancy*, pp. 133–42. Ed. R. G. Edwards. Serono Symposium 66. Raven Press, New York.

JONES, R. J., CALENO, P., SHARKIS, S. J. & SENSENBRENNER, L. L. (1989) Two phases of engraftment established by serial bone marrow transplantation in mice. *Blood*, **73**, 397–401.

JOYNER, A. L., SKARNES, W. C. & ROSSANT, J. (1988) Production of a mutation in mouse *En-2* gene by homologous recombination in embryonic stem cells. *Nature*, **338**, 153–6.

KELLER, R. E. (1986) The cellular basis of amphibian development. In: *Developmental Biology, A Comprehensive Synthesis*, pp. 241–327. Ed. L. W. Browder. Plenum Press, New York.

KELLY, S. J., MULNARD, J. G. & GRAHAM, C. F. (1978) Cell division and cell allocation in early mouse development. *Journal of Embryology & Experimental Morphology*, **48**, 37–51.

KIDDER, G. M. & McLACHLIN, J. R. (1985) Timing of transcription and protein synthesis underlying morphogenesis in preimplantation mouse embryos. *Developmental Biology*, **112**, 265–75.

KIM, H-S. & SMITHERS, O. (1988) Recombinant fragment assay for gene targetting based on the polymerase chain reaction. *Nucleic Acid Research*, **16**, 8887–903.

KIMELMAN, D. & KIRSCHNER, M. (1987) Synergistic induction of mesoderm by FGF and TGF-β and the identification of an mRNA coding for FGF in the early *Xenopus* embryo. *Cell*, **51**, 869–77.

KITAMURA, D., ROES, J., KÜHN, R. & RAJEWSKY, K. (1991) A β-cell deficient mouse by targetted disruption of the membrane exon of the immunoglobulin μ-chain. *Nature*, **350**, 423–6.

KRASNOW, M. A., CUMBERLEDGE, S., MANNING, G., HERZEN-BERG, L. A. & NOLAN, G. P. (1991) Whole animal cell sorting of *Drosophila* embryos. *Science*, **251**, 81–5.

LASKEY, R. A., FAIRMAN, M. P. & BLOW, J. J. (1989) S phase of the cell cycle. *Science*, **246**, 609–13.

LEESE, H. J., HUMPHERSON, P. G., HARDY, K., HOOPER, M. A. K., WINSTON, R. M. L., & HANDYSIDE, A. H. (1991) Profiles of hypoxanthine guanine phosphoribosyl transferase and adenosine phosphoribosyl transferase activities measured in single preimplantation human embryos by high-performance liquid chromatography. *Journal of Reproduction & Fertility*, **91**, 197–202.

LENARDO, M. J., STANDT, L., ROBBINS, P., KUANG, A., MULLI-GAN, R. C. & BALTIMORE, D. (1989) Repression of the Ig H enhancer in teratocarcinoma cells associated with a novel octamer factor. *Science*, **243**, 544–6.

LEWIN, B. (1980) Complexity of mRNA populations. In: *Gene Expression. II. Eukaryotic Chromosomes*, pp. 697–727. Ed. B. Lewin, Wiley & Sons, New York.

LOPATA, A. & HAY, D. L. (1989) The potential of early human embryos to form blastocysts, hatch from their zona and secrete HCG in culture. *Human Reproduction*, **4**, Supplement 1, 87–94.

LORD, R. I. (1983) In: *Haemopoietic Stem Cells*. Ed. C. S. Potten. Churchill Livingston, London.

LUCKETT, W. P. (1978) Origin and differentiation of the yolk sac and extraembryonic mesoderm in presomite human and rhesus monkey embryos. *American Journal of Anatomy*, **152**, 59–98.

McMAHON, A. P. & BRADLEY, A. (1990) The *Wnt-1(int-1)* proto-oncogene is required for development of a large region of the mouse brain. *Cell*, **62**, 1073–85.

MAGNUSON, T. (1986) Mutations and chromosomal abnormalities: How are they useful for studying genetic control of early mammalian development? In: *Experimental Approaches to Mammalian Embryonic Development*. pp. 437–74. Eds. J. Rossant & R. A. Pedersen. Cambridge University Press, Cambridge.

MAGNUSON, T. & EPSTEIN, C. J. (1987) Genetic control of very early mammalian development. *Biological Reviews*, **56**, 369–408.

MAKABE, S., NOTTOLA, S. A. & MOTTA, P. M. (1989) Life history of the human female germ cell: ultrastructural aspects. In: *Ultrastructure of Human Gametogenesis and Early Embryogenesis*, p. 33. Eds. J. van Blerkon & P. M. Motta. Kluwer, Boston.

MANES, C., BYERS, M. J. & CARVER, A. S. (1981) Mobilization of genetic information in the early rabbit trophoblast. In: *Cellular and Molecular Aspects of Implantation*, pp. 113–24. Eds. S. R. Glasser & D. W. Bullock. Plenum Press, New York.

MANES, C. & MENZEL, P. (1981) Demethylation of CpG sites of DNA in early rabbit trophoblast. *Nature*, **293**, 589–90.

MANSOUR, S. L., THOMAS, K. R. & CAPECCHI, M. R. (1988) Disruption of the proto-ocogene *int*-2 in mouse embryo-derived stem cells: a general strategy in targeting mutations to non-selectable genes. *Nature*, **336**, 348–52.

MARO, B., JOHNSON, M. H., PICKERING, S. J. & FLACH, G. (1984) Changes in actin distribution during fertilization of the mouse egg. *Journal of Embryology & Experimental Morphology*, **81**, 211–37.

MARTIN, G. R., EPSTEIN, C. J., TRAVIS, B., TUCKER, G., YATZIV, S., MARTIN, D. W. Jr, CLIFT, S. & COHEN, S. (1977) X-chromosome inactivation during differentiation of female teratocarcinoma stem cells *in vitro*. *Nature*, **271**, 329–33.

MARUO, T. & MOCHIZUKI, M. (1987) Immunohistochemical localization of epidermal growth factor receptor and myc oncogene product in human placenta: implication for trophoblast proliferation and differentiation. *American Journal of Obstetrics & Gynecology*, **156**, 721–7.

MASSAGUE, J. (1983) Epidermal growth factor-like transforming growth factor. II. Interaction with epidermal growth factor receptors in human placental membranes and A431 cells. *Journal of Biological Chemistry*, **258**, 13614–20.

MATSUI, Y., ZSEBO, K. M. & HOGAN, B. L. M. (1990) Embryonic expression of a haematopoietic growth factor encoded by the S1 locus and the ligand for c-kit. *Nature*, **347**, 667–9.

MERCOLA, M. & STILES, C. D. (1988) Growth factor superfamilies and mammalian embryogenesis. *Development*, **102**, 451–60.

METCALF, D. & MOORE, M. A. S. (1971) Haemopoietic cells. In: *Frontiers of Biology*, Volume 24. Eds. A. Neuberger & E. L. Tatum. North Holland, Amsterdam.

MOORE, K. L. (1988) *The Developing Human*. W. B. Saunders, Philadelphia.

MOORE, M. A. S. & METCALF, D. (1970) Ontogeny of the haemopoietic system: yolk sac origin of in vivo and in vitro colony forming cells in the developing mouse embryo. *British Journal of Haematology*, **18**, 279–86.

45

MOURY, J. D. & JACOBSON, A. G. (1990) The origin of neural crest cells in the axolotl. *Developmental Biology*, **141**, 243–53.

MURAMATSU, H., ISHIHARA, H., MIYAUCHI, T., GACHELIN, G., FUJISAKA, T., TEJIMA, S. & MURAMATSU, T. (1983) Glycoprotein-bound large carbohydrates of early embryonic cells: structural characteristic of the glycan isolated from F9 embryonal carcinoma cells. *Journal of Biochemistry*, **94**, 799–810.

MURGITA, R. A. & TOMASI, T. B. (1975) Suppression of the immune response by α-fetoprotein I and II. *Journal of Experimental Medicine*, **141**, 269 and 440.

NEW, D. A. T. (1991) The culture of post-implantation embryos. *Human Reproduction*, **6**, 58–63.

NICHOLAS, J. S. & HALL, B. B. (1940) Experiments on developing rats. II: The development of isolated blastomeres and fused eggs. *Journal of Experimental Zoology*, **90**, 441–59.

NICHOLAS, N. S. & PANAGI, G. S. (1985) Inhibition of interleukin-2 production by retroplacental sera: a possible mechanism for human fetal allograft survival. *American Journal of Reproductive Immunology & Microbiology*, **9**, 6.

NICHOLLS, R. D., KNOLL, J. H. M., BUTLER, M. G., KARAM, S. & LALONDE, M. (1989) Genetic imprinting suggested by maternal heterodisomy in non-deletion Prader-Willi syndrome. *Nature*, **342**, 281–5.

NICHOLS, D. H. (1981) Neural crest formation in the head of the mouse embryo as observed using a new histological technique. *Journal of Embryology & Experimental Morphology*, **64**, 105–20.

NUCCITELLI, R. & WILEY, L. M. (1985) Polarity of isolated blastomeres from morulae: detection of transcellular ion currents. *Developmental Biology*, **109**, 452–63.

OKAMOTO, K., OKAZAWA, H., OKUDA, A., SAKAI, M., MURAMATSU, M. & HAMADA, H. (1990) A novel octamer binding transcription factor is differentially expressed in mouse embryonic cells. *Cell*, **60**, 461–72.

O'NEILL, C., COLLIER, M., AMMIT, A. J., RYAN, J. P., SAUNDERS, D. M. & PIKE, I. L. (1989) Supplementation of *in-vitro* fertilisation culture medium with platelet activating factor. *Lancet*, **ii**, 769–72.

O'RAHILLY, R. & MULLER, F. (1987) *Developmental Stages in Human Embryos*. Carnegie Institute of Washington, publication 637.

OVERSTROM, E. W., BENOS, D. J. & BIGGERS, J. D. (1989) Synthesis of Na^+/K^+ ATPase by the preimplantation rabbit blastocyst. *Journal of Reproduction & Fertility*, **85**, 283–95.

OZIL, J.-P. (1983) Production of identical twins by bisection of blastocysts in the cow. *Journal of Reproduction & Fertility*, **69**, 463–8.

PALMITER, R. D., BRINSTER, R. L., HAMMER, R. E., TRUMBAUER, M. E., ROSENFELD, M. G., BIRNBERG, N. C. & EVANS, R. M. (1982) Dramatic growth of mice that develop from eggs microinjected with metallothionein-growth hormone fusion genes. *Nature*, **300**, 611–15.

PARIA, B. C. & DEY, S. K. (1990) Preimplantation embryo development *in vitro*: Cooperative interactions among embryos and role of growth factors. *Proceedings of the National Academy of Sciences, USA*, **87**, 4756–60.

PAYNTON, B. V., REMPEL, R. & BACHVAROVA, R. (1988) Changes in state of adenylation and time course of degradation of maternal mRNAs during oocyte maturation and early embryonic development in the mouse. *Developmental Biology*, **129**, 304–14.

PERA, M. F., COOPER, S., BENNET, W. & CRAWFORD-BRYCE, I. (1990) In vitro models for the study of human peri-implantation development. *Human Reproduction*, **6**, Supplement, Abstract no 103.

PERAH, G. & FELDMAN, M. (1976) In vitro activation of the in vivo colony-forming units of the mouse yolk sac. *Journal of Cellular Physiology*, **91**, 193–200.

PERONA, R. M. & WASSARMAN, P. M. (1986) Mouse blastocysts hatch *in vitro* by using trypsin-like proteinase associated with cells of mural trophectoderm. *Developmental Biology*, **114**, 42–52.

PIKO, L. & CLEGG, K. B. (1982) Quantitative changes in total RNA, total poly (A), and ribosomes in early mouse embryos. *Developmental Biology*, **89**, 362–78.

PLOEMACKER, R. E. & BRONS, N. H. (1989) Separation of CFU-S from primitive cells responsible for reconstitution of the bone marrow hemopoietic stem cell compartment following irradiation: evidence for a pre-CFU-S cell. *Experimental Haematology*, **17**, 263–6.

RAPPOLEE, D. A., BRENNER, C. A., SCHULTZ, R., MARK, D. & WERB, Z. (1988) Developmental expression of PDGF, TGF-α, and TFG-β genes in preimplantation mouse embryos. *Science*, **241**, 1823–5.

RAPPOLEE, D. A., STURM, K. S., SCHULTZ, G. A., PEDERSEN, R. A. & WERB, Z. (1989) In: *Early Embryonic Development and Paracrine Relationships*. Eds. S. Heyner & L. Wiley, UCLA Symposia on Molecular and Cellular Biology. New Series 117. A. R. Liss Inc., New York.

RICHA, J. & SOLTER, D. (1986) Role of cell surface molecules in early mammalian development. In: *Experimental Approaches to Mammalian Embryonic Development*, pp. 293–320. Eds. J. Rossant & R. A. Pedersen. Cambridge University Press, Cambridge.

RIZZINO, A. (1988) Transforming growth factor-β: Multiple effects on cell differentiation and extracellular matrices. *Developmental Biology*, **130**, 411–22.

ROBERTSON, E. J. & BRADLEY, A. (1986) Production of permanent cell lines from early embryos and their use in studying developmental problems. In: *Experimental Approaches to Mammalian Embryonic Development*, pp. 475–508. Eds. J. Rossant & R. A. Pedersen. Cambridge University Press, Cambridge.

ROSNER, M. H., VIGANO, M. A., OZATO, K., TIMMONS, P. M., POIRIER, F., RIGBY, P. W. J. & STANDT, L. M. (1990) A POU-domain transcription factor in early stem cells and germ cells of the mammalian embryo. *Nature*, **345**, 686–92.

ROSSANT, J. (1986) Development of extraembryonic cell lineages in the mouse embryo. In: *Experimental Approaches to Mammalian Embryonic Development*, pp. 97–120. Eds. J. Rossant & R. A. Pedersen. Cambridge University Press, Cambridge.

RUSSELL, E. S. & BERNSTEIN, S. S. (1966) Blood and blood formation. In: *Biology of the Laboratory Mouse*, pp. 351–72. Ed. E. L. Green. McGraw-Hill, New York.

RUSSELL, E. S., SMITH, L. J. & LAWSON, E. A. (1956) Implantation of normal blood-forming tissue in radiated genetically anaemic hosts. *Science*, **124**, 1076–7.

SAGATA, N., OSKARSSON, M., COPELAND, T., BRUMBAUGH, J. & VANDE WOUDE, G. G. (1988) Function of c-*mos* proto-oncogene product in meiotic maturation of *Xenopus* oocytes. *Nature*, **335**, 519–25.

SAWICKI, J. A., MAGNUSSON, T. & EPSTEIN, C. J. (1982) Evidence for the expression of the paternal genome in the two-cell mouse embryo. *Nature*, **294**, 450–1.

SCHÖLER, H. R., RUPPERT, S., SUZUKI, N., CHOWDHURY, K., & GRUSS, P. (1990) New type of POU domain in germ line-specific protein *oct*-4. *Nature*, **344**, 435–9.

SCHROEDER, T. E. (1986) The egg cortex in early development of sea urchins and starfish. In: *Developmental Biology, A Comprehensive Synthesis*, pp. 59–100. Ed. L. W. Browder. Plenum Press, New York.

SCHULTZ, R. M. (1986) Molecular aspects of mammalian oocyte growth and maturation. In: *Experimental Approaches to Mammalian Embryonic Development*, pp. 195–265. Eds. J. Rossant & R. A. Pedersen. Cambridge University Press, Cambridge.

SEIDEL, F. (1952) Die Entwicklungspotenzen einer isolierten Blastomere des Zweizellenstadiums im Saugetierei. *Naturwissenschaften*, **39**, 355–6.

SELLER, M. J. (1968) Transplantation of anaemic mice of the W-series with haemopoietic tissue bearing marker chromosomes. *Nature*, **220**, 300–1.

SEPPÄ, H., GROTENDORST, G., SEPPÄ, S., SCHIFFMANN, E. & MARTIN, G. R. (1982) Platelet-derived growth factor is chemotactic for fibroblasts. *Journal of Cellular Biology*, **92**, 584–8.

SHUR, B. D. (1977) Cell surface glycosyltransferases in gastrulating chick embryos. I. Temporally and spatially specific patterns of four endogenous glycosyltransferase activities. *Developmental Biology*, **58**, 23–39.

SKREB, N. & SVAJGER, A. (1975) Experimental teratomas in rats. In: *Teratomas and Differentiation*, pp. 83–97. Ed. D. Solter. Academic Press, London.

SMITH, A. G., HEATH, J. K., DONALDSON, D. D., WONG, G. G., MOREAU, J., STAHL, M. & ROGERS, D. (1988) Inhibition of pluripotential embryonic stem cell differentiation by purified polypeptides. *Nature*, **336**, 688–90.

SMITH, E. P., SADLER, T. W. & D'ERCOLE, A. J. (1987) Somatomedins/insulin-like growth factors, their receptors and binding proteins are present during mouse embryogenesis. *Development*, **101**, 73–82.

SOLURSH, M. (1986) Migration of sea urchin primary mesenchyme cells. In: *Developmental Biology, A Comprehensive Synthesis*, pp. 391–431. Ed. L. W. Browder. Plenum Press, New York.

SPANGRUDE, G. J., HEIMFELD, S. & WEISSMAN, I. L. (1988) Identification and characterisation of mouse hemopoietic stem cells. *Science*, **241**, 58–62.

SPIEGEL, E. & SPIEGEL, M. (1986) Cell–cell interactions during sea urchin morphogenesis. In: *Developmental Biology, A Comprehensive Synthesis*, pp. 195–240. Ed. L. W. Browder. Plenum Press, New York.

STEVENS, L. C. & LITTLE, C. C. (1954) Spontaneous testicular tumours in an inbred strain of mice. *Proceedings of the National Academy of Sciences, USA*, **40**, 1080–7.

STEVENS, L. C. & VARNUM, D. S. (1974) The development of teratomas from parthenogenetically activated ovarian mouse eggs. *Developmental Biology*, **37**, 369–80.

STEWART, C. L. (1982) Formation of viable chimaeras by aggregation between teratocarcinomas and preimplantation mouse embryos. *Journal of Embryology & Experimental Morphology*, **67**, 167–79.

STIMSON, W. H. (1972) Transplantation – nature's success. *Lancet*, **i**, 684.

SURANI, M. A., ALLEN, N. D., BARTON, S. C., FUNDELE, R., HOWLETT, S. K., NORRIS, M. L. & REIK, W. (1990) Developmental consequences of imprinting of parental chromosomes by DNA methylation. *Philosophical Transaction of the Royal Society, B*, **326**, 313–27.

SVAJGER, A., LEVAK-SVAJGER, B., KOSTOVIC-KNEZEVIC, L. & BRADAMANTE, Z. (1981) Morphogenetic behaviour of the rat embryonic ectoderm as a renal homograft. *Journal of Embryology & Experimental Morphology*, Suppl, **65**, 243–67.

TAKAGI, N. & MARTIN, G. R. (1984) Studies of the temporal relationship between the cytogenetic and biochemical manifestations of X-chromosome inactivation during the differentiation of LT-1 teratocarcinoma stem cells. *Developmental Biology*, **103**, 425–33.

TAKAGI, N., SUGAWARA, O. & SASAKI, M. (1982) Regional and temporal changes in the pattern of X-chromosome replication during the early post-implantation development of the female mouse. *Chromosoma, Berlin*, **85**, 275–86.

TARKOWSKI, A. K. & WROBLEWSKA, J. (1967) Development of blastomeres of mouse eggs isolated at the 4- and 8-cell stage. *Journal of Embryology & Experimental Morphology*, **18**, 155–80.

TESARIK, J. (1992) Metabolism of human preimplantation embryos. In: *Preimplantation Diagnosis of Human Genetic Disease*. Ed. R. G. Edwards. Cambridge University Press, Cambridge, in press.

TESARIK, J., KOPECNY, V., PLACHOT, M. & MANDELBAUM, J. (1987) Ultrastructural and auroradiographic observations on multinucleated blastomeres of human cleaving embryos obtained by in vitro fertilization. *Human Reproduction*, **2**, 127–36.

THOMAS, K. R. & CAPECCHI, M. R. (1987) Site-directed mutagenesis by gene targeting in mouse embryo-derived stem cells. *Cell*, **51**, 503–12.

THOMAS, K. R. & CAPECCHI, M. R. (1990) Targeted disruption of the murine *int*-1 proto-oncogene resulting in severe abnormalities in midbrain and cerebellar development. *Nature*, **346**, 847–50.

TILL, J. E. & McCULLOCH, E. A. (1961) A direct measurement of the radiation sensitivity of normal bone marrow cells. *Radiation Reviews*, **14**, 213–22.

TIMOR-TRITSCH, I. E. & ROTTEM, S. (eds.) (1988) *Transvaginal Sonography*. Heinemann Medical, London.

TOMLINSON, J. W. (1989) *Transplantation of foetal haemopoietic stem cells into lethally X-irradiated and beta-thalassaemic mice*. Thesis, Monash University, Victoria.

UPHOFF, D. E. (1958) Preclusion of secondary phase of irradiation syndrome by inoculation of foetal haemopoietic tissue following lethal total body X-irradiation. *Journal of the National Cancer Institute*, **20**, 625–32.

VEIGA, A., CALDERON, G., SANTALO, J., BARRI, P. N. & EGOZCUE, J. (1987) Chromosome studies in oocytes and zygotes from an IVF programme. *Human Reproduction*, **2**, 425–30.

WAGNER, E. F. (1990) On transferring genes into stem cells and mice. *EMBO Journal*, **9**, 3025–92.

WAGNER, E. F. & STEWART, C. L. (1986) Integration and expression of genes introduced into mouse embryos. In: *Experimental Approaches to Mammalian Embryonic Development*, pp. 509–49. Eds. J. Rossant & R. A. Pedersen. Cambridge University Press, Cambridge.

WASSARMAN, P. M. (1990) Biochemistry and functions of mouse zona pellucida glycoproteins. In: *Establishing a Successful Human Pregnancy*, pp. 103–14. Ed. R. G. Edwards. Serono Symposium 66. Raven Press, New York.

WATANABE, N., VANDE WOUDE, G. F., IKAWA, Y. & SAGATA, N. (1990) Specific proteolysis of the c-*mos* proto-oncogene product by calpain on fertilization of *Xenopus* eggs. *Nature*, **342**, 505–11.

WEISSMAN. X., PAPAIOANNOU, V. & GARDNER R. L. (1978) Fetal haemopoietic origins of the haematolymphoid system. In: *Differentiation of Normal and Neoplastic Haemopoietic Cells*, pp. 33–47. Eds. B. Clarkson, T. Marks & J. Till. Cold Spring Harbor, New York.

WILEY, L. M. (1984) The cell surface of the mammalian embryo during early development. In: *Ultrastructure of Reproduction*, pp. 190–204. Eds. J. van Blerkon & P. M. Motta. Martinus Nijhoff, The Hague.

WILLADSEN, S. (1979) A method for culture of micromanipulated sheep embryos and its use to produce monozygotic twins. *Nature*, **277**, 298–300.

WILLIAMS, D. A., LEMISCHKA, I. R., NATHAN, D. G. & MULLIGAN, R. C. (1984) Introduction of new genetic material into pluripotent haemopoietic stem cells of the mouse. *Nature*, **310**, 476–80.

WILLIAMS, R. L., COURTNEIDGE, S. A. & WAGNER, E. F. (1988) Embryonic lethalities and endothelial tumors in chimeric mice expressing polyoma virus middle T oncogene. *Cell*, **52**, 121–31.

WINKEL, G. K. & PEDERSEN, R. A. (1988) Fate of the inner cell mass in mouse embryos as studied by microinjection of lineage markers. *Developmental Biology*, **127**, 143–56.

WITTE, O. N. (1990) *Steel* locus defines new multipotent growth factor. *Cell*, **63**, 5–6.

WOLF, S. & MIGEON, B. R. (1985) Clusters of CpG dinucleotides implicated by nuclease hypersensitivity as control elements in housekeeping genes. *Nature*, **314**, 467–69.

WOOD, S. A. & KAYE, P. L. (1989) Effects of epidermal growth factor on preimplantation mouse embryos. *Journal of Reproduction & Fertility*, **85**, 575–82.

WYLIE, C. C., STOTT, D. & DONOVAN, P. J. (1986) Primordial germ cell migration. In: *Developmental Biology: A Comprehensive Synthesis*, pp. 433–48. Ed. L. W. Browder. Plenum Press, New York.

YACHNIN, S. & LESTER, E. (1976) Inhibition of human lymphocyte transformation by human alpha fetoprotein (HAFP); comparison of foetal and hepatoma HAFP and kinetic studies of in vitro immunosuppression. *Clinical and Experimental Immunology*, **26**, 484–90.

YAMAZAKI, K. & KATO, Y. (1989) Sites of zona pellucida shedding by mouse embryos other than mural trophectoderm. *Journal of Experimental Zoology*, **249**, 347–9.

YANAGIMACHI, R. (1988) Mammalian fertilization. In: *The Physiology of Reproduction*, pp. 135–85. Eds. E. Knobil & J. Neill. Raven Press, New York.

ZIOMEK, C. A. (1982) The roles of phenotype and position in guiding the fate of 16-cell mouse blastomeres. *Developmental Biology*, **91**, 440–7.

CHAPTER 2

Organogenesis and central nervous system development

T. W. SADLER

CONTENTS

ORGANOGENESIS BEGINS in the third week of gestation (postfertilization) with the process of gastrulation and ends in the eighth week. During this six-week period, known as the time of embryogenesis, primordia for most of the organ systems are established and the conceptus becomes recognizable as a human fetus. These six weeks are also marked as the period of greatest sensitivity for induction of major congenital malformations and each organ system experiences its own peak(s) of susceptibility to insult during this time frame. By the ninth week, the conceptus enters the fetal period, which is characterized by the growth and continued differentiation of the tissues and organs that were established previously. Thus, most of the tissues and organs are established early in gestation as a result of cell–cell interactions, including inductive events. The remainder of pregnancy is then characterized by continued cell differentiation and growth.

Gastrulation

Gastrulation is the process that establishes the three germ layers, ectoderm, mesoderm, and endoderm, that are responsible for formation of all embryonic structures. Prior to this process, the embryo consists of two cell layers comprising the epiblast dorsally and the hypoblast ventrally (Figure 2.1). On the fourteenth to fifteenth day of gestation, the caudal half of the epiblast becomes marked by a shallow depression, the primitive streak. Its cephalic end is marked by a slight elevation, the primitive node (of Henson), surrounding the primitive pit. Cells of the epiblast migrate toward the streak, detach from this cell

Figure 2.1. Schematic drawing of a 14-day embryo (postfertilization) at the initiation of gastrulation. The inset (arrow) shows a sagittal view of the 2 cell layers, epiblast (dorsally) and hypoblast (ventrally) that comprise the embryonic disc at this stage. In the large view the amnion (A) and primitive yolk sac (YS) have been cut away to reveal a dorsal view of the epiblast, which is marked by the primitive streak in the caudal half and the prochordal plate in the cephalic region. (Reproduced from T. Sadler, *Langman's Medical Embryology*, 6th edition, © (1990), the Williams & Wilkins Co., Baltimore.)

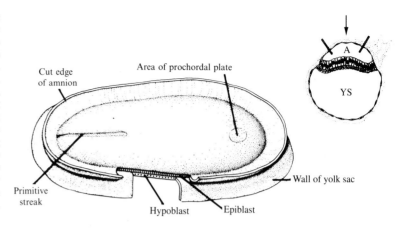

layer, and turn inward to lie between the hypoblast and remaining epiblast (Figure 2.2). The first cells to migrate displace the hypoblast and form the embryonic endoderm; later arriving cells form the mesoderm; and cells remaining in the epiblast form the ectoderm. Thus, all three germ layers and, ultimately, all tissues of the embryo are derived from the epiblast layer.

Ectoderm gives rise to the central and peripheral nervous systems; sensory epithelium of the ear, nose, and eye; subcutaneous glands, mammary glands, pituitary, and enamel of the teeth. Mesoderm provides: blood and lymph cells; endothelium of blood vessels and the heart; kidneys and gonads; cortical portion of the suprarenal glands; and the spleen. It also provides muscle, cartilage and bone, except in the facial region where the cells of the neural crest, which is a derivative of the neurectoderm, form the bone and connective tissue (Noden, 1988). Derivatives of the endoderm include: the epithelial lining of the respiratory tract; parenchyma of the thyroid, parathyroid, liver, and pancreas; reticular stroma of the tonsils and thymus; epithelial lining of

Figure 2.2. Schematic drawing of a 16-day embryo that is undergoing gastrulation; the process that establishes 3 germ layers (ectoderm, mesoderm, and endoderm) from which all organ systems will form. The primitive streak is marked cephalically by the primitive node (of Henson) and through these regions cells of the epiblast will migrate to form the endoderm and mesoderm. Cells remaining in the epiblast layer will form the ectoderm. (Reproduced from T. Sadler, *Langman's Medical Embryology*, 6th edition, © (1990), the Williams & Wilkins Co., Baltimore.)

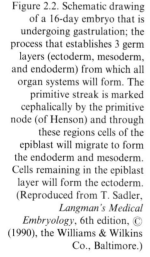
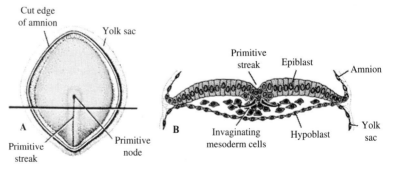

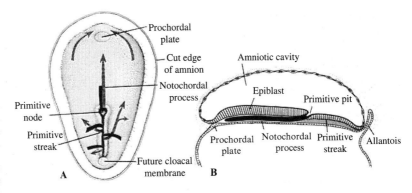

Figure 2.3. Schematic view showing paths of cell migration in a 16-day embryo undergoing gastrulation (A). The embryonic disc is slipper shaped, being larger at the cephalic end, and is marked by areas of fusion between epiblast and hypoblast cells in the cranial and caudal regions representing the prochordal and cloacal plates, respectively. Later these plates (membranes) will break down to provide openings to the oral and anal cavities. In a midsagittal section (B), the notochordal plate, which at this time is intercalated with the endoderm (see also Figure 2.4) can be observed. The primitive streak exists in the caudal portion of the embryo and will continue in existence until neural tube closure is completed on approximately day 27. (Reproduced from T. Sadler, *Langman's Medical Embryology*, 6th edition, © (1990), the Williams & Wilkins Co., Baltimore.)

the bladder and urethra; and the epithelial lining of the tympanic cavity.

As gastrulation proceeds, some cells turn inward in the region of the primitive pit and migrate in the midline to the prochordal plate (a fused region of epiblast and hypoblast at the cranial end of the embryo (Figure 2.3). Later it becomes the buccopharyngeal membrane). This central line of mesoderm cells first intercalates with the endoderm to form the notochordal plate (Figure 2.4) and later detaches to form the definitive notochord, which will serve as the basis for the axial skeleton. The notochord extends from the prochordal plate to the primitive pit and lengthens as the pit and primitive streak assume a more posterior position.

Gastrulation proceeds in a cephalocaudal direction, such that the cranial portion of the embryo is populated with cells prior to more caudal segments. The process is not completed until the end of the fourth week when the streak regresses and disappears. By this time neurulation has occurred and the primitive brain vesicles have been established. Thus, germ layers in the cranial end of the embryo begin their differentiation, while these layers continue their formation in caudal segments.

Molecular signals responsible for mesoderm formation during gastrulation are becoming better defined, but have been investigated primarily in non-mammalian species. The most popular organism for these studies is the frog *Xenopus*, which undergoes gastrulation by invagination of cells through the blastopore, a pore-like structure analogous to the primitive streak in humans (Figure 2.5). Interactions between animal pole cells (epiblast?) and cells of the vegetal hemisphere (hypoblast?) during the blastula stage establish the embryonic mesoderm and the dorsoventral and anterior–posterior axes (Spemann & Mangold, 1924; Nieuwkoop, 1969; Gurdon *et al.*, 1989; Smith, 1989).

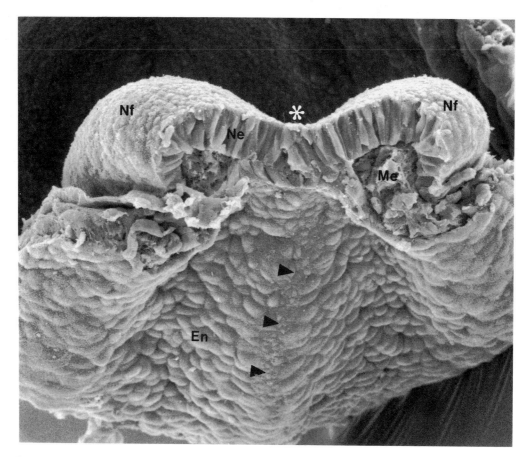

Figure 2.4. Scanning electron micrograph of the ventral surface of a mouse embryo equivalent to 16-day human conceptus. The notochordal plate (arrowheads) is intercalated with endoderm cells (En) in the midline. Neuroepithelial cells (Ne); neural folds (Nf); neural groove (asterisk); mesoderm (Me). (Courtesy Dr K. K. Sullik, Department of Cell Biology and Anatomy, University of North Carolina).

The vegetal cells produce mesoderm inducing factors (MIFs) including members of the TGF-β (transforming growth factor) family (Smith, 1987; Rosa et al., 1988; Smith et al., 1988), and basic fibroblast growth factor (bFGF) (Kimelman & Kirschner, 1987; Slack et al., 1987; Kimelman et al., 1988; Slack & Isaacs, 1989). These two factors are responsible for mesoderm induction, although different tissues are induced by each and are concentration dependent. Thus, TGF-β-like factors induce muscle, whereas bFGF induces the formation of mesenchyme and mesothelium (Green et al., 1990).

In addition to the initial process of mesoderm induction, the dorsal lip of the blastopore together with mesoderm cells, including the notochord (chordamesoderm), in the embryo are responsible for induction of neural tissue. This property of the dorsal lip has been known for many years and is present in amphibians, where it is known as the 'organizer' (Spemann & Mangold, 1924), and is also present in the primitive node surrounding the primitive pit in birds and mammals

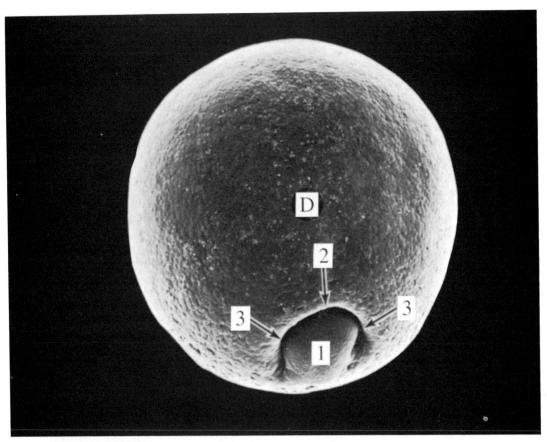

Figure 2.5. Scanning electron micrograph of the dorsal (D) surface of a frog embryo (*Xenopus*) undergoing gastrulation. The dorsal (2) and lateral (3) lips of the blastopore partially surround the yolk plug (1) and are equivalent to the primitive streak region of human embryos. Thus, cells migrate inward through this groove to form the germ layers. The dorsal lip region, together with cells of the notochord, induce the formation of neurectoderm. (Reproduced from Watterson & Schoenwolf (1984). *Laboratory Studies of Chicken, Pig, and Frog Embryos: Guide and Atlas of Vertebrate Embryology*, 5th edition, Burgess Publishing Company, Minneapolis).

(Waddington, 1933). Unfortunately, the factors responsible for this inductive process have not been identified. However, when they are discovered it is likely that they, or similar factors, will play a role in all epithelial–mesenchymal interactions, since these associations are the basis for the formation of virtually all organ systems.

Neurulation and central nervous system development

Neurulation

Under the inductive influence of the primitive node and chordamesoderm, the overlying epiblast cells are transformed into the neurectoderm, which forms the neural plate. This process begins in the head region at approximately day 17 of gestation and results in the overlying ectoderm cells becoming tall and columnar. This 'thickening' creates the neural plate which is identical to placodes found in formation of other ectodermally derived structures (Figure 2.6). Once the neural

Figure 2.6. Scanning electron micrographs of a mouse embryo at the early stages of neurulation (approximately day 18 human). The dorsal surface (A) is marked by the neural groove that separates the cranial neural folds (CF). The primitive streak is present in the caudal portion of the embryo, but is out of view in the specimen. A cross section (B) at the level of the line in Figure 2.6A shows columnar epithelium of the neurectoderm (Ec), fibroblast-like cells of the middle germ layer, the mesoderm (Me), and the endoderm (En). Cells of the neurectoderm are induced by the notochord and surrounding mesoderm (chordamesoderm) to form the neural plate, which represents a large placode. Mitotic cells (asterisks). (Reproduced from T. Sadler, *Langman's Medical Embryology*, 6th edition, © (1990), the Williams & Wilkins Co., Baltimore.)

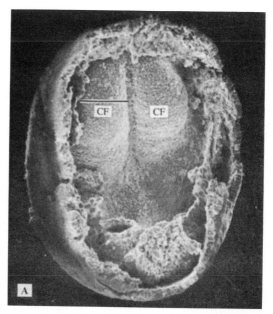

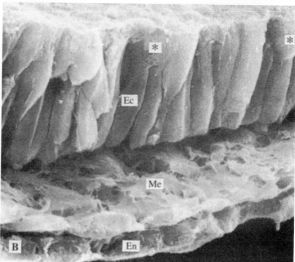

plate is formed, it elevates to create the neural folds and then fuses in the midline to surround a central lumen and thereby forms the brain and spinal cord.

Initial elevation of the plate is produced by proliferation of the underlying mesenchyme and synthesis of extracellular matrix by the same cells (Solursh & Morriss, 1977; Morriss & Solursh, 1978). The matrix is first composed of hyluronic acid, but is then altered so that it contains sulfated proteoglycans (Solursh & Morriss, 1977). The

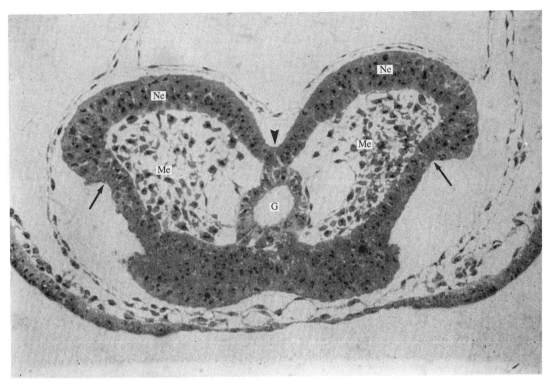

Figure 2.7. Cross section through the cranial neural folds of a mouse embryo at approximately 22 days of human development. At this stage, the neural folds are everted into a biconvex configuration such that the tips, which eventually must elevate around the neural groove (arrowhead) and fuse in the midline, are widespread. The folds have been raised from the neural plate by proliferation and synthesis of ECM by underlying mesenchyme cells (Me); neuroepithelium (Ne); neurectoderm–ectoderm junction (arrows); gut tube (G).

combination of cell proliferation and matrix production, and perhaps contraction of microfilament bundles in the basal aspects of the overlying neuroepithelial cells (Sadler *et al.*, 1982), elevates the cranial neural folds into a butterfly or biconvex configuration (Figure 2.7). From this point on, the folds must continue to rise and then bend toward each other to fuse in the midline. These morphogenetic movements are effected by the neuroepithelial cells via cytoskeletal contraction and differential rates of proliferation (Sadler *et al.*, 1982, 1986; Schoenwolf & Smith, 1990) and by the underlying mesenchyme through matrix production and increase in cell number.

Once the cranial neural folds have elevated to the biconvex stage, microfilament bundles increase in number in the apices of the neuro-epithelial cells (Baker & Schroeder, 1967; Burnside, 1973; Karfunkel, 1974; Sadler *et al.*, 1982). These filaments bind meromyosin (Nagele & Lee, 1980) and are themselves bound to the cell membrane by actin binding proteins (Sadler *et al.*, 1986) (Figure 2.8). Their contraction serves to roll the neural folds into a tube-like structure. However, the central nervous system is not just a tube and the variations in the shape of the neural folds is caused by intrinsic and extrinsic forces, including differential rates of mitosis in the neuroepithelium (for

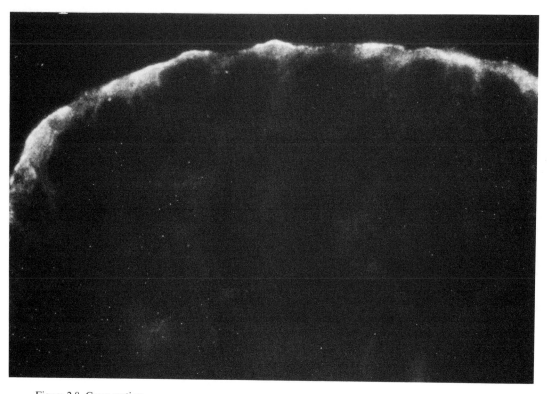

Figure 2.8. Cross section through one cranial neural fold of a mouse embryo at the biconvex stage (see Figure 2.7) of neural tube formation (approximately day 22 human) showing immunocytochemical staining of the actin binding protein, spectrin, in the apices of the neuroepithelial cells. Spectrin and other linkage proteins provide an anchor between the cell membrane and actin microfilaments which contract to assist in pulling the neural folds around the neural lumen toward closure of the neural tube.

review, see Schoenwolf & Smith, 1990). Thus, the headfolds are much larger than the folds forming the spinal cord, where elevation and fusion occur in a simpler fashion like the closing of a book (Figure 2.9).

Fusion of the folds occurs first in the cervical region at the level of the fifth somite (Figure 2.10) and involves the synthesis of surface glycoproteins (Moran & Rice, 1975; Sadler, 1978) that serve as a glue to hold the folds together until stronger cell–cell contacts are established (Figure 2.11). Closure proceeds in a zipper-like fashion in rostral and caudal directions, and regions where the folds remain open are known as the cranial and caudal neuropores (Figure 2.10). A secondary site of fusion appears in the forebrain and closure of the anterior neuropore, which occurs on approximately the twenty fifth day of gestation (18–20 somite stage), is effected by an expansion of this fusion zone cranially and caudally (Geelen & Langman, 1977). Closure of the posterior neuropore is completed by approximately day 27 (25 somite stage).

Differentiation of the central nervous system

As neurulation proceeds, differentiation of the central nervous system begins and, in fact, regionalization of the brain into forebrain

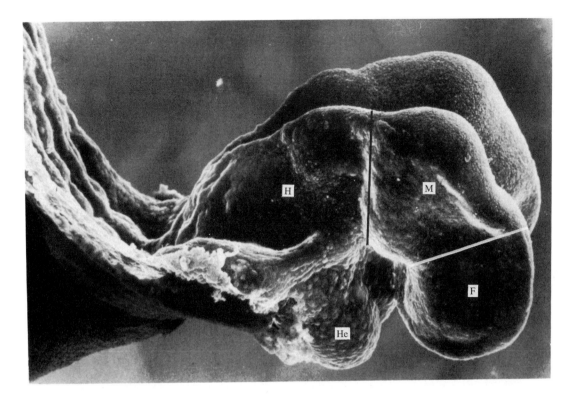

Figure 2.9. Lateral view of the headfolds of a mouse embryo in scanning electron microscopy at approximately 23 days of human gestation. Cranial neural folds are larger, elevated to a higher level, and more complex than folds of the spinal cord (see Figure 2.10). Even prior to closure, the boundaries of the primary brain regions, i.e. prosencephalon (forebrain, F) mesencephalon (midbrain, M), and rhombencephalon (hindbrain, H), can be distinguished. The heart (He) is also shown.

(prosencephalon), midbrain (mesencephalon), and hindbrain (rhombencephalon) areas occurs prior to fusion of the neural folds (Figure 2.9). The midbrain and hindbrain regions form from the original neural plate, whereas the forebrain arises primarily by a flow of cells cranially from the midbrain–rostral hindbrain areas (Morriss-Kay & Tuckett, 1987).

Molecular mechanisms regulating these events are not known, although recent evidence suggests that putative regulatory genes are expressed in a coordinated fashion with morphogenetic events in the hindbrain. Proliferation centers form in the neuroepithelium in the hindbrain (Kallen, 1962; Lumsden, 1990) which, subsequently, becomes segmented into eight spatially distinct regions known as rhombomeres and pairs of these structures give rise to specific motor nerves (Figure 2.12). The pattern is visible by day 25 of development and each segment represents a domain of cell lineage restriction (Fraser et al., 1990). Interestingly, this metameric pattern is presaged by segmentation of the underlying mesenchyme into somitomeres and it has been suggested that patterning in this mesenchyme 'instructs' the overlying epithelium (Fraser et al., 1990).

Two genes that may play a role in establishing a pattern in the hindbrain are:

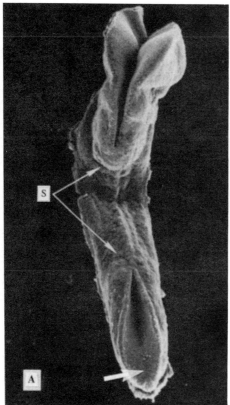
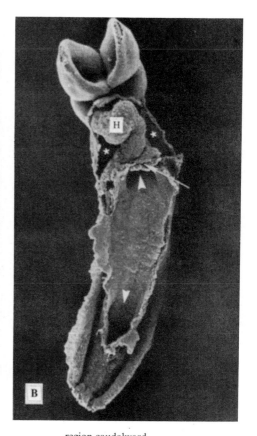
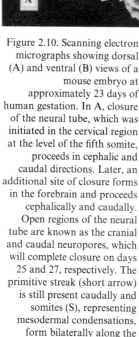

Figure 2.10. Scanning electron micrographs showing dorsal (A) and ventral (B) views of a mouse embryo at approximately 23 days of human gestation. In A, closure of the neural tube, which was initiated in the cervical region at the level of the fifth somite, proceeds in cephalic and caudal directions. Later, an additional site of closure forms in the forebrain and proceeds cephalically and caudally.

Open regions of the neural tube are known as the cranial and caudal neuropores, which will complete closure on days 25 and 27, respectively. The primitive streak (short arrow) is still present caudally and somites (S), representing mesodermal condensations, form bilaterally along the neural tube from the occipital region caudalward. (Reproduced from Sadler, 1990.)

In B, the lateral body wall is folding ventrally toward the midline. By now the heart (H) is undergoing its looping process and is flanked by primitive pleural cavities (asterisk). The septum transverum (arrow), a layer of mesoderm that contributes to formation of the diaphragm, partially separates the pleural–pericardial cavity from the abdominal cavity. Openings from the unfused midgut into the foregut and hindgut regions are also present (arrowheads). (Reproduced from T. Sadler, *Langman's Medical Embrology*, 6th edition, © (1990), the Williams & Wilkins Co., Baltimore.)

60

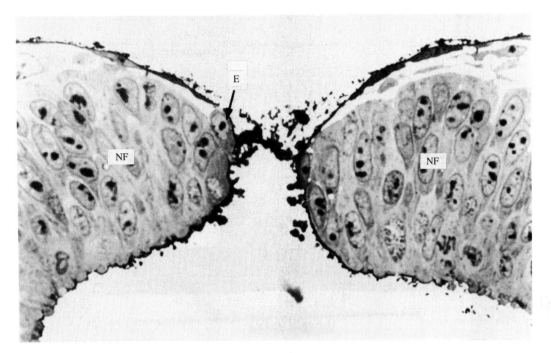

Figure 2.11. Histological section of mouse neural folds (NF) from the midbrain region immediately prior to fusion. The folds have been stained with ruthenium red to illustrate the glycoprotein-rich surface-coat material that provides the 'glue' to hold the folds together until cell to cell contacts can be established. The coat is formed in all areas of the neural tube, is most prominent at the site of fusion, and disappears once the process is completed. With the exception of the most cephalic portion of the forebrain, overlying ectoderm cells (E) make initial contact, not the neuroepithelium. In spinal cord regions and the cephalic part of the forebrain, neuroepithelial cells make the initial contact.

1 Krox 20, a segmentation gene and possible transcription factor whose expression precedes the morphological appearance of rhombomeres 3 and 5

2 the Hox 2 homeobox gene cluster, which contains homologues of the *Drosophila* Antp homeotic gene (Wilkinson & Krumlauf, 1990)

Hox 2.6, 2.7, and 2.8 are expressed in the hindbrain, but their expression has different anterior limits at the boundaries of rhombomeres 6/7, 4/5, and 2/3, respectively. In contrast, Hox 2.9 is expressed only in rhombomere 4 (Wilkinson *et al.*, 1989). Therefore, the temporal and spatial patterns of expression for these genes is intriguing as is the fact that *Drosophila* segmentation genes, such as Krox 20, regulate homeotic genes, such as Hox 2. In fact, data showing that the Krox 20 encoded protein can bind to Hox gene promoter regions supports this hypothesis (Chavrier *et al.*, 1990), although the limited expression of Krox 20 in the hindbrain suggests that additional transcription factors must be involved. Also, the Hox 2 genes must be involved in regulating genes that control cell behavior and differentiation. In this regard, the proto-oncogene *int*-2 is expressed in conjunction with Hox 2 in rhombomeres 5 and 6 (Wilkinson & Krumlauf, 1990).

Thus, a complex sequence of gene expression patterns have been

T. W. Sadler

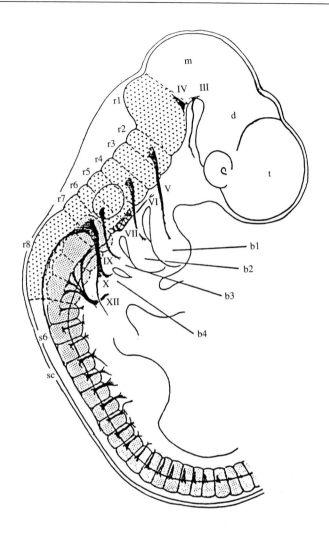

Figure 2.12. Schematic drawing showing embryonic segmentation patterns in the brain and mesoderm which appear by day 25 of development. The hindbrain (coarse stipple) is divided into eight rhombomeres (r1 to r8) and pairs of these structures give rise to the motor nerves (V, VI, VII, IX, X, XII). Mesoderm segmentation precedes the meristic series in the central nervous system. Thus, somitomeres form along the brain and somites (fine stipple) form along the spinal cord (sc). Telencephalon (t); diencephalon (d); mesencephalon (m); branchial arches (b1 to b4); somite 6 (s6); cranial nerves (III and IV). (Reproduced from Lumsden (1990) with the permission of Elsevier Trends Journals, Cambridge, UK.)

established for the hindbrain region. However, demonstrating functional roles for these genes has been difficult. One approach has been to 'knock out' genes using embryonic stem cells and homologous recombination techniques. Using this approach, it has been possible to disrupt hindbrain and midbrain development by eliminating expression of the proto-oncogene int-1 (Wnt-1) (McMahon & Bradley, 1990). Mechanisms responsible for the resulting dysmorphogenesis have not been delineated, but the defects occur in regions that normally express the gene (Wilkinson et al., 1987). Interestingly, genes and their patterns of expression for the midbrain and forebrain regions, which do not exhibit definitive segmentation patterns, have not been identified.

Near the thirty second day of development, the forebrain and hindbrain regions subdivide: the forebrain (prosencephalon) forms the

62

Figure 2.13. At the beginning of the 6th week the primary brain vesicles have subdivided into 5 regions (A, B and C). The prosencephalon (forebrain) forms the telencephalon and diencephalon; the mesencephalon fails to divide; and the rhombencephalon forms the metencephalon and myelencephalon. Since the regions do not grow at the same rates, flexures form as indicated in A and B. (Reproduced from T. Sadler, *Langman's Medical Embryology*, 6th edition, © (1990), the Williams & Wilkins Co., Baltimore.)

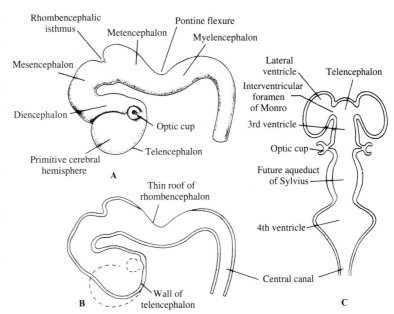

telencephalon and diencephalon, whereas the hindbrain (rhombence-phalon) forms the metencephalon and myelencephalon. The midbrain (mesencephalon) fails to divide. These regions do not all grow at the same rate, however, and so a number of flexures are produced that give the brain its characteristic appearance (Figure 2.13). Regardless of the region, the cellular organization is similar, initially. Thus, the neuroepithelial cells, which are organized into a pseudostratified columnar epithelium that is several nuclear layers thick, provide the germinal epithelium that is the source of neurons, glial, and other cell types of the central nervous system. Neurons begin to form soon after neural tube closure has occurred and become organized into the mantle layer, which then subdivides into a dorsal region, the alar plate containing sensory neurons, and a ventral region, the basal plate containing motor neurons (Figure 2.14). In the brain, the alar plates increase dramatically in size, whereas the basal plates undergo a relative decrease.

Brainstem

The myelencephalon, metencephalon and mesencephalon comprise the brainstem. In the regions of the myelencephalon and metencepha-lon, the alar and basal plates are everted (Figure 2.15). The roof of the myelencephalon remains thin and becomes vascularized to form the

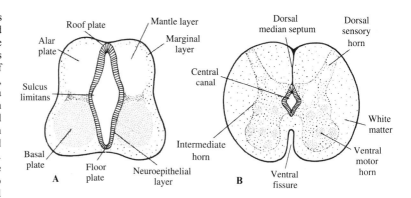

Figure 2.14. Schematic cross section of the spinal cord region soon after neural tube closure, neuroepithelial cells differentiate into a number of cell types including neurons, which become organized into a mantle layer that in turn segregates into alar and basal plates (A). Alar plates contain sensory neurons, whereas basal plates contain motor neurons.

In the spinal cord (B) these plates become organized into dorsal sensory horns and ventral motor horns. Similar regions form in the brain, but in the forebrain alar plates increase dramatically, whereas basal plates either do not form or become diminished in size. (Reproduced from T. Sadler, *Langman's Medical Embryology*, 6th edition, © (1990), the Williams & Wilkins Co., Baltimore.)

tela choroidea covering the fourth ventricle. The alar and basal plates in this region are well defined by 45 days of gestation and will form motor and sensory nuclei related to cranial nerves, medullary sensory nuclei, and autonomic nuclei as the regulatory centers for cardiac, respiratory and digestive functions. In addition, the olivary nucleus is derived by a ventral migration of cells from the alar plates (Figure 2.15).

The sensory and motor plates of the metencephalon contribute nuclei for cranial nerves and the pontine nuclei, which are derived from alar plate cells that migrate ventrally (Figure 2.16). The roof plate is derived from the dorsal aspects of the alar plates (the rhombic lips) and forms the cerebellum. Development of the cerebellum begins between

Figure 2.15. Dorsal view (A) of the myelencephalon, metencephalon, and mesencephalon (which form the brainstem) at approximately 40 days of gestation showing everted alar plates. B shows the thin roof over the fourth ventricle. Cells of the alar and basal plates in the myelencephalon form: motor and sensory nuclei related to cranial nerves; medullary sensory nuclei; and autonomic nuclei as regulatory centers for cardiac, respiratory, and digestive functions. In addition, cells of the alar plate migrate ventrally to form the olivary nucleus and the roof over the fourth ventricle forms the choroid plexus (C). (Reproduced from T. Sadler, *Langman's Medical Embryology*, 6th edition, © (1990), the Williams & Wilkins Co., Baltimore.)

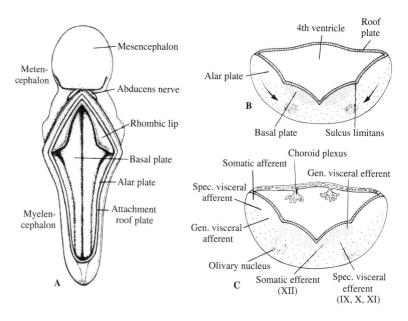

Figure 2.16. Cross section through the metencephalon. Alar and basal plates contribute nuclei for cranial nerves and the alar plates form the pontine nuclei and the rhombic lips from which the cerebellum is derived. (Reproduced from T. Sadler, *Langman's Medical Embryology*, 6th edition, © (1990), the Williams & Wilkins Co., Baltimore.)

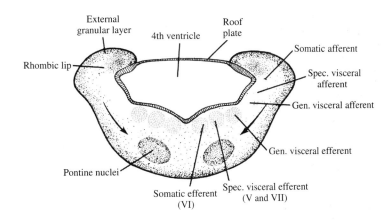

Figure 2.17. Schematic representation of formation of the cerebellum from the metencephalon at 8 weeks (A) and 12 weeks (B) of development. The alar plate forms the rhombic lips (see Figure 2.16) which are widespaced ridges caudally, but meet in the midline at the junction of the mesencephalon (A). As the pontine flexure deepens, the lips become compressed to form the cerebellar plate, which has a small midline portion, the vermis, and two hemispheres laterally. By 12 weeks, a transverse fissure separates the nodule from the vermis and the flocculonodular lobe from the hemispheres. Differentiation of the flocculus, vermis, and nodule is completed prior to birth, whereas the hemispheres complete development postnatally. (Reproduced from T. Sadler, *Langman's Medical Embryology*, 6th edition, © (1990), the Williams & Wilkins Co., Baltimore.)

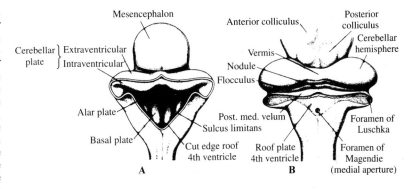

40 and 45 days of gestation and by the twelfth week it consists of a central portion, the vermis, and two lateral portions, the hemispheres (Figure 2.17). The nodule and flocculus are then separated from the vermis and hemispheres, respectively, by a transverse fissure. The flocculus, vermis, and nodule comprise the paleocerebellum, which is the most primitive part of the structure, and their maturation is complete prior to birth. The hemispheres constitute the neocerebellum and development of this structure parallels that of the cerebral cortex and is completed after birth.

As mentioned previously, the mesencephalon does not divide. The alar plates form the roof and give rise to the superior and inferior colliculi, which serve as reflex centers for ocular and auditory stimuli that are independent of conscious perception. The floor plate houses the nuclei for the third and fourth cranial nerves and also contains the nucleus ruber and substantia nigra, which represent nuclei of the extrapyramidal system. Large motor fibers, connecting the cerebral cortex with lower centers in the pons and spinal cord, thicken the

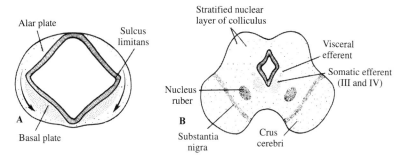

Figure 2.18. Cross sections through the mesencephalon which is the only primary brain vesicle that fails to subdivide. Alar and basal plates are well defined and form the superior and inferior colliculi and nuclei for cranial nerves III and IV, respectively (A). Cells from the alar plate also migrate ventrally to form the nucleus ruber and substantia nigra (B). Collections of motor fibers, running between cortex and lower centers in the pons and spinal cord, create swellings, the cerebral peduncles, on the ventral mesencephalon. (Reproduced from T. Sadler, *Langman's Medical Embryology*, 6th edition, © (1990), the Williams & Wilkins Co., Baltimore.)

marginal layer considerably to form the cerebral peduncles. The lumen of the mesencephalon becomes the aqueduct of Sylvius, connecting the third and fourth ventricles (Figure 2.18).

Prosencephalon

The prosencephalon is characterized by massive growth of the alar plates and regression of the basal plates as represented by the enlargement of the cerebral hemispheres and the absence of segmentation. Consequently, receptor and associative centers are emphasized. The diencephalon arises from the prosencephalon and is characterized by a large alar region, which gives rise to dorsal, lateral, and ventral derivatives. Dorsally, the roof plate becomes thin, closes the third ventricle, and gives rise to the choroid plexus for this region. It also differentiates into the habenular structures and the pineal gland. Ventrally, the neural primordia of the eye arise and the infundibulum and neurohypophysis are derived in the midline. Laterally, the walls of the diencephalon thicken to form the thalamus superiorly and the hypothalamus inferiorly. Primordia for these structures are apparent by the seventh week of gestation (Figure 2.19).

Figure 2.19. Sections through the prosencephalon (A) and diencephalon (B) at the 7-week stage illustrating structures derived from these regions. Derivatives of the prosencephalon arise from the alar plate and there is some question whether or not basal plate areas ever exist. As a result, receptor and associative centers are emphasized. (Reproduced from T. Sadler, *Langman's Medical Embryology*, 6th edition, © (1990), the Williams & Wilkins Co., Baltimore.)

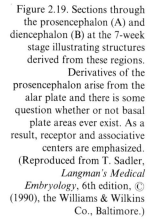
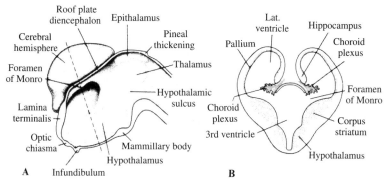

Figure 2.20. Mid-sagittal section through the forebrain of a 10-week embryo (A) and a transverse section (B) through the region indicated by the broken line in figure A. Cerebral hemispheres arise as outpocketings from the telencephalic vesicle at the fifth week of development. Their dorsal portion forms the pallium (cortex) and the ventral region forms the striatum. (Reproduced from T. Sadler, *Langman's Medical Embryology*, 6th edition, © (1990), the Williams & Wilkins Co., Baltimore.)

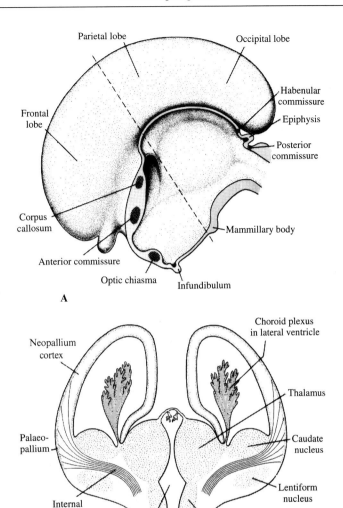

The cerebral hemispheres arise from the telencephalic vesicle of the prosencephalon in the fifth week of development. Each of the hemispheres has a dorsal portion, the pallium or future cortex, and a ventrolateral region, the future striatum. The pallium thickens and forms the neopallial, archeopallial, and paleopallial regions, which give rise to the cerebral cortex, hippocampus, and olfactory lobes, respectively. By the second month, the floor of the hemispheres bulges into the lumen of the lateral ventricle. This growth results from formation of the corpus striatum, which later divides into a dorsome-dial portion, the caudate nucleus, and a ventrolateral portion, the lentiform nucleus (Figure 2.20). Externally, in the sixth month, the

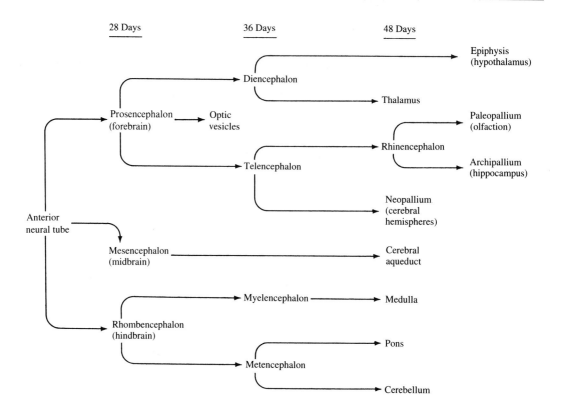

| 28 Days | 36 Days | 48 Days |

Anterior neural tube

Prosencephalon (forebrain)
→ Optic vesicles
→ Diencephalon
→ Epiphysis (hypothalamus)
→ Thalamus

→ Telencephalon
→ Rhinencephalon
→ Paleopallium (olfaction)
→ Archipallium (hippocampus)
→ Neopallium (cerebral hemispheres)

Mesencephalon (midbrain) → Cerebral aqueduct

Rhombencephalon (hindbrain)
→ Myelencephalon → Medulla
→ Metencephalon → Pons
→ Cerebellum

Figure 2.21. Chart indicating the timing of key events in brain development. (Reproduced from Gilbert (1988) with the permission of Sinauer Associates, Inc., Sunderland, Massachusetts.)

fissure of Rolando and then the parieto-occipital fissure appear. Fissure formation then continues until the patterns are well established at birth. Internally, the lumens of the lateral ventricles communicate with that of the diencephalon via the interventricular foramina of Monro.

Differentiation of cell types in the cortex begins in the third month. At about the sixth month, nerve processes form and by the seventh month motor, receptor, associative, and intermediary structures have been established. At birth, most of the cortical neurons have originated, although the connections of each neuron continue to be established to the order of 10 000 synapses per cell. (Key events in brain development are summarized in Figure 2.21.)

Epithelial–mesenchymal interactions

Organogenesis

Gastrulation and neurulation are not the only events that occur during the third and fourth weeks of development. For example, the lateral

Table 2.1. *Some organs formed by epithelial–mesenchymal*
interactions

Skin derivatives
Teeth, hair, sweat glands, mammary glands

Limbs

Gut derivatives
Lungs, pancreas, liver, gall bladder, thyroid, parathyroid, thymus, salivary
  glands

Kidneys

Facial structures

plate mesoderm and the endoderm fold ventrally to create the body
wall, body cavities, and gut tube (Figure 2.10). The heart, which begins
as a horseshoe-shaped structure cephalad to the prochordal plate, folds
into a tube and begins to beat (Figure 2.10). The paraxial mesoderm,
lying near the midline on either side of the notochord, condenses into
somitomeres in the head region and somites in the cervical and caudal
areas, thereby establishing the metameric pattern of the embryonic axis
(Meier & Tam, 1982). Also, the phenomena involved in gastrulation
and neurulation, i.e. epithelial–mesenchymal interactions, cell migration and proliferation, fusion of epithelial folds, etc., recur throughout organogenesis.

While the central nervous system is developing so are the other
organs of the body and most involve epithelial–mesenchymal interactions similar to those responsible for neural tube formation (see Table
2.1). Thus, in many cases, the mesenchyme induces the epithelium to
differentiate as, for example, in the classic experiments of Deuchar
(1975) who showed that lung epithelium could be induced to form
gastric mucosa, liver, intestine, or lungs depending upon the source of
mesenchyme with which it was cocultured. In addition to the initial
induction process, however, the two types of tissue undergo many
instructive interactions to establish an organ system, including those
controlling pattern formation. Perhaps the best studied example of
these interactions is limb development and it is also one in which a
putative inducer and potential molecular controls have been identified.

Retinoic acid and limb bud formation

Limb buds first appear as outgrowths from the flank of the embryo
during the fifth week. Lateral plate mesoderm from the flank induces

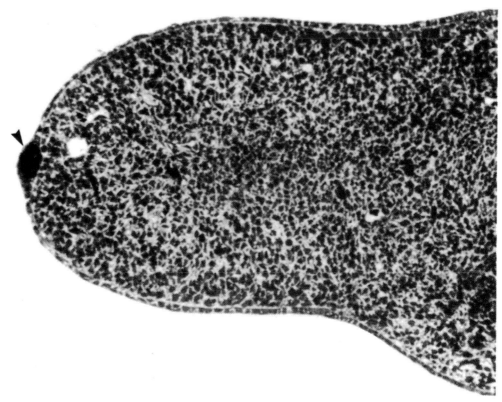

Figure 2.22. Sagittal section through a mouse forelimb at a stage equivalent to the fifth week of human development. The mesenchyme of the limb is covered by ectoderm that thickens at the distal tip to form the apical ectodermal ridge (AER) (arrowhead). (Reproduced from T. Sadler, *Langman's Medical Embryology*, 6th edition, © (1990), the Williams & Wilkins Co., Baltimore.)

the overlying ectoderm at the limb tip to thicken into the apical ectodermal ridge (AER) (Figure 2.22). In turn, the AER interacts with limb mesenchyme beneath the ridge to maintain a high proliferative rate and produce growth in a proximo-distal direction (Zwilling, 1955; Saunders *et al.*, 1957). However, this growth is not sufficient to result in the patterning characteristic of the limb where polarity in an anterior–posterior direction is essential for proper digit formation.

This positional information is controlled by the zone of polarizing activity (ZPA), a small population of mesoderm cells residing in the posterior part of the limb at its union with the flank. This tissue is responsible for the ordering of the digits and, in fact, if a second ZPA is transplanted to the anterior surface of the limb then duplication of the digits occurs and the order of the new digits is a mirror image of the normally produced structures (Saunders & Gasseling, 1968; Tickle *et al.*, 1975; Summerbell, 1979; Tickle, 1981). The mechanism of action of the ZPA appears to be to establish a gradient involving a morphogen to which the cells respond (Summerbell, 1979).

Several investigations provide evidence that the morphogen is retinoic acid including:

1   Implantation of retinoic acid soaked beads in the anterior margin of chick wing buds reproduces the mirror image duplication patterns produced by ZPA tissue (Tickle *et al.*, 1982)

2   A gradient of naturally occurring retinoic acid exists across the limb bud and its highest concentration is at the ZPA (Eichele & Thaller, 1987; Thaller & Eichele, 1987)

3   Retinoic acid receptors and binding proteins have been demonstrated in limb buds (Kwarta *et al.*, 1985; Madden & Summerbell, 1986; Dolle *et al.*, 1990)

It should be noted that recent evidence suggests that retinoic acid may not be *the* morphogen, but instead may participate in an orchestrated series of signals to produce pattern formation in the limb (Noji *et al.*, 1991; Wanek *et al.*, 1991).

Despite this contradictory evidence, a model for limb morphogenesis is emerging in which retinoic acid acts as a morphogen via the retinoic acid receptors which are known to act as transcription factors. The retinoid binding proteins serve to control the availability of retinoids for the receptors. Target genes for the retinoic acid receptors have not been identified, but recent evidence suggests that homeobox genes might be involved. For example, the spatial and temporal expression of genes from the Hox 5 complex in the limb is consistent with patterns established under the influence of the ZPA (Dolle *et al.*, 1989). Furthermore, it has been observed that retinoic acid induces the expression of homeobox genes in differentiating teratocarcinoma cells (Colberg-Poley *et al.*, 1985; Deschamps *et al.*, 1987; Schultze *et al.*, 1987; Dony & Gruss, 1988; LaRosa & Guden, 1988; Mavilio *et al.*, 1988) and cultures of embryonic brain (Deschamps *et al.*, 1987).

Do retinoic acid, its receptors and binding proteins, and homeobox genes regulate development in other organ systems involving epithelial–mesenchymal interactions, thereby acting as a common mechanism for pattern formation and differentiation? The answer is not known for certain, but evidence is accumulating that similar mechanisms might be operating in these systems. For example, retinoic acid binding proteins and receptors are expressed with regional specificity during gastrulation, neurulation, and brain development, including formation of the rhombencephalon (Ruberte *et al.*, 1991), where homeobox genes are predicted to play a role in morphogenesis, as discussed previously. Also, transplant experiments in chick embryos have demonstrated that the primitive (Henson's) node has polarizing activity when it is grafted into a chick wing bud (Hornbruch & Wolpert, 1986). Could the primitive node act to control expression of homeobox genes, and, subsequently, pattern formation along the cephalo-caudal axis (Dolle *et al.*, 1989)? Finally, it is interesting to note that exposure to retinoic acid during early stages of organogenesis induces developmental abnormalities in a variety of organ systems (Shenefelt, 1972), including the central nervous system, where spina bifida and exencephaly occur following exposure during the period of neurulation (Alles & Sulik, 1990).

Therefore, a common mechanism for organogenesis is an intriguing hypothesis that awaits further study. Undoubtedly, other participants, such as growth factors, proto-oncogenes etc., will be discovered that will play key roles in the complex orchestration of organ formation.

References

ALLES, A. J. & SULIK, K. K. (1990) Retinoic acid-induced spina bifida: Evidence for a pathogenetic mechanism. *Development*, **108**, 73–81.

BAKER, P. C. & SCHROEDER, T. E. (1967) Cytoplasmic filaments and morphogenetic movement in the amphibian neural tube. *Developmental Biology*, **15**, 432–50.

BURNSIDE, B. (1973) Microtubules and microfilaments in amphibian neurulation. *American Zoologist*, **13**, 989–1006.

CHAVRIER, P., VESQUE, C., GALLIOT, B., VIGNERON, M., DOLLE, P., DUBOULE, D. & CHARNAY, P. (1990) The segment specific gene Krox-20 encodes a transcription factor with binding sites in the promoter region of the Hox-1.4 gene. *EMBO Journal*, **9**, 1209–18.

COLBERG-POLEY, A. M., VOSS, S. D., CHOWDHURY, K. & GRUSS, P. (1985) Structural analysis of murine gene containing homeobox sequences and their expression in embryonal carcinoma cells. *Nature*, **314**, 731–8.

DESCHAMPS, J., DELAAF, R., VERRIJZEN, P., DeGOURO, M., DES-TREL, O. F. & MEIJLINK, F. (1987) The mouse Hox 2.3 homeobox containing gene: Regulation in differentiating pluripotent stem cells and expression pattern in embryos. *Differentiation*, **35**, 21–30.

DEUCHAR, E. M. (1975) *Cellular Interactions in Animal Development*. Chapman and Hall, London.

DOLLE, P., IZPISUA-BELMONTE, J. C., FALKENSTEIN, H., RENUCCI, A. & DUBOULE, D. (1989) Coordinate expression of the murine Hox-5 complex homeobox-containing genes during limb pattern formation. *Nature*, **342**, 767–72.

DOLLE, P., RUBERTE, E., LEROY, P., MORRISS-KAY, G. & CHAM-BON, P. (1990) Retinoic acid receptors and cellular retinoid binding proteins. I. A systematic study of their differential pattern of transcription during mouse organogenesis. *Development*, **110**, 1113–51.

DONY, C. & GRUSS, P. (1988) Expression of a murine homeobox gene precedes the induction of c-fos during mesodermal differentiation of P19 teratocarcinoma cells. *Differentiation*, **37**, 115–22.

EICHELE, G. & THALLER, C. (1987) Characterization of concentration gradients of a morphogenetically active retinoid in the chick limb bud. *Journal of Cell Biology*, **105**, 1917–23.

FRASER, S. E., KEYNER, R. J. & LUMSDEN, A. (1990) Segmentation in the chick embryo hindbrain is defined by cell lineage restrictions. *Nature*, **344**, 431–5.

GEELEN, J. A. G. & LANGMAN, J. (1977) Closure of the neural tube in the cephalic region of the mouse embryo. *Anatomical Record*, **189**, 625–39.

GILBERT, S. F. (1988) *Developmental Biology*, 2nd edition. Sinauer Associates, Inc., Sunderland, Massachusetts.

GREEN, J. B. A., HOWES, G., SYMES, K., COOK, J. & SMITH, J. C.

(1990) The biological effects of XTC-MIF: quantitative comparison with *Xenopus* bFGF. *Development*, **108**, 173–83.

GURDON, J. B., MOHUN, T. J., SHARPE, C. R. & TAYLOR, M. V. (1989) Embryonic induction and muscle gene activation. *Trends in Genetics*, **5**, 51–6.

HORNBRUCH, A. & WOLPERT, L. (1986) Positional signaling by Henson's node when grafted to the chick limb bud. *Journal of Embryology & Experimental Morphology*, **94**, 257–65.

KALLEN, B. (1962) Miotic patterning in the central nervous system of chick embryos; studied by a colchicine method. *Zeitschrift für Anatomie und Entwicklungsgeschichte*, **123**, 309–19.

KARFUNKEL, P. (1974) The mechanisms of neural tube formation. *International Review of Cytology*, **38**, 245–71.

KIMELMAN, D., ABRAHAM, J. A., HAAPARANTA, T., PALISI, T. M. & KIRSCHNER, M. (1988) The presence of FGF in the frog egg: its role as a natural mesoderm inducer. *Science*, **242**, 1053–6.

KIMELMAN, D. & KIRSCHNER, M. (1987) Synergistic induction of mesoderm by FGF and TGF-B and the identification of and mRNA coding for FGF in the early *Xenopus* embryo. *Cell*, **51**, 369–77.

KWARTA, R. F. Jr, KIMMEL C. A., KIMMEL, G. L. & SLIKKER, W., Jr (1985) Identification of the cellular retinoic acid binding protein (cRABP) within the embryonic mouse (CD-1) limb bud. *Teratology*, **32**, 103–11.

LAROSA, G. J. & GUDEN, L. J. (1988) Early retinoic acid-induced F9 teratocarcinoma stem cell gene ERA-1: Alternate splicing creates transcripts for a homeobox-containing protein and one lacking a homeobox. *Molecular & Cellular Biology*, **8**, 3906–17.

LUMSDEN, A. (1990) The cellular basis of segmentation in the developing hindbrain. *Trends in Neuroscience*, **13**, 329–35.

MADDEN, M. & SUMMERBELL, D. (1986) Retinoic acid binding protein in the chick limb bud: Identification at developmental stages and binding affinities of various retinoids. *Journal of Embryology & Experimental Morphology*, **97**, 239–50.

MAVILIO, F., SIMEONE, A., BONCINELLI, E. & ANDREWS, P. W. (1988) Activation of 4 homeobox gene clusters in human embryonal carcinoma cells induced to differentiate by retinoic acid. *Differentiation*, **37**, 73–91.

McMAHON, A. P. & BRADLEY, A. (1990) The *Wnt*-1 (*int*-1) proto-oncogene is required for development of a large region of the mouse brain. *Cell*, **62**, 1073–85.

MEIER, S. & TAM, P. P. L. (1982) Metameric pattern development in the embryonic axis of the mouse. I. Differentiation of the cranial segments. *Differentiation*, **21**, 95–108.

MORAN, D. & RICE, R. W. (1975) An ultrastructural examination of the role of cell membranes surface coat material during neurulation. *Journal of Cell Biology*, **64**, 172–86.

MORRISS, G. M. & SOLURSH, M. (1978) Regional differences in mesenchymal cell morphology and glycosaminoglycans in early neural-fold stage rat embryos. *Journal of Embryology & Experimental Morphology*, **46**, 37–52.

MORRISS-KAY, G. M. & TUCKETT (1987) Fluidity of the neural epithelium during forebrain formation in rat embryos. *Journal of Cell Science*, **8**, 433–49.

NAGELE, R. G. & LEE, H. Y. (1980) Studies on the mechanism of neurulation in the chick: Microfilament mediated changes in cell shape during uplifting of the neural folds. *Journal of Experimental Zoology*, **213**, 391–8.

NIEUWKOOP, P. D. (1969) The formation of the mesoderm in urodelian amphibians. I. The induction by the endoderm. *Wilhelm Roux Archiv. Ento. Mech. Org.*, **162**, 341–73.

NODEN, D. M. (1988) Interactions and fates of avian craniofacial mesenchyme. *Development*, **103**, 121–140.

NOJI, S., NOHNO, T., KOYAMA, E., MUTO, K., OHYAMA, K., AOKI, Y., TAMURA, K., OHSUGI, K., IDE, H., TANIGUCHI, S. & SAITO, T. (1991) Retinoic acid induces polarizing activity but is unlikely to be a morphogen in the chick limb bud. *Nature*, **350**, 83–6.

ROSA, F., ROBERTS, A. B., DANIELPOUR, D., DART, L. L., SPORN, M. B. & DAWID, I.B. (1988) Mesoderm induction in amphibians: The role of TGF-B2 like factors. *Science*, **329**, 783–785.

RUBERTE, E., DOLLE, P., CHAMBON, P. & MORRISS-KAY, G. (1991) Retinoic acid receptors and cellular retinoid binding proteins. II. Their differential patterns of transcription during early morphogenesis in mouse embryos. *Development*, **111**, 45–8.

SADLER, T. W. (1978) Distribution of surface coat material on fusing neural folds of mouse embryos during neurulation. *Anatomical Record*, **191**, 345–50.

SADLER, T. W. (1990) *Langman's Medical Embryology*, 6th edition. Williams & Wilkins, Baltimore.

SADLER, T. W., BURRIDGE, K. & YONKER, J. (1986) A potential role for spectrin during neurulation. *Journal of Embryology & Experimental Morphology*, **94**, 73–82.

SADLER, T. W., LESSARD, J. L., GREENBERG, D. & COUGHLIN, P. (1982) Actin distribution patterns in the mouse neural tube during neurulation. *Science*, **215**, 172–4.

SAUNDERS, J. W., Jr, CAIRNS, J. M. & GASSELING, M. T. (1957) The role of the apical ridge of ectoderm in the differentiation of the morphological structure and induction specificity of limb parts of the chick. *Journal of Morphology*, **101**, 57–88.

SAUNDERS, J. W., Jr. & GASSELING, M. T. (1968) Ectodermal–mesenchymal interactions in the origin of wing symmetry. In: *Epithelial Mesenchymal Interactions*, pp. 78–97. Eds. R. Flischmajer & R. E. Billingham. Williams & Wilkins, Baltimore.

SCHOENWOLF, G. C. & SMITH, J. L. (1990) Mechanisms of neurulation: Traditional viewpoint and recent advances. *Development*, **109**, 243–70.

SCHULTZE, F., CHOWDHURG, K., ZIMMER, A., DRESCHER, U. & GRUSS, P. (1987) The murine homeobox gene product, Hox 1.1 protein is growth controlled and associated with chromatin. *Differentiation*, **36**, 130–7.

SHENEFELT, R. E. (1972) Morphogenesis of malformations in hamsters caused by retinoic acid: relation to dose and stage at treatment. *Teratology*, **5**, 103–8.

SLACK, J. M. W., DARLINGTON, B. G., HEATH, J. K. & GODSAVE, S. F. (1987) Mesoderm induction in early *Xenopus* embryos by heparin-binding growth factors. *Nature*, **326**, 197–200.

SLACK, J. M. W. & ISAACS, H. (1989) Presence of basic fibroblast growth factor in the early *Xenopus* embryo. *Development*, **105**, 147–53.

SMITH, J. C. (1987) A mesoderm inducing factor is produced by a *Xenopus* cell line. *Development*, **99**, 3–14.

SMITH, J. C. (1989) Mesoderm induction and mesoderm-inducing factors in early amphibian development. *Development*, **105**, 665–77.

SMITH, J. C., YAQUOB, M. & SYMES, K. (1988) Purification, partial characterization, and biological properties of the XTC mesoderm-inducing factor. *Development*, **103**, 591–600.

SOLURSH, M. & MORRISS, G. M. (1977) Glycosaminoglycan synthesis in rat embryos during the formation of the primary mesenchyme and neural folds. *Developmental Biology*, **57**, 75–86.

SPEMANN, H. & MANGOLD, H. (1924) Induction of embryonic primordia by implantation of organizers from a different species. In: *Foundations of Experimental Embryology*, pp. 144–84. Eds. B. H. Wilkier & J. M. Oppenheimer. Hafner, New York.

SUMMERBELL, D. (1979) The zone of polarizing activity: Evidence for a role in abnormal chick limb morphogenesis. *Journal of Embryology & Experimental Morphology*, **50**, 217–33.

THALLER, C. & EICHELE, G. (1987) Identification and spatial distribution of retinoids in the developing chick limb bud. *Nature*, **327**, 625–8.

TICKLE, C. (1981) The number of polarizing region cells required to specify additional digits in the developing chick wing. *Nature*, **289**, 295–8.

TICKLE, C., ALBERTS, B., WOLPERT, L. & LEE, J. (1982) Local application of retinoic acid to the limb bud mimics the action of the polarizing region. *Nature*, **296**, 564–6.

TICKLE, C., SUMMERBELL, D. & WOLPERT, L. (1975) Positional signalling and specification of digits in chick limb morphogenesis. *Nature*, **254**, 199–202.

WADDINGTON, C. H. (1933) Induction of the primitive streak and its derivatives in the chick. *Journal of Experimental Biology*, **10**, 38–46.

WANEK, N., GARDINER, D. M., MUNEOKA, K. & BRYANT, S. V. (1991) Conversion by retinoic acid of anterior cells into ZPA cells in the chick wing bud. *Nature*, **350**, 81–3.

WATTERSON, R. L. & SCHOENWOLF, G. C. (1984) *Laboratory Studies of Chick, Pig and Frog Embryos: Guide and Atlas of Vertebrate Embryology*, 5th edition. Burgess Publishing Co., Minneapolis, Minnesota.

WILKINSON, D. G., BAILES, J. R. & MacMAHON, A. P. (1987) Expression of the proto-oncogene *int*1 is restricted to specific neural cells in the developing mouse embryos. *Cell*, **50**, 79–88.

WILKINSON, D. G., BHATT, S., COOK, M., BONCINELLI, E. & KRUMLAUF, R. (1989) Segmental expression of *Hox-2* homeobox-containing genes in the developing mouse hindbrain. *Nature*, **341**, 405–9.

WILKINSON, D. G. & KRUMLAUF, R. (1990) Molecular approaches to the segmentation of the hindbrain. *Trends in Neuroscience*, **13**, 335–8.

ZWILLING, E. (1955) Ectoderm–mesoderm relationship in the development of the chick embryo limb bud. *Journal of Experimental Zoology*, **128**, 423–41.

CHAPTER 3

Experimental human hematopoiesis in immunodeficient SCID mice engrafted with fetal blood-forming organs

B. PÉAULT, R. NAMIKAWA, J. KROWKA and

J. M. McCUNE

CONTENTS

THE MATURE HEMATOPOIETIC SYSTEM retains conspicuous embryonic features: extensive stem cell production, migration and differentiation ensure in the adult a permanent supply of myeloid and lymphoid elements. This enormous capacity for regeneration provides a unique opportunity for the investigator who can controllably reconstitute animals whose blood system has been ablated with cytotoxic drugs or ionizing radiation. Such experimental approaches in the mouse have been seminal in the study of stem cell biology, hematopoietic differentiation in blood-forming organs and 'self' restriction of T lymphocyte function. Similar studies in man are, of course, deontologically unacceptable. Therefore, our understanding of human blood cell physiology still relies largely on animal paradigms or on the evaluation of in vitro cultured cells.

These approaches are of uncertain relevance and useful only in limited areas of investigation. Growing intact human organ pieces in a laboratory animal could obviously offer a key for the experimental study of living tissues in man. Transplantation is ideally achieved between histocompatible, syngeneic individuals, but xenogeneic chimeras can be constructed if the recipient is unable to mount a graft-rejecting immune response. This condition can be met if the host is either an embryo, whose immune system has not developed yet (see LeDouarin (1978) for a review), or a congenitally immunodeficient adult. For example, human fetal tissues such as brain and pancreas have been implanted into athymic, partially immunodeficient rodents (Tuch *et al.*, 1984; Stromberg *et al.*, 1989). In a further step, lymphocyte-free mice, affected by the SCID (severe combined immunodeficiency) mutation, were used as recipients for human fetal blood-forming tissues (McCune *et al.*, 1988) or isolated hematopoietic cells (Mosier *et al.*, 1988).

Homozygous C.B.-17 *scid/scid* mutants, referred to hereafter as SCID, lack functional T and B lymphocytes as a consequence of defective rearrangements in antigen receptor genes (Bosma *et al.*, 1983; Schuler *et al.*, 1986). The prediction that human fetal tissue and SCID mice should be tolerant of each other was realized beyond expectations: fetal thymus was observed not only to survive in the mouse but to grow, differentiate and sustain hematopoietic activity. This discovery prompted attempts to approximate the cycle of human lymphopoiesis in the SCID mouse more closely by supplying the grafted thymus with hematopoietic precursor cells. This chapter will summarize the results of experiments that have led to the construction, in a laboratory animal, of a replica of the human hematopoietic system that we now use routinely to study the normal and pathologic development of human blood cells.

Growing human fetal thymus in SCID mice

Human thymus obtained from elective abortions (9–23 weeks of gestation) is cut into pieces, generally about one cubic millimeter in size, and surgically implanted under the kidney capsule of one to two-month-old SCID mice. In that location, the thymus undergoes considerable growth, frequently reaching the size of the mouse kidney after two to three months. A vascular network irrigates the white, full, typically lymphoid-looking implant (McCune *et al.*, 1988) (Figure 3.1). The growth potential of the thymus is optimal before the twenty second week of gestation; in contrast, implants of postnatal and adult human thymus can be maintained viable but demonstrate only minimal evidence of growth and differentiation in the SCID mouse (our unpublished observations; Barry *et al.*, 1991).

Upon histological analysis, early thymus grafts (up to one month) exhibit the typical anatomical features of a fresh, age-matched thymus,

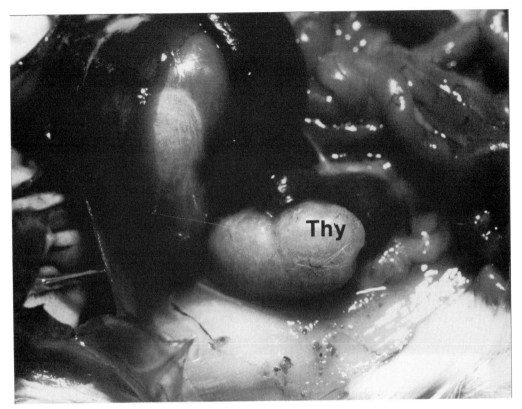

Figure 3.1. Anatomy of a human fetal thymus implant in the SCID mouse. One lobe from a 9 weeks of gestation thymus (about 0.5 mm × 0.5 mm × 2 mm in size) was implanted for thirteen weeks under the left kidney capsule of a SCID mouse. The graft size at autopsy was 10 mm × 5 mm × 5 mm.

with a well-demarcated cortex and medullary areas replete with Hassal's corpuscles (Figure 3.2) (McCune *et al.*, 1988). When mechanically dispersed, stained and analyzed on the fluorescence-activated cell sorter (FACS), the densely packed lymphocytes seen on graft sections are found to include, in the expected proportions, the three major thymocyte subsets, i.e. immature $CD4^+$ $CD8^+$ and mature $CD4^+$ or $CD8^+$ cells.

Surface major histocompatibility complex (MHC) class I antigen expression by graft thymocytes also reflects the normal differentiative hierarchy of thymus lymphocytes, with a large proportion of immature cortical cells expressing no, or low amounts of, class I molecules and a smaller population of high class I-expressing T cells corresponding to mature medullary-type lymphocytes (Figure 3.3A).

After longer periods of engraftment, modifications in the cellularity of the grafts are noted. Gross observation reveals that thymus implants become more translucent and fibrous. Mechanical disruption yields a lower relative number of lymphocytes. Upon histological analysis, aging thymus grafts show a much smaller cortical compartment.

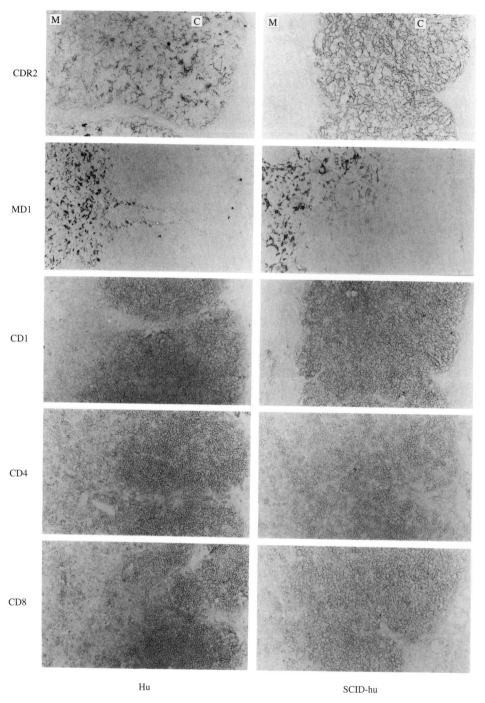

Hu

SCID-hu

Figure 3.2.
Immunohistochemical analysis of the human fetal thymus (20 weeks of gestation) before (Hu) and after (SCID-hu) a four week-long engraftment in the SCID mouse. Tissue sections were stained by the avidin-biotin-peroxydase method with the following antibodies:

CDR2, anti-human cortical epithelial cells; MD1, anti-human medullary, subcapsular and Hassal's corpuscle-associated epithelium; CD1, antihuman cortical thymocytes, CD4 and CD8, anti-T lymphocyte markers M: medulla; C: cortex.

Figure 3.3. HLA class I antigen expression on the surface of fresh human fetal thymocytes (A) and after engraftment of the thymus for 1 month (B) and 2 months (C) in the SCID mouse. Cells in suspension were stained in a two-color indirect immunofluorescence assay for T lymphocytes markers (CD3, CD4, CD8) and for HLA class I antigens, then analyzed by FACS.

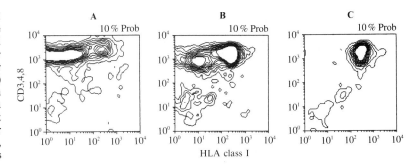

Eventually, after about six months of engraftment, the thymic cortex virtually disappears and only medullary lymphoid tissue, containing numerous Hassal's corpuscles, is observed.

FACS analysis reveals that the involution of the thymus graft with time is accompanied by a progressive disappearance of the pool of immature, cortical-type, MHC class I-negative T lymphocytes (Figure 3.3B, C). The majority of these cells has likely died as a result of clonal deletion events. A subset of them has further differentiated and contributed to the population of mature, medullary class I-high thymus lymphocytes (Figure 3.3).

These observations clearly confirm that the thymus normally does not harbor long-lived hematopoietic stem cells but depends upon an inflow of extrinsic stem cells to maintain continued lymphocyte production (Owen & Ritter, 1969; LeDouarin & Jotereau, 1975). In the absence of a blood-borne precursor cell supply, the pool of intrathymic pre-T cells becomes progressively exhausted. As a result, long-term engrafted human thymuses contain terminally differentiated T lymphocytes only. Advantage was taken of these cell population dynamics for the thymus repopulation experiments that are described in the following sections.

Long-term thymus hematopoiesis in the SCID-hu mouse

Implantation of human fetal thymus into SCID mice created an experimental model, the 'SCID-hu' mouse, in which T cell progenitors can proliferate and differentiate (McCune *et al.*, 1988). However, the decrease in the number of cortical thymocytes after transplantation suggested that hematopoietic progenitor cells and/or their supportive microenvironment were required for long-term reconstitution of SCID-hu mice. Since liver is known to be one of the major hematopoietic organs in fetal life, we have constructed SCID-hu mice that contain fragments of both human fetal thymus and liver (thus including the hematopoietic precursors and their stromal microenvironment) (Namikawa et al., 1990).

Small fragments of fetal thymus (14–23 weeks of gestation) and liver (18–23 weeks of gestation) were implanted in close association under the kidney capsule of SCID mice. This approach provides for long-term maintenance of human progenitor cells in the thymus grafts and stable generation of circulating human T cells. In some cases, the conjoint thymus plus liver (Thy/Liv) implants develop foci of extramedullary hematopoiesis ('thymic isles') which are indistinguishable from those seen in normal human bone marrow.

The circulation of human T cells in peripheral blood persists over long periods of time (up to fifteen months) under these conditions. When SCID-hu mice that had a thymus graft alone (Thy/–) were compared with mice that had a Thy/Liv graft, a clear difference was observed. More than 50% of mice with Thy/Liv grafts were found to be positive for human cells in peripheral blood up to six to eleven months after transplantation, whereas only 10% or fewer of the mice with Thy/– grafts were positive for human cells at five to six months after transplantation. The histological analysis of Thy/Liv grafts at six to eleven months after transplantation showed a structure which was indistinguishable from that of a normal human thymus (Figure 3.4A). The cortex was filled with thymocytes, indicating active T lymphopoiesis, whereas cortical lymphocyte depletion was a common observation in grafts of thymus alone. The surface phenotypes of those cells were also very similar to those of normal thymocytes. These findings strongly suggested the presence of long-lasting human T cell progenitors in the Thy/Liv grafts.

In addition, structures similar to bone marrow, consisting of blast cells, immature and mature forms of myelomonocytic cells, and megakaryocytes were observed inside the Thy/Liv grafts (Figure 3.4B). This suggested that multipotent progenitor cells and the environment which supports their maintenance and differentiation were present. These thymic isles were localized in the septal areas of the thymus. Human multipotent hematopoietic progenitor cell activity inside the Thy/Liv grafts was directly evidenced by colony-forming units in methylcellulose culture (CFU-C) assay (Namikawa et al., 1990). Colony-forming units for granulocyte-macrophages (CFU-GM) and burst-forming units for erythrocytes (BFU-E) were observed in the CFU-C assay with cells obtained from Thy/Liv grafts five to eleven months after transplantation, indicating the presence of progenitor cells for the myeloid and erythroid lineages. The human origin of these cells was confirmed with specific antibodies.

The histological findings described above and the results of the

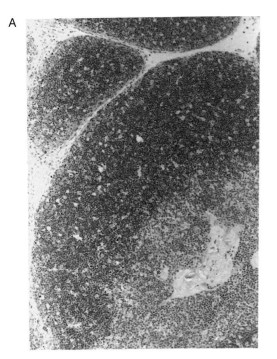

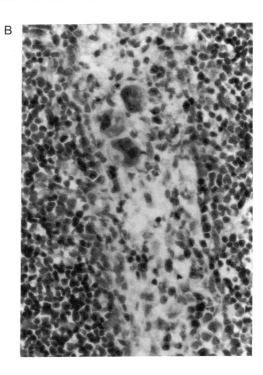

Figure 3.4. Histological features of fetal human thymus/liver (Thy/Liv) grafts in the SCID mouse. A. Typical histology of a Thy/Liv graft, 6 months after implantation. The structure of the thymus is indistinguishable from that of a normal thymus. (Giemsa staining, × 80.) B. Structure of a thymic isle. Blast cells, mature and immature forms of myelomonocytic cells and megakaryocytes are present in the septal area of the thymus graft. (Giemsa staining, × 320.)

CFU-C assays clearly demonstrate that long-term reconstitution of the SCID-hu mouse with human hematopoietic progenitor cells occurs following conjoint implantation of human fetal liver and thymus. Since these phenomena were observed much more frequently in Thy/Liv constructs than in Thy/– grafts, it was obvious that implanted liver fragments play an important role. To evaluate this point more closely, SCID-hu mice were prepared with combinations of human fetal liver and thymus that were allogeneic with respect to human MHC class I antigens. Monoclonal antibodies against marker antigens were used to trace cell movement later. The MHC type of the liver donor was found on T cells and macrophages in the Thy/Liv graft. Cells grown in the methylcellulose colony assay and cells in the bone marrow-like thymic isle structure were also found to express the HLA type of the liver donor. Thus, coimplantation of fetal liver and thymus was associated with long-term maintenance and differentiation of multilineage hematopoietic progenitor cells of fetal liver origin. The mechanisms that underlie the formation of thymic isles, such as the origin and the function of the stromal elements, require further analysis.

The SCID-hu mouse harboring Thy/Liv implants is the first animal model in which human hematopoietic function is actively maintained. It should provide a powerful tool to analyze the pathology and pathophysiology of human hematopoiesis *in vivo*.

Identification of human hematopoietic stem cells using SCID mice

Development in SCID mice of thymus rudiments colonized in vitro *by selected precursor cell populations*

The founders of the hematopoietic system are rare cells that are found in the yolk sac and liver in early fetal development and in the bone marrow at later stages. These morphologically banal elements had long been evidenced only indirectly, once they had already expanded and differentiated into blood cells in irradiated hosts (Till & McCulloch, 1961). Numerous attempts to characterize these stem cells on physical or biological criteria (see Spangrude, 1989, for a review) culminated when Spangrude *et al.* (1988) used sophisticated immunoselection methods to isolate a minute population of mouse bone marrow cells displaying a unique combination of surface antigens and exhibiting the expected properties of multipotential blood stem cells. These cells read out at a near unit efficiency in assays for clonogenic myeloerythroid and thymic progenitors. At low numbers, they also restore the whole blood system of lethally irradiated animals. The demonstrated feasibility of physically isolating blood cell precursors opened the way for the purification of human hematopoietic stem cells, a goal of considerable fundamental and therapeutic importance. However, such a search was hampered by the lack of appropriate assay systems; most of the tests devised to identify animal blood stem cells are ethically unacceptable for use in the human species.

It is true that the interactions between progenitor cells and stromal elements required for the production of hematopoietic cells can be, in some instances, reproduced experimentally *in vitro*. Cultured bone marrow cells support myelopoiesis and B lymphocyte production, yielding in vitro stem cell assays in mice (see Whitlock *et al.*, 1985, for a review) and in humans (Toogood *et al.*, 1980; C. Baum & A. Tsukamoto, 'SyStemix Inc.' submitted for publication). In contrast, the maintenance of the three-dimensional structure of the thymic reticulum appears to be a prerequisite for driving the full differentiation of stem cells into mature T lymphocytes. In the mouse, experimental T cell differentiation can be achieved in a quantitative manner by transfer of precursor cell candidates into irradiated hosts, either systemically (Ezine *et al.*, 1984) or by direct intrathymic injection (Goldschneider *et al.*, 1986; Guidos *et al.*, 1989). Similar physiologic assays of putative T cell precursors in man are, of course, impossible.

Therefore, we reasoned that human blood-forming organs, and especially thymus, transplanted into SCID mice could provide a unique model for testing putative human stem cells. The hematopoietic precursor cells that were first analyzed for their T cell potentialities in the SCID-hu system express the CD34 surface antigen and represent about 1–4% of bone marrow and fetal liver mononucleated cells. CD34$^+$ cells include colony-forming units endowed with myeloid (Civin *et al.*, 1984; Andrews *et al.*, 1986; Strauss *et al.*, 1986; Lu *et al.*, 1987) and pre-B cell activity (C Baum & A. Tsukamoto, 'SyStemix Inc.' submitted for publication); they also give rise to colonies of blast cells on bone marrow stroma capable of self-renewal and multilineage commitment (Brandt *et al.*, 1988). These observations suggest that the CD34$^+$ cell pool may include multipotential hematopoietic stem cells.

In vitro colonization of the human thymus with sorted stem cells

Conceptually, the full cycle of thymus physiology can be observed in the SCID-hu model: the 'homing' of blood-borne stem cells into the graft followed by differentiation and then peripheralization of mature lymphocytes. Supplying the grafted thymus with precursor cells injected into the mouse circulation is, however, difficult. When fetal liver cells were injected intravenously, they homed to the human thymus implants in a few cases only (McCune *et al.*, 1988). In order to circumvent these limitations, it was decided to supply the thymus with stem cells prior to its engraftment in the mouse.

Since a lymphocyte-free thymus is a much better candidate for experimental colonization, individual lobules dissected from fresh human fetal thymus were first depleted of hematopoietic cells by a week-long in vitro organ culture at 24 °C (Robinson & Jordan, 1983). Graded numbers of sorted CD34$^+$ cells that were to be tested for their potential pre-T activity were then transferred, using a microinjection device, into HLA-dissimilar, thymocyte-depleted thymus fragments, which were virtually reduced to an epithelial network.

Development of chimeric human thymuses in the SCID mouse

Even after in vitro organ culture for a week and stem cell microinjection, the human fetal thymus was found to grow and differentiate when implanted into the SCID mouse, albeit at a slightly slower rate than its fresh counterpart. At intervals, grafts of the conditioned thymus were dissected out, reduced into cell suspensions and analyzed for chimerism in the T lymphocyte compartment, i.e. for the presence of T cells derived from the donor CD34$^+$ precursors. Using MHC class I antigens as a marker for the progeny of injected cells, donor-derived immature T lymphocytes could be first detected at three weeks after engraftment; within six weeks, they expanded to yield mature, class I-high T cells (Figure 3.5). Similar to the kinetics of development of endogenous thymocytes (see section above: 'Growing human fetal thymus in SCID mice'), donor cells thus evolved through the whole cycle of intrathymic differentiation, ending up as mature T lymphocytes (Péault *et al.*, 1991).

In addition to T cells, the thymus includes an hematopoietic cell compartment composed of macrophages and interdigitating cells (Wong *et al.*, 1982). These 'accessory' cells, which play a major role in lymphocyte education, are derived from blood-borne precursors (Barclay & Mayrhofer, 1981; Guillemot *et al.*, 1984). These elements are tightly intricated in the thymic epithelial network and therefore not readily dispersable by mechanical means. To identify their origin in chimeric thymuses, graft sections were stained with antibodies specific for either host or donor HLA antigens. Numerous donor-derived dendritic cells were observed in the medulla and in the cortex (Péault *et al.*, 1991).

These results extended the differentiation capacities of bone marrow $CD34^+$ cells to thymus lymphocytes and myelomonocytic cells. As few as 100 of these precursors were shown to repopulate fully the engrafted thymus (Péault *et al.*, 1991). These experiments also revealed that it is technically possible to reconstitute the human hematopoietic system in SCID mice with selected precursor cell populations, an important step towards the characterization of blood stem cells in man.

Phenotypes and functional capabilities of human lymphocytes in SCID-hu mice

In addition to its value as a basic research tool and in the testing of anti-HIV drugs *in vivo*, the SCID-hu mouse may be useful in the evaluation of candidate vaccines for the generation of therapeutically-useful human monoclonal antibodies and for immunotoxicological testing. As a prerequisite for these applications, it was necessary to demonstrate that human lymphocytes in SCID-hu mice are functionally competent and qualitatively similar to their counterparts in humans. The phenotypic and functional characteristics of human lymphocytes in Thy/Liv grafts and peripheral blood of SCID-hu mice will be discussed in the following sections.

Human T cells in SCID-hu Thy/Liv grafts

The coimplantation of human fetal thymus and liver tissue under the kidney capsule of SCID mice results in the establishment of a

Figure 3.5. Top: Lymphoid reconstitution of the human fetal thymus following *in vitro* transfer of 3500 CD34$^+$ donor cells sorted from fetal bone marrow and 2-month engraftment in the SCID mouse. The majority of T lymphocytes in the graft are donor-derived. Bottom: As a control: an unreconstituted thymus from the same experiment.

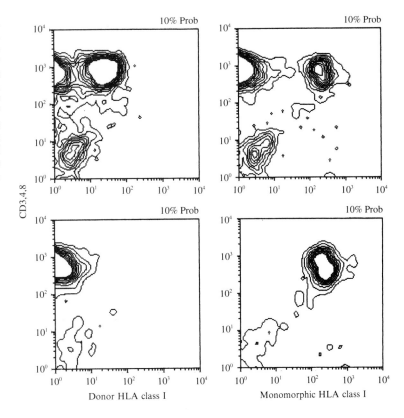

functional Thy/Liv graft and long-term T lymphopoiesis (Namikawa *et al.*, 1990), as discussed previously in this chapter. The phenotypes of human cells in the Thy/Liv grafts and their organization closely resemble human thymus tissue (Namikawa *et al.*, 1990). Between 50% and 80% of cells from SCID-hu Thy/Liv grafts are immature T cells that express both CD4 and CD8. Approximately 20% are CD4$^+$8$^-$ and between 4% and 15% of these cells are CD4$^-$8$^+$. Functional studies have demonstrated that cells from SCID-hu Thy/Liv grafts are also similar to fetal human thymocytes in their proliferative responses to mitogens and human alloantigens (Krowka *et al.*, 1991). Studies are currently in progress to determine if all T cell subsets from SCID-hu Thy/Liv grafts are functionally similar to their counterparts in the human thymus.

Phenotypes of human lymphocytes in SCID-hu peripheral blood

Within approximately two months after the coimplantation of human fetal thymus and liver tissue, low levels of human T cells, generally less than 5% of total peripheral blood lymphocytes (PBL), can be detected

87

in the peripheral blood of SCID-hu mice (Krowka *et al.*, 1991). Virtually all the human cells in the peripheral blood of SCID-hu mice are CD3$^+$ cells that express $\alpha\beta$ type T cell receptors. The ratio of CD4$^+$ to CD8$^+$ cells is approximately 2:1, which is similar to the ratio of these T cell subsets in humans (Krowka *et al.*, 1991). Approximately 60% of circulating human T cells in SCID-hu mice express Leu 8, the human equivalent of the mouse MEL14 antigen that is involved in organ-specific homing of lymphocytes (Gallatin *et al.*, 1983; Camerini *et al.*, 1989). Similar to normal human PBL, 1% or fewer human T cells in the peripheral blood of SCID-hu mice express the activation antigens CD25 or CD69, suggesting that graft-versus-host disease (GVHD) is not occurring. Approximately 74% of human SCID-hu PBL express CD45RA, a marker of relatively immature or 'naive' T cells (Serra *et al.*, 1988). Approximately 18% of human SCID-hu PBL express CD29, a marker of relatively mature or memory cells. The predominance of CD45RA$^+$ T cells in SCID-hu peripheral blood is similar to the levels of these cells in children (Pilarski *et al.*, 1991) and may reflect the limited exposure to foreign antigens that SCID-hu mice have experienced in their contained environment. These studies demonstrate that human T cells in SCID-hu peripheral blood are phenotypically similar to peripheral blood T cells from healthy human donors.

Functional capabilities of human T cells in SCID-hu peripheral blood

Owing to the relatively small numbers of human lymphocytes in the peripheral blood of SCID-hu mice, sensitive flow-cytometric assays were necessary to show that they are similar to adult human T cells in their responses to mitogens and antigens. The PBL from SCID-hu mice were cultured overnight *in vitro* in the presence or absence of antigens or mitogens and then analyzed for the coexpression of the human pan-leucocyte marker CD45 and the CD69 activation marker. Previous studies have demonstrated that CD69 is expressed within hours after activation of T cells, B cells, and natural killer (NK) cells but is not expressed on resting lymphocytes (Hara *et al.*, 1986; Lanier *et al.*, 1988). Figure 3.6 shows CD45 and CD69 expression 24 hours after stimulation of PBL from a SCID-hu mouse that had been constructed approximately nine months previously with human fetal thymus and liver tissue under the kidney capsule. Approximately 7% of the PBL from this mouse were human. In the absence of mitogens or antigens in culture less than 1% of the CD45$^+$ human T cells expressed CD69. After culture with Sepharose-conjugated CD3 antibody, 62% of the CD45$^+$ cells expressed the activation marker CD69. SCID-hu PBL have also been observed to respond to human alloantigens (Krowka *et*

Figure 3.6. CD69 and CD45 expression on SCID-hu PBL after *in vitro* stimulation. (PE is phycoerythrin; FITC is fluorescein isothiocyanate.)

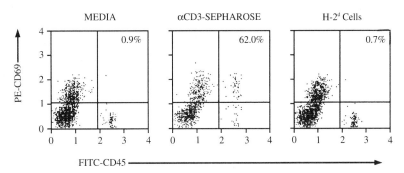

al., 1991). In contrast, after stimulation of SCID-hu PBL with inactivated mouse (H-2^d) cells, less than 1% of the human SCID-hu PBL expressed CD69 (Figure 3.6).

These studies demonstrate that SCID-hu PBL are similar to adult human PBL in their ability to be activated by mitogens or alloantigens. They are not, however, responsive to the xenogeneic histocompatibility antigens of the mouse. Clonal analysis has also confirmed the presence of alloreactive human T cells (Vandekerckhove *et al.*, 1991) and the apparent absence of xenoreactive (antimouse) human T cells in SCID-hu mice (our unpublished observations). In addition, the organs of SCID-hu mice with circulating human T cells for more than six months did not show any histological evidence for GVHD (Namikawa *et al.*, 1990). These studies indicate that graft-versus-host reactivity is *not* detectable in SCID-hu mice which are constructed with fetal lymphoid tissue. In contrast, recent reports indicate that GVHD and Epstein–Barr virus-induced lymphomas occur frequently when adult human lymphoid cells are introduced into immunodeficient mice (Bankert *et al.*, 1989; Krams *et al.*, 1989; Purtilo *et al.*, 1991). The processes by which progenitor cells from fetal liver mature in the SCID-hu Thy/Liv graft into functionally competent CD4$^+$ or CD8$^+$ T cells remain to be defined.

It is unclear whether the human T cells in SCID-hu mice are truly 'tolerant' of their murine environment or are merely unresponsive. Mouse cells with a dendritic morphology have been detected in subcapsular and cortical areas of SCID-hu Thy/Liv grafts (McCune *et al.*, 1988). It is possible that these murine cells within the Thy/Liv graft tolerize and perhaps delete any human T cells that recognize H-2^d or other antigens of the host C.B.-17 *scid/scid* mouse.

Conclusions

Almost three decades ago, the now classical studies of Moore & Owen (1965) on blood cell ontogeny in parabiosed embryos and the famous demonstration, by Till & McCulloch (1961), of bone marrow stem cell expansion and differentiation in irradiated hosts pioneered the use of experimental chimeras in the study of hematopoiesis. Since then, animal chimeras have been key models for the delineation of the complex cellular interactions involved in the development of blood-forming organs. As a recent extension in this experimental trend, in this chapter we have presented the successful replication of human hematopoiesis in immunodeficient mice.

Relying on our experience with almost 10 000 transplantations to date, we show that the human fetal thymus can grow and function in the SCID mouse. The SCID-hu mouse also provides a unique model for the study of HIV infection (Namikawa et al., 1988) and is now routinely used for preclinical trials of anti-HIV drugs (McCune et al., 1990; Kaneshima et al., 1991).

The kinetics of thymocyte development in SCID-engrafted human thymuses confirmed the inability of that organ to sustain long-term lymphopoiesis in the absence of an extrinsic stem cell supply. Conversely, prolonged T cell production ensued when fetal liver was coengrafted as a source of hematopoietic stem cells (Namikawa et al., 1990). To further characterize thymus-repopulating precursor cells, pre-engraftment colonization was performed with sorted stem cell populations (Péault et al., 1991). This experimental method, the only one that allows for the study of human thymus development from selected precursors, revealed T lymphocyte potentialities among the bone marrow $CD34^+$ (but not $CD34^-$) cell compartment, and also a subpopulation of bone marrow cells defined by a new differentiation marker, J1.43 (Y. Aihara, B. Péault, C. Baum, I. L. Weissman & A. Tsukamoto, submitted for publication). These are important steps towards the characterization and purification of human hematopoietic stem cells for genetic modification and clinical use (reviewed in Weatherall, 1991). The possibility of constructing human chimeric thymuses may facilitate the study of positive selection (MHC restriction) and negative selection (self-tolerance) of developing human thymocytes. Also, this system will permit studies of potential human precursor cell targets of pathogenic viruses such as HIV and cytomegalovirus (CMV).

Our studies also demonstrate that human T lymphocytes developing in SCID-hu mice are phenotypically normal and functionally competent (Krowka et al., 1991). Furthermore, immunization of SCID-hu mice can elicit the production of specific antibodies (our unpublished observations). SCID-hu mice could be used to produce an almost limitless variety of antibodies for therapeutic applications in neoplastic, infectious, or autoimmune diseases. The prophylactic and therapeutic effects of active or passive immunization could also be analyzed in this test system. Clearly, SCID-hu mice may be utilized for multiple applications in the development of prophylactic or therapeutic strategies in a variety of human diseases. Additional studies are in progress to test the feasibility of these approaches.

The present report has emphasized the transfer of human thymus and T cell development in SCID mice. This does not mean that the model is limited to these aspects of human hematopoiesis. Current exploratory experiments address the growth of other human organs in the SCID mouse. Encouraging preliminary results suggest that this human/mouse chimera will facilitate analysis of many more aspects of the normal and pathologic development of the human blood system.

Acknowledgments
The authors would like to acknowledge Yukoh Aihara, Dennis Sasaki, Ben Chen, Susan Mayo, Reina Mebius, Sujata Sarin, Phil Streeter, Paul von Hoegen, Kathy Weilbaecher, Hideto Kaneshima, Charles Baum, Ann Tsukamoto, Henry Outzen, Edwin Yee, Brian Ford, Alicia Mizerek-Erhart (Systemix, Inc.), Irving Weissman and Miriam Lieberman (Stanford University) for their various contributions to this work; and Nita Chapman and Kristina Cranias for assistance in preparing this document.

References

ANDREWS, R. G., SINGER, J. W. & BERNSTEIN, I. D. (1986) Monoclonal antibody 12–8 recognizes a 115 kd molecule present on both unipotent and multipotent colony-forming cells and their precursors. *Blood* **67**, 842.

BANKERT, R. B., UMEMOTO, T., SUGIYAMA, T., CHEN, F. A., REPASKY, E. & YOKOTA, S. (1989) Human lung tumors, patient peripheral blood lymphocytes and tumor infiltrating lymphocytes propagated in Scid mice. *Current Topics in Microbiology and Immunology*, **152**, 201

BARCLAY, N. & MAYRHOFER, G. (1981) Bone marrow origin of Ia-positive cells in the medulla of the rat thymus. *Journal of Experimental Medicine*, **153**, 1666.

BARRY, T. S., JONES, D. M., RICHTER, C. B. & HAYNES, B. F. (1991) Successful engraftment of human postnatal thymus in severe combined immune deficient (SCID) mice: differential engraftment of thymic components with irradiation versus anti-asialo GM1 immunosuppressive regimens. *Journal of Experimental Medicine*, **173**, 167

BOSMA, G. C., CUSTER, R. P. & BOSMA, M. J. (1983) A severe combined immunodeficiency mutation in the mouse. *Nature*, **301**, 527.

BRANDT, J., BAIRD, N., LU, L., SROUR, E. & HOFFMAN, R. J. (1988) Characterization of a human hematopoietic progenitor cell capable of forming blast cell containing colonies *in vitro*. *Clinical Investigation*, **82**, 1017.

CAMERINI, D., JAMES, S. P., STAMENKOVIC, I. & SEED, B. (1989) Leu-8/TQ1 is the human equivalent of the Mel-14 lymph node homing receptor. *Nature*, **342**, 78.

CIVIN, C. I., STRAUSS, L. C., BROVALL, C., FACKLER, M. J., SCHWARTZ, J. F. & SHAPER, J. H. (1984) Antigenic analysis of hematopoiesis III. A hematopoietic progenitor cell surface antigen defined by a monoclonal antibody raised against KG-1a cells. *Journal of Immunology*, **133**, 157.

EZINE, S., WEISSMAN, I. & ROUSE, R. (1984) Bone marrow cells give rise to distinct clones within the thymus. *Nature*, **309**, 629.

GALLATIN, W. M., WEISSMAN, I. L. & BUTCHER, E. C. (1983) A cell surface molecule involved in organ-specific homing of lymphocytes. *Nature*, **304**, 30.

GOLDSCHNEIDER, I., KOMSCHLIES, K. L. & GRENIER, D. L. (1986) Studies of thymocytopoiesis in rats and mice. I. Kinetics of appearance of thymocytes using a direct intrathymic adoptive transfer assay for thymocyte precursors. *Journal of Experimental Medicine*, **163**, 1.

GUIDOS, C. J., WEISSMAN, I. L. & ADKINS, B. J. (1989) Development potential of CD4$^-$ 8$^-$ thymocytes. Peripheral progeny include mature CD4$^-$ 8$^-$ T cells bearing $\alpha\beta$ T cell receptor. *Journal of Immunology*, **142**, 3773.

GUILLEMOT, F. P., OLIVER, P. D., PÉAULT, B. & LeDOUARIN, N. M. (1984) Cells expressing Ia antigens in the avian thymus. *Journal of Experimental Medicine*, **160**, 1803.

HARA, T., JUNG, L. K., BJORNDAHL, J. M. & FU, S. M. (1986) Human T cell activation. III. Rapid induction of a phosphorylated 28 KD/32 KD disulfide-linked early activation antigen (EA1) by 12-O-tetradecanoyl phorbol-13-acetate, mitogens, and antigens. *Journal of Experimental Medicine*, **164**, 1988.

KANESHIMA, H., SHIH, C-C., NAMIKAWA, R., RABIN, L. & McCUNE, J. M. (1991) Human immunodeficiency virus infection of human lymph nodes in the SCID-hu mouse. *Proceedings of the National Academy of Sciences, USA*, **88**, 4523.

KRAMS, S. M., DORSHKIND, K. & GERSHWIN, M. E. (1989) Generation of biliary lesions after transfer of human lymphocytes into severe combined immunodeficient (SCID) mice. *Journal of Experimental Medicine*, **170**, 1919.

KROWKA, J. F., SARIN, S., NAMIKAWA, R., McCUNE, J. M. & KANESHIMA, H. (1991) Human T cells in the SCID-hu mouse are phenotypically normal and functionally competent. *Journal of Immunology*, **146**, 3751.

LANIER, L. L., BUCK, D. W., RHODES, L., DING, A., EVANS, E., BARNEY, C. & PHILLIPS, J. J. (1988) Interleukin 2 activation of natural killer cells rapidly induces the expression and phosphorylation of the Leu-23 activation antigen. *Journal of Experimental Medicine*, **167**; 1572.

LeDOUARIN, N. M. (1978) Ontogeny of hematopoietic organs studied in avian embryo interspecific chimaeras. *Cold Spring Harbor Conference on Cell Proliferation*, **5**, 5–31.

LeDOUARIN, N. M. & JOTEREAU, F. V. (1975) Tracing of cells of the avian thymus through embryonic life in interspecific chimaeras. *Journal of Experimental Medicine*, **142**, 17.

LU, L., WALKER, D., BROXMEYER, H. E., HOFFMAN, R., HU, W. & WALKER, E. J. (1987) Characterization of adult human marrow hematopoietic progenitors highly enriched by two-color cell sorting with MY-10 and major histocompatibility class II monoclonal antibodies. *Journal of Immunology*, **139**, 1823.

McCUNE, J. M., NAMIKAWA, R., KANESHIMA, H., SHULTZ, L. D., LIEBERMAN, M. & WEISSMAN, I. L. (1988) The SCID-hu mouse: murine model for the analysis of human hematolymphoid differentiation and function. *Science*, **241**, 1632.

McCUNE, J. M., NAMIKAWA, R., SHIH, C-C., RABIN, L. & KANESHIMA, H. (1990) Suppression of HIV infection in AZT-treated SCID-hu mice. *Science*, **247**, 564.

MOORE, M. A. S. & OWEN, J. J. T. (1965) Chromosome marker studies on the development of the hemopoietic system in the chick embryo. *Nature*, **208**, 956.

MOSIER, D. E., GULIZIA, R. J., BAIRD, S. & WILSON, D. B. (1988) Transfer of a functional human immune system to mice with severe combined immunodeficiency. *Nature*, **335**, 256.

NAMIKAWA, R., KANESHIMA, H. LIEBERMAN, M., WEISSMAN, I. L. & McCUNE, J. M. (1988) Infection of the SCID-hu mouse by HIV-1. *Science*, **242**, 1684.

NAMIKAWA, R., WEILBAECHER, K. N., KANESHIMA, H., YEE, E. J. & McCUNE, J. M. (1990) Long-term hematopoiesis in the SCID-hu mouse. *Journal of Experimental Medicine*, **172**, 1055.

OWEN, J. J. T. & RITTER, M. A. (1969) Tissue interactions in the development of thymus lymphocytes. *Journal of Experimental Medicine*, **129**, 431.

PÉAULT, B., WEISSMAN, I., BAUM, C. & TSUKAMOTO, A. (1991) Lymphoid reconstitution of the human fetal thymus in SCID mice with CD34$^+$ precursor cells. *Journal of Experimental Medicine*, **174**, 1283.

PILARSKI, L. M., YACYSHYM, B. R., JENSEN, G. S., PRUSKI, E. & PABST, H. F. (1991) *B*1 Integrin (CD29) expression on human postnatal T cell subsets defined by selective CD45 isoform expression. *Journal of Immunology*, in press.

PURTILO, D. T., FALK, K., PIRRUCELLO, S. J. *et al.* (1991) SCID mouse model of Epstein–Barr virus-induced lymphomagenesis of immunodeficient humans. *International Journal of Cancer*, **47**, 510.

ROBINSON, J. H. & JORDAN, R. K. (1983) Thymus *in vitro*. *Immunology Today*, **4**, 41.

SCHULER, W., WEILER, I. J., SCHULER, A., PHILIPS, R. A., ROSEN-BERG, N., MAK, T., KEARNEY, J. F., PERRY, R. P. & BOSMA, M. J. (1986) Rearrangement of antigen receptor genes is defective in mice with severe combined immunodeficiency. *Cell*, **46**, 963.

SERRA, H. M., KROWKA, J. F., LEDBETTER, J. A. & PILARSKI, L. M. (1988) Loss of CD45R (Lp220)represents a post-thymic T cell differentiation event. *Journal of Immunology*, **140**, 1435.

SPANGRUDE, G. J. (1989) Enrichment of murine hematopoietic stem cells: diverging roads. *Immunology Today*, **10**, 344.

SPANGRUDE, G. J., HEIMFELD, S. & WEISSMAN, I. L. (1988) Purification and characterization of mouse hematopoietic stem cells. *Science*, **241**, 58.

STRAUSS, L. C., ROWLEY, S. D., LaRUSSA, V. F., SHARKIS, S. J., STUART, R. K. & CIVIN, C. I. (1986) Antigenic analysis of hematopoiesis V. Characterization of MY-10 antigen expression by normal lymphohematopoietic progenitor cells. *Experimental Hematology*, **14**, 878.

STROMBERG, I., *et al.* (1989) Human fetal mesencephalic tissue grafted to dopamine-denervated striatum of athymic rats: light- and electron-microscopical histochemistry and in vivo chronoamperometric studies. *Journal of Neuroscience*, **9**, 614.

TILL, J. E. & McCULLOCH, E. A. (1961) A direct measurement of the radiation sensitivity of normal mouse bone marrow cells. *Radiation Research*, **14**, 213.

TOOGOOD, I. R. G., DEXTER, T. M., ALLEN, T. D., SUDA, T. & LAJTHA, L. G. (1980) The development of a liquid culture system for the growth of human bone marrow cultures. *Leukemia Research*, **4**, 449.

TUCH, B. E., NG, A. B. P., JONES, A. & TURTLE, J. R. (1984) Histologic differentiation of human fetal pancreatic explants transplanted into nude mice. *Diabetes*, **33**, 1180.

VANDEKERCKHOVE, B. A., KROWKA, J. F., McCUNE, J. M., deVRIES, J. E. & RONCAROLO, M. G. (1991) Clonal analysis of the peripheral T cell compartment of the SCID-hu mouse. *Journal of Immunology*, **146**, 4173.

WEATHERALL, D. J. (1991) Gene therapy in perspective. *Nature*, **349**, 275.

WHITLOCK, C., DENIS, K., ROBERTSON, D. & WITTE, O. (1985) In vitro analysis of murine B-cell development. *Annual Reviews in Immunology*, **3**, 213.

WONG, T. W., KLINKERT, W. E. F. & BOWERS, W. E. (1982) Immunological properties of thymus cell subpopulations: rat dendritic cells are potent accessory cells and stimulators in a mixed leukocyte culture. *Immunobiology*, **160**, 413.

CHAPTER 4

Ontogeny of human T- and B-cell immunity

M. ELDER, M. S. GOLBUS and M. J. COWAN

CONTENTS

THE ONTOGENY OF THE HUMORAL and the cell-mediated immune responses, which are the primary mediators of successful organ and hematopoietic stem cell transplantation, is reviewed in this chapter. With the growing interest in using the fetus either as the source or as the recipient of stem cell or organ transplants, it is imperative that we understand the ontogeny of these two aspects of the immune system. Humoral immunity results from the antigenic stimulation of bone-marrow-derived or B lymphocytes and their subsequent differentiation into plasma cells capable of secreting neutralizing antibodies. Cellular immunity is the consequence of antigenic stimulation of thymus-derived or T lymphocytes, which then function to kill cellular targets or to help B cells or cytotoxic T cells to respond appropriately to antigenic exposure.

Antibody- and cell-mediated immunity develop during fetal life and the ontogeny of the immune system is currently under intensive study (Figure 4.1). Hematopoietic stem cells originate in the yolk sac and within a few weeks of gestation are found in the human fetal liver. During midgestation the bone marrow becomes the primary organ of hematopoiesis. The maturation and differentiation of hematopoietic stem cells into B lymphocytes is much better understood than that of T cells; the characterization of both pathways has benefitted greatly by recent advances in molecular biological techniques that have allowed the identification of cell surface molecules and gene rearrangement events that are expressed sequentially in differentiating precursor populations.

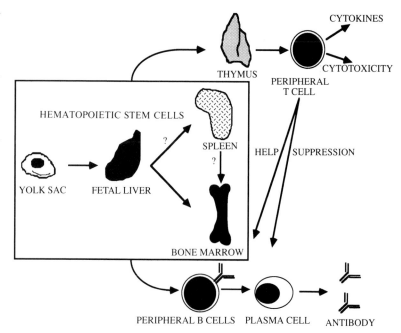

Figure 4.1. Development of hematopoietic stem cells into T and B cells. Stem cells are first found in the yolk sac in the first few weeks of human ontogeny. By 4–6 weeks of gestation hematopoiesis originates in the liver and by 20 weeks can be found in the bone marrow. The role of the spleen in ontogeny of hematopoiesis is not well defined.

B-cell immune system

B lymphocytes

B lymphocytes are the precursors of antibody-producing plasma cells and are responsible for the humoral immune response. Antibodies are antigen-specific immunoglobulins that are essential for host protection against bacteria and many viruses. Immunoglobulin production occurs in response to the binding of antigen to receptors on the B-cell surface membrane. This process usually requires the cooperation of helper T lymphocytes to secrete soluble factors, referred to as lymphokines, that are important for B-cell activation, proliferation and differentiation. However, antibody synthesis by some B cells does not require helper T cells, particularly those B cells producing antibodies against encapsulated organisms. Such T-cell-independent B cells are not present during gestation, do not become functional until the second year of life (Davie, 1985), and will not be discussed in detail here.

B cells are distinguished from other cells by the presence of membrane-bound immunoglobulin molecules, which function as antigen-specific receptors. Following the binding of antigen to these receptors, the B cell is activated to proliferate and differentiate into plasma cells. Plasma cells secrete antibodies having an antigen-specificity identical with that of the original membrane-bound immunoglobulin molecules on the B cell from which the plasma cells developed.

The immunoglobulins

Antibodies are classified by their heavy chain isotype into one of five classes: IgM, IgD, IgG, IgA and IgE (Natvig & Kunkel, 1973). Each heavy chain isotype designates a distinct 'effector function', which is specified by the Fc portion of the immunoglobulin molecule. IgM antibodies are the first immunoglobulins to be synthesized by a developing B cell and are expressed initially on the surface of immature B lymphocytes. IgM production predominates in primary immune responses and usually indicates exposure to new antigens. Secreted IgM antibodies have a structure distinct from that of surface IgM, existing as a pentamer of IgM molecules with a molecular weight (MW) of 950 000. These antibodies are found mainly in the peripheral blood and function to clear organisms by opsonization, activation of the classical complement pathway and stimulation of the reticuloendothelial system (Natvig & Kunkel, 1973; Winkelhake, 1978).

IgD antibodies function primarily as antigen receptors and are coexpressed with IgM on the surface of mature B cells (Cooper & Burrows, 1989). IgD is present in trace levels in the serum and has no known role as a secreted immunoglobulin.

IgG represents approximately 75% of the total serum immunoglobulins and is also the predominant extravascular antibody class. IgG antibodies mediate the secondary or anamnestic immune response and are the most frequent immunoglobulin molecules found on the surface of memory B cells. IgG molecules have a molecular weight (MW) of 150 000 and are also involved in the activation of the complement cascade and phagocytosis of antigen by the reticuloendothelial system (Natvig & Kunkel, 1973; Burton, 1985). IgG antibodies belong to one of four subclasses: IgG1, IgG2, IgG3, and IgG4, which have distinct functions. IgG1 and IgG3 antibodies are produced primarily against protein antigens, require lymphokines secreted by T lymphocytes for synthesis and are the first IgG subclasses to appear in B-cell ontogeny. IgG2 and IgG4 antibodies are produced primarily upon exposure to polysaccharide antigens, do not necessarily require T-cell help for production and are not usually detected until birth (Davie, 1985).

Approximately 15% of serum immunoglobulins and the majority of antibodies found in bodily secretions are IgA molecules. Secretory IgA exists primarily as a dimer of 500 000 MW in contrast to membrane-bound and serum IgA which are monomers of 160 000 MW (Tomasi,

1972; Natvig & Kunkel, 1973). Secretory IgA is felt to play a critical role in host defense of mucosal tissues (Underdown, & Schiff, 1986). Antibodies of the IgA1 subclass are found predominantly in the blood and protease-resistant IgA2 antibodies are detected mainly in secretions.

IgE is a rare circulating antibody and is associated with atopy. In allergic individuals, large amounts of IgE are synthesized and bound to the cell membranes of basophils and mast cells, where these molecules can stimulate degranulation and anaphylactoid responses after binding of antigen (Ishizaka & Ishizaka, 1975).

Immunoglobulin structure

The antibody molecule is composed of paired identical heavy chains and paired light chains, which are joined by several interchain disulfide bonds (Hilschmann & Craig, 1965; Nisonoff *et al.*, 1975). The antigen specificity of the immunoglobulin molecule is determined by the antigen-combining site located in the Fab portion of the molecule; the sequences of this portion vary considerably from one antibody molecule to another and result in antibody diversity and the ability to bind most of the antigens encountered by humans (Edelman & Gall, 1969; Capra & Kehoe, 1975; Nisonoff *et al.*, 1975). This antibody diversity is the result of rearrangement and alteration of the DNA sequences encoding the immunoglobulin heavy chains and light chains.

By recombinant DNA techniques, the DNA sequences coding for the immunoglobulin heavy chain have been found to be discontinuous, dispersed along the chromosome as multiple gene fragments, which are neither functionally transcribed into RNA nor subsequently translated into protein in this germline configuration (Ravetch *et al.*, 1981; Siebenlist *et al.*, 1982; Kodaira *et al.*, 1986; Honjo *et al.*, 1989; Rathburn *et al.*, 1989). The light chain loci are arranged similarly (Hieter *et al.*, 1981; Zachau, 1989). Before antibody synthesis can occur, the developing B lymphocyte must join representative gene fragments encoding segments of the heavy chain and light chain by a specialized process called immunoglobulin gene rearrangement (Seidman & Leder, 1978; Ravetch *et al.*, 1981; Yancopoulos & Alt, 1986; Rathburn *et al.*, 1989). Pairs of identical heavy chains and light chains are then assembled to form functional antibody molecules in the Golgi apparatus of the B cell.

The extensive antibody diversity required for host protection against the vast numbers of antigens that may be encountered is provided by the ability of multiple B cell precursors to create unique immunoglobu-

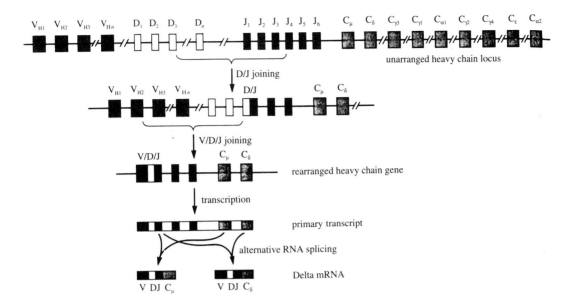

Figure 4.2. Rearrangement and expression of the H chain locus. Unlike the L chain genes, assembly of an H chain V region exon requires 2 sequential DNA rearrangement events involving 3 different types of gene segments. The D_H and J_H segments are joined first and are then fused to a V_H segment. Nine alternative C region sequences are present; of these, however, only the C_μ and C_δ sequences are initially transcribed. The primary transcript can be spliced in either of 2 ways to generate mRNAs that encode μ or δ H chains with identical V domains. This diagram is highly schematic: each C_H sequence is actually composed of multiple exons whose aggregate length is more than 3 times longer than that of the V/D/J exon. (Reprinted with permission from Stites & Terr, *Basic and Clinical Immunology*, 7th edition, © Appleton & Lange 1991.)

lin genes by fusion of different immunoglobulin DNA sequences (Seidman & Leder, 1978; Yancopoulos & Alt, 1986; Cooper & Burrows, 1989). This rearrangement occurs sequentially during ontogeny: immunoglobulin heavy chain genes are rearranged and joined prior to light chain genes (Yancopoulos & Alt, 1986; Cooper & Burrows, 1989; Rathbun *et al.*, 1989). An example of the complexity of heavy (H) chain rearrangement is shown in Figure 4.2. This specialized process of immunoglobulin gene rearrangement commits cells of the B-cell lineage to production of antibodies (Cooper & Burrows, 1989).

B-cell ontogeny

The B-cell differentiation pathway has been elucidated primarily by the observed stages of immunoglobulin gene rearrangement and the presence of other cell surface markers on developing B lymphocytes. The maturation of the hematopoietic stem cell to the terminally differentiated plasma cell is shown in Figure 4.3.

Hematopoietic stem cell. Hematopoiesis develops initially in the blood islands of the yolk sac, where proliferation and differentiation of primitive hematopoietic stem cells is seen in the second and third week of gestation in humans (Figure 4.1) (Stites *et al.*, 1975; Owen, 1977; Kincade & Phillips, 1985; Cooper & Burrows, 1989). These precursors of the erythroid, monocyte, granulocyte, megakaryocyte and

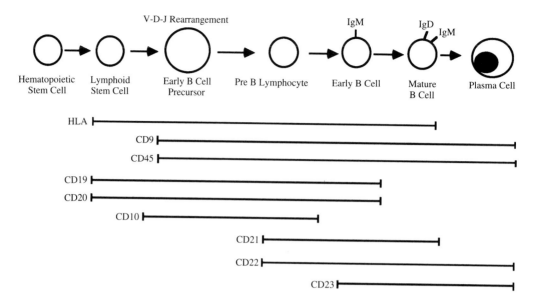

Figure 4.3. Development of B-cell immune system. HLA, human leukocyte antigens; CD, cluster of differentiation antigens expressed on the cell surface (Zola, 1987).

lymphoid lineages migrate into the fetal liver by the sixth week of gestation and begin to express markers unique to each lineage (Cooper & Burrows, 1989).

Lymphoid stem cells destined to become T and B cells have not been recognized morphologically in the fetal liver, but can be detected by the presence in their nuclei of terminal deoxynucleotide transferase (TdT) (Janossy et al., 1979; Cooper & Burrows, 1989). This enzyme is responsible for the insertion of additional nucleotide residues into rearranging immunoglobulin genes in B cells, contributing to anti-body-combining site diversity (Baltimore, 1974; Cooper & Burrows, 1989). These stem cells also have detectable expression of major histocompatibility complex (MHC) class II or HLA DR antigens on their cell surface (Baltimore, 1974). HLA DR molecules are present on all cells of the B-cell lineage and are critical for antigen presentation and interactions with antigen-presenting cells and T lymphocytes. HLA A, B and C antigens (MHC class I molecules) are also expressed on cells of the lymphoid lineage.

Other surface molecules initially expressed by the most primitive B-cell precursors include clusters of differentiation molecules CD19 and CD20 (Hokland et al., 1985; Zola, 1987). (See Table 4.1 for more details of CD molecules.) CD19 defines a common B-cell surface molecule whose function is unknown (Zola, 1987). CD20 is expressed on most B cells and is involved in activation of resting B lymphocytes (Zola, 1987).

Table 4.1. *Cluster of differentiation (CD) for T and B Cells*

Designation	Primary cell reactivity	Features[a]	References[b]
CD1 (T6)	Cortical thymocytes	MW 49 000	1, 2
CD2 (T11)	Thymocytes, T cells	MW 50 000; sheep rbc receptor	2, 3–6
CD3 (T3)	Thymocytes, T cells	5 chain complex with TCR	7–11, 12
CD4 (T4)	Helper T cells	MW 55 000; binds HLA class II molecule	13–18
CD5 (T1)	B cell subset, thymocytes	MW 67 000	19–22
CD7	T cells, thymocytes	MW 40 000	5
CD8 (T8)	Cytotoxic/suppressor T cells	Monomer MW 34 000; dimer binds HLA class I molecule	13, 14, 23, 24, 18
CD9	Pre-B cells	MW 24 000	25
CD10	Pre-B cells, ALL subset	MW 100 000; cALLA	25
CD19	B cells	MW 95 000	25, 26
CD20	B cells	MW 35 000	25, 26
CD21	Pre-B and most B cells	MW 140 000; C3d/EBV receptor	25
CD22	Pre-B and most B cells	Monomer MW 135 000	25
CD23	Activated B cells	MW 45 000; IgE-Fc receptor	25, 27
CD38 (T10)	Lymphoid progenitors	MW 45 000	1, 2
CD45	B and T cells	MW 180–240 000; protein tyrosine phosphatase	28–30
CD71 (T9)	Lymphoid progenitors	Transferrin receptor	1, 2

Notes:
[a] Apparent molecular weight (MW) by electrophoretic gel analysis.
C3d/EBV is C3d/Epstein–Barr virus; rbc is red blood cell.
[b] Key
1, Reinherz & Schlossman (1980); 2, Rosenthal *et al.* (1983); 3, Reinherz (1985); 4, Haynes *et al.* (1988); 5, Haynes *et al.* (1989); 6, Kabelitz (1990); 7, Borst *et al.* (1983); 8, Meuer *et al.* (1983); 9, Acuto & Reinherz (1985); 10, Samelson *et al.* (1985); 11, Fowlkes & Pardoll (1989); 12, Reis *et al.* (1989); 13 Meuer *et al.* (1982); 14, Swain (1983); 15 Blue *et al.* (1985); 16 Ashwell *et al.* (1986); 17, Doyle & Strominger (1987); 18, Campana *et al.* (1989); 19, Wu *et al.* (1976); 20, Antin *et al.* (1986); 21, Gadol & Alt (1986); 22, Hardy & Hayakawa (1986); 23, Fleischer & Wagner (1986); 24, Norment *et al.* (1988); 25, Zola (1987); 26, Hokland *et al.* (1985); 27, Wang *et al.* (1987); 28, Abe (1989); 29, Clark & Ledbetter (1989); 30, Pilarski & Deans (1989).

Committed B-cell progenitor. Early B-cell lineage precursors are the least differentiated lymphocytes to undergo immunoglobulin heavy chain gene rearrangements. These cells, as seen in fetal liver cultures at six to eight weeks of gestation, appear as large basophilic lymphocytes (Landreth *et al.*, 1982; Cooper & Burrows 1989), and express nuclear TdT, corresponding to the initiation of immunoglobulin heavy chain gene rearrangement (Baltimore, 1974; Cooper & Burrows, 1989). No rearrangement of light chain genes occurs in these B-cell lineage precursors (Yancopoulos & Alt, 1986; Cooper & Burrows, 1989).

In addition to the cell surface molecules mentioned previously, B-cell precursors also begin to express CD45, CD9 and CD10 molecules (Hokland *et al.*, 1985; Zola, 1987; Abe, 1989; Clark & Ledbetter, 1989; Pilarski & Deans, 1989). CD45 (B220) is expressed on all cells of the B-cell lineage; other forms of this protein are found on T cells (Clark & Ledbetter, 1989; Pilarski & Deans, 1989). CD45 is a protein tyrosine phosphatase and may function in signal transduction of the antigen-binding event into the cytoplasm of the B cell and in interactions with other membrane-associated molecules (Korsmeyer *et al.*, 1982; Abe, 1989). CD9 is encoded on chromosome 12 and is expressed on early B cells, as well as on non-T acute lymphoblastic leukemia (ALL) cells, other B-cell malignancies and multiple other non-B-cell types. Its function is also unclear, but may be associated with cell proliferation and differentiation (Zola, 1987). CD10 or the common acute lympho-blastic leukemia antigen (cALLA) is also expressed on a subclass of non-T ALL cells, some B-cell lymphomas and on other non-lymphoid tissues (Zola, 1987). CD10 expression is subsequently lost with further B-cell differentiation.

Pre-B lymphocytes. Pre-B cells are distinguished by the presence of μ heavy chains in their cytoplasm. These lymphocytes synthesize μ chains encoded by the rearranged μ heavy chain gene (Rathburn *et al.*, 1989). At this early pre-B-cell stage, the μ chains remain bound to retention proteins in the endoplasmic reticulum of the cell and are not expressed on the plasma membrane (Cooper & Burrows, 1989).

Morphologically, early pre-B cells are large, but rapidly differentiate into small, mature pre-B lymphocytes after the commencement of light chain gene rearrangement (Korsmeyer *et al.*, 1982; Cooper & Burrows, 1989). The successful assembly of an individual heavy chain gene and light chain gene in the pre-B cell results in the subsequent production of a single type of immunoglobulin molecule in the B lymphocyte. This phenomenon dictates that all immunoglobulins produced by any B-cell clone have identical light chains and antigen-combining sites, which is referred to as 'clonal restriction' (Korsmeyer *et al.*, 1982; Yancopoulos & Alt, 1986; Cooper & Burrows, 1989). Enhancement of antibody diversity after immunoglobulin gene rearrangement has been completed is thought to occur at the pre-B-cell stage as a result of 'somatic hypermutation' in which point mutations in the DNA sequences occur at high frequencies resulting in gene alteration (Rathburn *et al.*, 1989).

Approximately 0.2% of fetal liver cells at seven to eight weeks of gestation are cytoplasmic μ^+ by immunofluorescence; this frequency increases to approximately 4% of fetal liver cells at twelve to thirteen weeks of gestation (Gathings *et al.*, 1977; Hayward, 1981). These pre-B lymphocytes are not detected in the bone marrow until fourteen weeks of gestation, at which time they constitute about 10% of the nucleated cells. Throughout the rest of gestation, pre-B-cell proliferation occurs almost exclusively in the bone marrow and is antigen-independent (Lawton *et al.*, 1972). Pre-B lymphocytes are rarely found (fewer than 2% of cells) in the fetal spleen or peripheral blood throughout fetal life (Gathings *et al.*, 1977; Hayward, 1981).

CD22 is first expressed on pre-B cells, but is subsequently found on a majority of peripheral blood and lymph nodal B cells (Zola, 1987). The function of CD22 is not presently known. Expression of CD21 is seen at this stage as well. It is a 140 000 MW protein detected on mature pre-B cells and also on a majority of peripheral blood and lymph nodal B lymphocytes. This molecule appears to function as the receptor for both Epstein–Barr virus and the complement C3d component (Zola, 1987).

B cells. Pre-B cells differentiate into definitive B lymphocytes only after heavy chain gene rearrangements are completed and cytoplasmic μ heavy chains are expressed (Cooper & Burrows, 1989). Once sufficient quantities of light chains are also synthesized, the retention proteins bound to the cytoplasmic μ heavy chains are displaced; intact IgM molecules are then assembled in the Golgi apparatus and transported to the cell surface for expression, but are not secreted to any appreciable extent (Cooper & Burrows, 1989). These surface immunoglobulin molecules will serve as the first antigen receptors. However, immature surface-IgM$^+$ B cells appear to be tolerized rather than activated by binding of antigen to their receptors, which is thought to be related to the absence of membrane-bound IgD (Nossal, 1983).

Surface-IgM$^+$ lymphocytes are first detected in the fetal liver at about nine weeks of gestation (Lawton *et al.*, 1972; Gathings *et al.*, 1977; Cooper & Burrows, 1989). Approximately 2% of cells in the fetal liver and 10% of cells in the spleen between twelve to thirteen weeks of gestation are surface-IgM$^+$ B cells (Gathings *et al.*, 1977; Cooper & Burrows, 1989). With further proliferation and migration, the frequency of these early B lymphocytes increases to approximately 5% in the liver, 8% in the bone marrow, 35% in the spleen, 13% in lymph nodes and 30% in peripheral blood at fourteen to seventeen weeks of gestation (Gathings *et al.*, 1977). Similar results have been reported by other investigators (Lawton *et al.*, 1972; Vossen, 1975).

These surface-IgM$^+$ cells subsequently differentiate into mature B cells, which synthesize and express membrane-bound IgD as well as IgM (Cooper & Burrows 1989). The IgD molecule will possess an antigen-combining site, and thus antigen specificity, identical with the

IgM receptor (Cooper & Burrows, 1989; Honjo et al., 1989). This process apparently does not require exposure to antigen nor a requirement for T-cell help. Surface-IgM$^+$ IgD$^+$ B lymphocytes appear shortly after surface-IgM$^+$ cells and are able to proliferate and differentiate into plasma cells upon binding of antigen to their immunoglobulin receptors (Cooper & Burrows, 1989). IgM$^+$ IgD$^+$ B lymphocytes constitute approximately 0.4% of cells in the fetal liver and 9% of cells in the spleen at twelve to thirteen weeks of gestation (Gathings et al., 1977). The frequency of IgM$^+$ IgD$^+$ B lymphocytes increases to approximately 2% of liver cells, 3% of bone marrow cells, 29% of spleen cells, 9% of nodal lymphocytes, and 22% of nucleated cells in the peripheral blood of fetuses at fourteen to seventeen weeks of gestation (Gathings et al., 1977).

Additional cell surface molecules initially expressed at the B-cell stage include the IgG-Fc receptor and CD23 or IgE-Fc receptor (Wang et al., 1987; Zola, 1987). The IgG-Fc receptor is important for opsonization and stimulation of the reticuloendothelial system. CD23 is a human B-cell specific differentiation antigen possibly involved in B-cell growth and differentiation and in responses to the lymphokine, interleukin-4 (IL-4) (Wang et al., 1987; Zola, 1987). CD19, CD20, and CD10 expression are lost at the B-cell stage of differentiation.

As stated previously, the differentiation of B lymphocytes into memory B cells and antibody-secreting plasma cells requires binding of antigen to membrane-bound immunoglobulin molecules and, in most cases, the cooperation of helper T lymphocytes (Cooper & Burrows, 1989). Helper T cells are CD4$^+$ T cells and release IL-4, IL-6, interferon-γ, as well as other lymphokines, which stimulate B-cell proliferation and differentiation, heavy chain class switching and immunoglobulin secretion (Jelinek & Lipsky, 1987). For some B-cell responses, actual physical contact with the CD4$^+$ T cell is required. In addition, the helper T lymphocyte and the B cell must share identical HLA DR molecules for cooperation to occur.

Antigenic stimulation of IgM$^+$ IgD$^+$ B cells results in loss of expression of surface IgD and the initiation of a process termed 'isotype or class switch' whereby other classes of antibody molecules are expressed on the B-cell surface (Jelinek & Lipsky, 1987; Honjo et al., 1989). These antibodies will have a different effector function as specified by the Fc region of the molecule, but an antigen-binding site and antigen specificity identical with the initially expressed IgM and IgD molecules.

Surface-IgG$^+$ and IgA$^+$ B cells have been detected at as early as ten to twelve weeks of gestation in fetal liver by several investigators (Lawton et al., 1972; Gathings et al., 1977), suggesting that B-cell differentiation is spontaneous and independent of antigenic stimulation *in utero* (Cooper & Burrows, 1989). However, the actual mechanisms controlling B-cell activation, proliferation and differentiation in the fetus are not known. In fetuses of fourteen to twenty weeks of gestation, surface-IgG$^+$ B lymphocytes represent approximately 1% of liver cells, 2% of bone marrow cells, and 6–9% of peripheral blood, spleen and lymph nodal cells (Gathings *et al.*, 1977). Surface-IgA$^+$ B cells are detected at a much lower frequency of 0.1–2% of nucleated cells in these fetal tissues (Gathings *et al.*, 1977). The frequencies of IgG$^+$ B cells and IgA$^+$ B lymphocytes in various lymphoid tissues at fifteen to twenty weeks of gestation are comparable to those seen in adult peripheral blood, spleen and lymph nodes (Lawton *et al.*, 1972, Gathings *et al.*, 1977).

Plasma cells. The terminally differentiated antibody-producing cell appears morphologically as a large lymphocyte with an eccentric nucleus, and a well-developed Golgi apparatus, consistent with its active protein synthetic machinery (Siverstein & Lukes, 1962; Zucker-Franklin *et al.*, 1981). These cells have very low levels of membrane-bound immunoglobulin and are detected primarily by the presence of cytoplasmic antibodies, which are secreted in large quantities (Van Furth *et al.*, 1965; Hayward, 1981). CD21 expression is lost at this stage (Zola, 1987).

Memory B cells and plasma cells are rare in the non-infected fetus (Lawton *et al.*, 1972; Hayward, 1981). Exuberant lymphoid tissue development and plasma cell proliferation have been noted in fetuses of greater than twenty weeks' gestational age who were exposed to intrauterine infections such as syphilis and toxoplasmosis (Siverstein & Lukes, 1962; Lawton *et al.*, 1972).

Immunoglobulin synthesis

Depending on the experimental procedures used, the timing of immunoglobulin production in the fetus is found to be variable. IgM synthesis has been detected *in vitro* in fetal spleen cultures of ten to twelve weeks of gestation (Gitlin & Biasucci, 1969; Miler, 1983), but is not usually detected in the serum of healthy fetuses until approximately seventeen weeks of gestation (Van Furth *et al.*, 1965; Hayward, 1981; Miler, 1983). IgG synthesis has been seen in fetal liver and spleen cultures *in vitro* in the eleventh to twelfth week of gestation (Gitlin & Biasucci, 1969; Miler, 1983) and in the serum from the sixteenth week of gestation (Gitlin & Biasucci, 1969; Miler, 1983). However, other studies have not detected serum IgG until after twenty weeks of gestation in healthy fetuses (Lawton *et al.*, 1972; Goldman &

Goldman, 1977). IgA synthesis has not been demonstrated *in vitro* until after thirty weeks of gestation (Van Furth *et al.*, 1965; Lawton *et al.*, 1972), but has been detected in trace levels in the serum of fourteen week and twenty-seven week fetuses (Cederquist & Litwin, 1974; Miler, 1983).

Although these results suggest that the fetus has normally functioning B cells, serum immunoglobulin levels do not reach those of adults until well after birth. Adult levels of serum IgM, IgG and IgA are not obtained until about one year, five years and greater than ten years of age, respectively (Buckley *et al.*, 1968). The delayed production of serum immunoglobulins probably reflects the immaturity of the requisite CD4$^+$ T lymphocytes (Cooper & Burrows, 1989). This possibility has been suggested by in vitro studies in which stimulation of proliferation and immunoglobulin synthesis by fetal and neonatal B cells was restored to mature levels after replacement of the fetal T cells with mature T lymphocytes by immunization with pokeweed mitogen (PWM) (Wu *et al.*, 1976).

CD5 (Leu-1) B cells

CD5$^+$ B lymphocytes were originally discovered in patients with chronic lymphocytic leukemia and are thought to arise from a stem cell lineage distinctly different from that of the classical B lymphocyte (Antin *et al.*, 1986; Gadol & Alt, 1986; Hardy & Hayakawa, 1986). CD5$^+$ B cells appear to constitute a major subpopulation of B cells in the fetus, in cord blood and in bone marrow transplant recipients, but their function is unknown at this time (Wu *et al.*, 1976; Antin *et al.*, 1986; Gadol & Alt, 1986).

T-cell immune system

T lymphocytes

Thymus-derived or T lymphocytes are responsible for cellular immunity. T cell-mediated immune responses include graft rejection, delayed-type hypersensitivity reactions, regulation of antibody synthesis and host protection against viruses, fungi and certain obligate intracellular organisms. Antigen recognition is mediated through the surface T-cell receptor (TCR). Unlike B cells, which can respond to soluble free antigen, the T lymphocyte recognizes a complex, consisting of antigen bound to a self MHC class I (HLA, A,B,C) or class II (HLA DR,DQ,DP) molecule expressed on the surface of an antigen-presenting cell (APC: Meuer *et al.*, 1982; Swain, 1983; Unanue, 1984). Whole antigens must first be degraded, processed and then presented to the T cell as immunogenic peptides by the APC before TCR binding and T-cell recognition can result (Allen *et al.*, 1984; Unanue, 1984). Binding of the peptides to the appropriate self MHC molecules occurs in the cytoplasm of the APC prior to transport of the peptide–MHC complex to the cell surface (Unanue, 1984). Most APC are macrophages or epithelial dendritic cells.

This 'MHC restriction' dictates which T-cell subpopulation will respond to antigen bound to a self MHC molecule: $CD4^+$ T cells recognize peptide in association with MHC class II gene products on the APC, and $CD8^+$ T lymphocytes react to antigen bound to class I molecules on the surface of their target cell (Meuer *et al.*, 1982; Swain, 1983). CD4 and CD8 molecules are thought to bind invariant amino acid sequences present in the MHC class II and class I proteins, respectively (Doyle & Strominger, 1987; Blue *et al.*, 1988; Norment *et al.*, 1988, Table 4.1). The majority of $CD4^+$ cells are helper T lymphocytes, whose primary function is the secretion of various lymphokines necessary for antibody synthesis by B cells and target cell killing by cytotoxic/suppressor T cells (Morimoto *et al.*, 1985a, b; Fleischer & Wagner, 1986). However, a small subset of $CD4^+$ T cells are cytotoxic T lymphocytes (Fleischer & Wagner, 1986). Cytotoxic/suppressor T lymphocytes usually express CD8 molecules and function largely through physical contact with their target cell (Fleischer & Wagner, 1986). The targets recognized by cytotoxic/suppressor T lymphocytes are usually virally infected, malignant or allogeneic transplanted cells.

T-cell receptor–CD3 complex

The classical TCR is a disulfide-linked heterodimer composed of two glycoproteins, an α chain of approximately 39 000–46 000 MW and a 40 000–44 000 MW β chain (Reinherz *et al.*, 1983; Acuto & Reinherz, 1985; Fowlkes & Pardoll, 1989; Reis *et al.*, 1989). The TCR-αβ is expressed on the T-cell plasma membrane as part of a macromolecular complex with CD3 (Borst *et al.*, 1983; Meuer *et al.*, 1983; Acuto & Reinherz, 1985; Fowlkes & Pardoll, 1989; Reis *et al.*, 1989). Analogous to immunoglobulin molecules, amino acid sequences within both chains generate the antigen-combining site and TCR diversity, which is comparable to that of antibodies (Adkins *et al.*, 1987; Toribio *et al.*, 1988; Chan & Mak, 1989; Fowlkes & Pardoll, 1989). Recently, a small population of T cells has been characterized that expresses a distinct TCR in association with CD3 (Lanier & Weiss, 1986). This TCR-γδ consists of a 35 000 MW to 55 000 MW γ chain and an approximately 40 000 MW δ subunit (Bank *et al.*, 1986; Brenner *et al.*, 1986; LeFranc,

1988; Chan & Mak, 1989). The TCR-$\gamma\delta$ structure is similar to that of the TCR-$\alpha\beta$. However, in most cases, γ/δ T lymphocytes do not express either CD4 or CD8 nor do they appear to have MHC-restricted function, in contrast to α/β T cells (Bank *et al.*, 1986; Adkins *et al.*, 1987; LeFranc, 1988).

TCR expression on the T-cell surface requires the non-covalent binding of the TCR heterodimer to CD3. Detailed structural analysis of CD3 reveals that it is actually a complex of four or five proteins, consisting of a single γ chain (CD-γ), a δ molecule (CD-δ), a nonglycosylated ϵ chain (CD-ϵ) and a ζ chain, which can exist on the cell membrane as either a homodimer (CD-$\zeta\zeta$) or as a heterodimer with a η molecule (CD-$\zeta\eta$) (Borst *et al.*, 1983; Samelson *et al.*, 1985; Fowlkes & Pardoll, 1989). Assembly of the TCR–CD3 proteins occurs in the endoplasmic reticulum of the T lymphocyte and is required for transport and cell surface expression of the TCR–CD3 complex. T-cell mutants lacking a TCR or CD3 protein do not transport or express a TCR–CD3 complex on their cell surface and thus cannot recognize and respond to antigen (Allison & Lanier, 1987; Cooper & Burrows, 1989; Reis *et al.*, 1989).

The binding of peptide to the TCR–CD3 complex initiates multiple intracellular events, including hydrolysis of phosphatidylinositol 4,5-bisphosphate, a rise in intracellular free calcium and activation of protein kinase C (Weiss & Imboden, 1987). These events are involved in T-cell activation by unknown mechanisms. The CD3 complex is felt to be pivotally involved in signal transduction and coupling of antigen-binding to intracellular biochemical pathways, resulting in T-cell activation. In summary, the TCR–CD3 complex has at least two critical functions: (1) specific antigen recognition by the TCR-$\alpha\beta$ in association with a self MHC molecule; (2) CD3 mediation of signal transduction necessary for activation of the T cell and a cellular immune response. CD4 and CD8 molecules are loosely associated but not structurally bound to the TCR–CD3 complex and are required for recognition of antigen by the appropriate TCR-$\alpha\beta^{+}$ cell subset.

TCR-$\alpha\beta$ and TCR-$\gamma\delta$ genes

The genomic arrangement of the TCR-$\alpha\beta$ and TCR-$\gamma\delta$ genes is very similar to that of the immunoglobulin sequences, suggesting that both have evolved from a common ancestral gene. Analogous to immunoglobulin genes, rearrangement and juxtaposition of TCR-α and TCR-β DNA sequences is required to produce functional TCR genes (Kronenberg *et al.*, 1986; Chan & Mak, 1989; Fowlkes & Pardoll, 1989; Raulet, 1989). Consequently, diversity of the α and β chains produced by the possible joining of multiple different gene segments results in increased numbers of possible antigen-combining sites. α Chain diversity is further increased by the random insertion of nucleotides at the junctions of gene fragments during DNA rearrangement, changing the DNA sequences encoding the antigen-combining site (Adkins *et al.*, 1987; Chan & Mak, 1989; Fowlkes & Pardoll, 1989). This process may be the function of TdT present in early T cells. Assembly of the TCR α and β chains to form a TCR-αβ with an unique antigen-combining site then occurs in the endoplasmic reticulum and is transported to the cell membrane after non-covalent binding to CD3 (Adkins *et al.*, 1987; Fowlkes & Pardoll, 1989).

The TCR-γ chain locus and the TCR-δ locus also rearrange similarly to TCR-α and TCR-β genes (LeFranc, 1988; Fowlkes & Pardoll, 1989; Raulet, 1989). T lymphocytes express either TCR-αβ or TCR-γδ, but not both molecules (Denning *et al.*, 1989). Due to the genomic organization of the TCR genes, the TCRs produced by gene rearrangement and expressed on any T-cell clone will have identical antigen-combining sites and antigen specificity.

HLA molecules

Class I molecules. Human class I molecules, referred to as HLA (human leukocyte antigen) A,B,C antigens, are expressed on all nucleated cells and are composed of two chains: $β_2$-microglobulin encoded on chromosome 15 and a single 45 000 MW α chain encoded by one gene in one of three loci (HLA-A, -B and -C) on chromosome 6 (Bjorkman *et al.*, 1987; Dupont, 1989a, b). Two gene products of each class I locus are present on the cell surface, since molecules encoded by both parental chromosomes are expressed. $CD8^+$ T cells, which represent approximately 40% of peripheral T lymphocytes, are restricted in their function by class I molecules and are thought to recognize foreign peptides bound to self MHC class I antigens on target cells. As mentioned previously, CD8 binds an invariant region of the MHC class I molecule.

By serological detection with monoclonal antisera, the gene products of the HLA-A, -B and -C loci exhibit extensive sequence or polymorphism of the α chain; $β_2$-microglobulin is considered invariant. The α chain polymorphism can be attributed to the multiple alternative gene forms or alleles present in the human genome for the α chain of each class I locus. Currently, approximately twenty three HLA-A alleles, at least forty seven HLA-B alleles and ten HLA-C alleles have been detected serologically (Dupont, 1989a, b).

Differences in the amino acid sequences of MHC class I proteins are recognized by CD8$^+$ T lymphocytes and are the primary stimulus for vigorous graft rejection and the in vitro cell-mediated lympholysis reaction (CML), as well as partially responsible for alloantibody production and graft versus host disease (Sondel *et al.*, 1975; Mason *et al.*, 1984; Mason, 1986; Forman, 1987). The recognition of non-self or allogeneic class I MHC molecules is thought to be mediated by the identical pool of cytotoxic T cells that recognizes foreign peptides bound to self MHC class I molecules (Sondel *et al.*, 1975; Mason, 1986; Allison & Lanier, 1987). This phenomenon of 'alloreactivity' is not well understood, since, theoretically, a CD8$^+$ T cell would not bind a non-self MHC molecule. Current models for the recognition of foreign MHC class I molecules suggest that alloreactive CD8$^+$ T cells could recognize either a peptide–non-self MHC complex or non-self MHC determinants alone without bound peptide (Matzinger & Bevan, 1977; Bevan, 1984; Mason, 1986; Townsend & Bodmer, 1989). Since the TCR–CD3 complex can bind a variety of peptides with different affinities, it has been proposed that alloreactive cytotoxic T lympho-cytes recognize non-self MHC class I antigens as possibly a foreign peptide–self MHC complex. Currently, alloreactivity and graft rejec-tion are poorly understood and much work needs to be done in these areas.

Class II molecules. MHC class II molecules are encoded by the HLA DR, DQ and DP loci located on chromosome 6. Structurally, each of these class II molecules are dimers of one approximately 25 000–33 000 MW α chain and an approximately 24 000–29 000 MW β chain, which are non-covalently associated (Dupont, 1989*a*, *b*). The HLA DR α chain is encoded by one gene; in contrast, HLA DQ and DP α chains are encoded by one of two possible genes in each locus. The HLA DR β chain is encoded by one of several possible genes in the DR locus; the DQ and DP β chains are each encoded by one of two genes in both the DQ and DP loci (Dupont, 1989*a*, *b*). Each parental chromosome encodes an HLA DR, DQ and DP gene product and both parental products are expressed on the cell surface. These proteins are expressed primarily on APC, cells of the B-cell lineage and some activated T lymphocytes. As stated previously, CD4$^+$ T cells, which are primarily, but not exclusively, helper T cells, recognize and are activated by foreign peptides bound to MHC class II molecules. CD4 binds a non-polymorphic region of the MHC class II molecule, dictating that only CD4$^+$ cells are involved in recognition of antigens in association with class II molecules (Meuer *et al.*, 1982; Swain, 1983; Blue *et al.*, 1985; Ashwell *et al.*, 1986).

Extensive polymorphism is found in all MHC class II molecules and, in particular, in HLA DR antigens. HLA DR molecules have marked

Table 4.2. *Recognized HLA specificities*

A		B	C	D	DR	DQ	DP
A1	B5	B51(5)	Cw1	Dw1	DR1	DQw1	DPw1
A2	B7	Bw52(5)	Cw2	Dw2	DR2	DQw2	DPw2
A3	B8	Bw53	Cw3	Dw3	DR3	DQw3	DPw3
A9	B12	Bw54(w22)	Cw4	Dw4	DR4	DQw4	DPw4
A10	B13	Bw55(w22)	Cw5	Dw5	DR5	DQw5(w1)	DPw5
A11	B14	Bw56(w22)	Cw6	Dw6	DRw6	DQw6(w1)	DPw6
Aw19	B15	Bw57(17)	Cw7	Dw7	DR7	DQw7(w3)	
A23(9)	B16	Bw58(17)	Cw8	Dw8	DRw8	DQw8(w3)	
A24(9)	B17	Bw59	Cw9(w3)	Dw9	DR9	DQw9(w3)	
A25(10)	B18	Bw60(40)	Cw10(w3)	Dw10	DRw10		
A26(10)	B21	Bw61(40)	Cw11	Dw11(w7)	DRw11(5)		
A28	Bw22	Bw62(15)		Dw12	DRw12(5)		
A29(w19)	B27	Bw63(15)		Dw13	DRw13(w6)		
A30(w19)	B35	Bw64(14)		Dw14	DRw14(w6)		
A31(w19)	B37	Bw65(14)		Dw15	DRw15(2)		
A32(w19)	B38(16)	Bw67		Dw16	DRw16(2)		
Aw33(w19)	B39(16)	Bw71(w70)		Dw17(w7)	DRw17(3)		
Aw34(10)	B40	Bw70		Dw18(w6)	DRw18(3)		
Aw36	Bw41	Bw72(w70)		Dw19(w6)			
Aw43	Bw42	Bw73		Dw20	DRw52[a]		
Aw66(10)	B44(12)	Bw75(15)		Dw21	DRw53[a]		
Aw68(28)	B45(12)	Bw76(15)		Dw22			
Aw69(28)	Bw46	Bw77(15)		Dw23			
Aw74(w19)				Dw24			
	Bw48	Bw4[a]		Dw25			
	B49(21)	Bw6[a]		Dw26			
	Bw50(21)						

Notes:
Numbers in parentheses indicate the common HLA antigen from which the designated antigens are split.
[a] Bw4, Bw6, DRw52, and DRw53 are 'public' antigens i.e. they are determinants that are common to several HLA molecules each of which expresses a distinct HLA 'private' antigen.
Source: Dupont (1989a,b).

variability in the amino acid sequences of the β chain; in contrast, the DR α chain is encoded by one gene and is invariant. Consequently, the HLA DR polymorphism is due to the numbers and multiple possible allelic forms of the β chain genes. Each HLA DR β chain is coded by an allelic form of one β gene; all haplotypes express an HLA DR molecule with an HLA DR β_1 gene product, which is referred to as the private specificity by serological detection. Presently, approximately eighteen HLA DR private specificities have been detected, designated HLA DR1–18 (Dupont, 1989a, b; Table 4.2). However, depending on the HLA DR private specificity expressed, a second HLA DR molecule with a β chain encoded by one of several other available β genes may also be found on the cell surface (Dupont, 1989a, b). For example, cells expressing HLA DR3 additionally express HLA DRw52, which has a β chain encoded by the HLA DR β_3 gene. In contrast, HLA DR4$^+$ cells also express HLA DR53, with a β chain encoded by the β_2 gene.

Two α and two β genes are encoded within the HLA DQ loci; however, only one gene product is expressed, that of DQ α_1 and DQ β_1. Limited polymorphism exists in both the DQ α and β chains, with about nine allelic forms able to be detected by monoclonal antisera at the present time. Similarly, two HLA DP α and two HLA DP β genes exist, but only one gene product of limited polymorphism is expressed on the cell surface. In summary, cells expressing MHC class II antigens have one or two detectable HLA DR molecules, one HLA DQ molecule and one HLA DP molecule encoded by each parental chromosome, the products of which are found on the cell membranes of diploid cells (Dupont, 1989a, b).

CD4$^+$ T lymphocytes have been characterized that can recognize the polymorphic sequences of each type of class II molecule. Alloreactive CD4$^+$ T cells respond vigorously to MHC class II differences, and are primarily involved in graft versus host disease, but can also participate in transplant rejection (Mason $et\ al.$, 1984; Mason, 1986; Ashwell $et\ al.$, 1986; Wheelahan & McKenzie, 1987; Toribio $et\ al.$, 1988; Fowlkes & Pardoll, 1989).

Historically, the in vitro mixed leukocyte culture (MLC) was felt to assay peripheral blood lymphocyte stimulation to MHC class II differences and, therefore, primarily reflect proliferation of CD4$^+$ cells (Chan $et\ al.$, 1974; Reinherz & Schlossman, 1980; Fowlkes & Pardoll, 1989). However, it is now known that CD8$^+$ T cells can also proliferate in MLC to MHC class I differences (Hayry & Defendi, 1970). Comparable to alloreactive CD8$^+$ T cells, it has been hypothesized that alloreactive CD4$^+$ T cells may be 'fooled' into recognizing a foreign peptide bound to a non-self MHC class II molecule as a variant of foreign peptide bound to a self MHC class II molecule (Hunig & Bevan, 1981, Bevan, 1984). Currently, evidence is lacking to support this or other models (Matzinger & Bevan, 1977; Bevan, 1984; Mason, 1986), especially in the field of human transplantation.

T-cell ontogeny

$Thymic\ development.$ The thymus is derived from three primitive germ layers: the thymic cortical epithelium is formed from the endoderm of the third pharyngeal pouch; the thymic medullary epithelium is derived from the ectoderm of the third branchial cleft; and mesenchymal

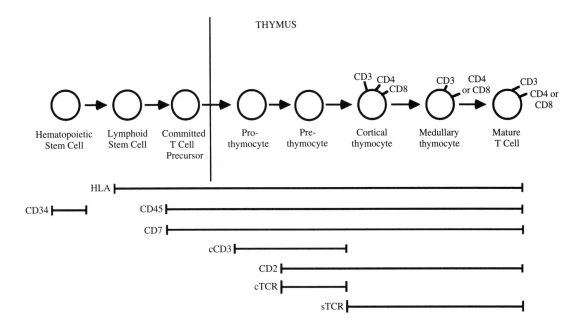

THYMUS

Figure 4.4. Development of T-cell immune system. HLA, human leukocyte antigens; CD, cluster of differentiation antigens; c, cytoplasmic; s, surface; TCR, T-cell receptor (Haynes *et al.*, 1989).

elements contribute to the formation of the fibrous capsule, stroma and vessels (Hayward, 1981; Haynes *et al.*, 1984). Lymphoid cells begin to populate the thymus between the eighth and ninth weeks of gestation and are induced to begin differentiation into T cells. Thymic differentiation is required for the development of mature, immuno-competent T cells. The organization of the thymus is completed by ten to twelve weeks of gestation, at which time a well-demarcated cortex and medulla populated by T-lineage cells in various stages of differentiation is seen (Prindull, 1974; Hayward, 1981). The development of monoclonal antisera that react with subpopulations of thymocytes has led to better understanding of intrathymic differentia-tion and the development of immunocompetence (Figure 4.4).

Committed T-cell precursors. Lymphoid precursors entering the thymus express the cell surface markers T9 (or CD71) and probably CD38, formerly designated T10 (Reinherz & Schlossman, 1980; Rosenthal *et al.*, 1983). These two molecules are not T-cell specific, being found on immature, dividing cells of various lineages and are not thought to have important functions in the maturation of T cells. In addition, these precursor cells may express the surface molecules CD45 and CD7.

CD7 is felt to be involved in early T-cell development and is expressed on some multipotent stem-cell and TdT[+] acute myelogenous leukemia cells, but is otherwise specific for the T-cell lineage (Haynes *et al.*, 1989). CD45, which was previously described in the section on B cells, is a protein tyrosine phosphatase with several isoforms that is felt to be important for T-cell development and signalling of antigen-binding events (Clark & Ledbetter, 1989; Pilarski & Deans, 1989). These lymphoid precursors, which are referred to as early pro-thymocytes by some authors, also express MHC class I molecules (designated here as HLA-A$^+$) and are located primarily in the thymic subcapsular cortex (Prindull, 1974; Rosenthal *et al.*, 1983).

Pro-thymocytes. Cytoplasmic CD3 (cCD3) expression is the earliest recognizable event in thymic differentiation (Rosenthal *et al.*, 1983; Furley *et al.*, 1986; Toribio *et al.*, 1988; Campana *et al.*, 1989; Haynes *et al.*, 1989). Once entry into the thymic cortex has occurred, pro-thymocytes with detectable cCD3 may be seen by immunofluores-cence. Pro-thymocytes are otherwise distinguished by non-rearrange-ment of their TCR genes. Pro-thymocytes arise from the rapidly dividing CD7$^+$ CD45$^+$ precursor population and are detected by $8\frac{1}{2}$ weeks of gestation. Cytoplasmic and then surface expression of CD2 occurs shortly thereafter (Rosenthal *et al.*, 1983; Haynes *et al.*, 1989). CD2, formerly called T11, is the sheep erythrocyte receptor, and its expression is critical for T-cell differentiation (Reinherz, 1985; Haynes *et al.*, 1988; Kabelitz, 1990). CD5, which is also found on some B cells, is first expressed at the pro-thymocyte stage and has no defined function in T cells.

In summary, mature pro-thymocytes are HLA-A$^+$ CD7$^+$ CD45$^+$ CD2$^+$ CD5$^+$ cells and constitute approximately 10% of lymphoid cells in the thymus (Reinherz, 1985; Haynes *et al.*, 1988, 1989).

Pre-thymocytes. The next stage of T-cell precursor differentiation is that of the pre-thymocyte, which can be distinguished by the onset of TCR gene rearrangement events, but without cell surface expression of TCR. At $9\frac{1}{2}$ weeks' gestation, cytoplasmic TCR β chains (cTCR-β) and TCR γ chains (cTCR-γ) can be detected in distinct cells, suggesting that the divergence of TCR-$\alpha\beta$ and TCR-$\gamma\delta$ lymphocyte pools from a common T-cell precursor occurs at this time (Haynes *et al.*, 1988, 1989; Toribio *et al.*, 1988; Campana *et al.*, 1989). Receptors for IL-2 (IL-2R), a lymphokine with potent T-cell growth properties, are also expressed initially by pre-thymocytes (Toribio *et al.*, 1988).

Pre-thymocytes are thus designated HLA-A$^+$ CD7$^+$ CD45$^+$ CD2$^+$ CD5$^+$ IL-2R$^+$ cCD3$^+$ cTCR-β^+ or HLA-A$^+$ CD7$^+$ CD45$^+$ CD2$^+$ CD5$^+$ IL-2R$^+$ cCD3$^+$ cTCRγ^+ cells and have been referred to as 'double-negative cells', due to the absence of cell-membrane-bound CD4 and CD8 (Toribio *et al.*, 1988; Campana *et al.*, 1989; Haynes *et al.*, 1989). Pre-thymocytes constitute approximately 5% of the thymic lymphoid population and are also found in the thymic cortex.

Cortical thymocytes. Cortical thymocytes are the first T-cell precursors to express TCR and, thus, to be exposed to antigenic stimulation. TCR β chain synthesis initially occurs at $9\frac{1}{2}$ to 10 weeks' gestation, resulting in low level surface expression of TCR-$\alpha\beta$ at that time (Haynes *et al.*, 1988, 1989; Campana *et al.*, 1989). Synthesis of TCR δ chains is also seen and TCR-$\gamma\delta$ can be detected on the cell membrane between $9\frac{1}{2}$ and $10\frac{1}{2}$ weeks of gestation (Campana *et al.*, 1989; Haynes *et al.*, 1989). The expression of CD4, CD8 and CD1 is seen at this time as well.

As detailed in earlier sections, CD4 and CD8 are accessory molecules expressed on T cells that are involved in MHC restriction of function. CD1, formerly known as T6, is found primarily on cortical thymocytes (Reinherz & Schlossman, 1980; Rosenthal *et al.*, 1983). Most cortical thymocytes are thus HLA-A$^+$ CD7$^+$ CD45$^+$ CD2$^+$ CD5$^+$ IL-2R$^+$ CD3$^+$ TCR-$\alpha\beta^+$ CD4$^+$ CD8$^+$ CD1$^+$ or, rarely, HLA-A$^+$ CD7$^+$ CD45$^+$ CD2$^+$ CD5$^+$ IL-2$^+$ CD3$^+$ TCR$\gamma\delta^+$ CD1$^+$. The TCR-$\alpha\beta^+$ cells are referred to as 'double positive' lymphocytes, since both CD4 and CD8 expression are seen (Toribio *et al.*, 1988; Campana *et al.*, 1989). CD4 and CD8 molecules are not found on most γ/δ T cells (Lanier & Weiss, 1986; Denning *et al.*, 1989; Fowlkes & Pardoll, 1989; Reis *et al.*, 1989). Double positive thymocytes are immunoincompetent and comprise approximately 80% of thymic lymphoid cells.

However, the vast majority of these immature thymocytes are not destined to differentiate further and instead are destroyed in the processes of 'positive' and 'negative selection' (Sha *et al.*, 1988; Teh *et al.*, 1988; Fowlkes & Pardoll, 1989). Current models favor that, during these processes, TCR-$\alpha\beta^+$ thymocytes are selected to survive if they possess a certain affinity for self MHC molecules. It is thought that the thymus selects T-cell precursors that recognize foreign peptides bound to self MHC class I or class II molecules. During 'positive selection', only α/β double-positive thymocytes that can bind either a self MHC class I or class II molecule expressed on the cortical thymic epithelium will be allowed to survive (Sha *et al.*, 1988; von Boehmer *et al.*, 1988; Fowlkes & Pardoll, 1989). Subsequently, these α/β double-positive cells lose expression of either the CD4 or CD8 molecule (theoretically, the molecule not able to bind a self MHC antigen) and emigrate to the thymic medulla. 'Negative selection' is thought to be mediated in the thymic medulla by dendritic cells and macrophages, but may occur in the thymic cortex and precede positive selection (Kappler *et al.*, 1987; Fowlkes & Pardoll, 1989).

In the highly theoretical process of 'negative selection', single-positive thymocytes expressing high affinity TCR-$\alpha\beta$ for self MHC molecules or other self antigens which may be autoreactive in the periphery undergo cell death. Only those thymocytes having a certain range of affinities for self MHC molecules bound to foreign peptides are allowed to exit the thymus as mature T cells. However, this model is one of several possibilities and has not been proven.

Medullary thymocytes. These mature thymocytes can be distinguished by the expression of either CD4 or CD8 molecules, but not both, and are referred to as 'single-positive' cells. Medullary thymocytes comprise about 10% of the thymic population of lymphoid cells.

Peripheral T cells. TCR-$\alpha\beta^+$ CD8$^+$ and CD4$^+$ T cells existing in the thymic medulla are immunocompetent and are able to recognize an antigenic peptide bound to a self MHC class I molecule or class II molecule, respectively. Seeding of the spleen, fetal liver and peripheral blood with immunocompetent T cells can be detected initially at about fifteen weeks of gestation (Prindull, 1974; Asma *et al.*, 1977; Rosenthal *et al.*, 1983).

After exiting the thymus, T cells lose the expression of several differentiation molecules; most peripheral T lymphocytes are HLA-A$^+$ CD7$^+$ CD45$^+$ CD2$^+$ CD3$^+$ CD4$^+$ TCR-$\alpha\beta^+$ or HLA-A$^+$ CD7$^+$ CD45$^+$ CD2$^+$ CD3$^+$ CD8$^+$ TCR-$\alpha\beta^+$. These α/β T cells constitute approximately 98% of peripheral blood T cells and most T cells of peripheral lymphoid organs. TCR-$\gamma\delta^+$ cells include a small population of thymocytes, dendritic epithelial cells and some intestinal epithelial cells, whose function is unknown (Hayward, 1981; Janeway *et al.*, 1988; Fowlkes & Pardoll, 1989).

T-cell function

In vivo evidence of fetal T-cell immunocompetence is limited and relates primarily to the ability of helper T lymphocytes to secrete lymphokines essential for B-cell differentiation and antibody synthesis. As discussed for B-cell immunity, despite the presence of normal numbers of IgM$^+$, IgG$^+$ and IgA$^+$ B cells in the fetus by approximately fifteen weeks of gestation, functional plasma cells are rare in the non-infected fetus and normal levels of serum immunoglobulins are not obtained until well after birth (Buckley *et al.*, 1968). Furthermore, plasmacytosis and appreciable antibody production are not seen in fetuses exposed to antigenic stimulation through in utero infection until twenty weeks of gestation (Siverstein & Lukes, 1962). These results suggest that helper T cells may be functionally immature throughout fetal life (Barrett *et al.*, 1981; Hayward, 1981).

In vitro tests of T-cell function include proliferative responsiveness to mitogenic stimulation and to allogeneic MHC determinants in MLC and CML assays. Phytohemagglutinin (PHA) is a plant lectin that is mitogenic for T cells, resulting in cell proliferation that can be measured by uptake of tritiated-thymidine in culture. Multiple studies have demonstrated PHA stimulation of T-cell proliferation in ten to twelve week gestational thymocytes and initially in cultures of peripheral blood and splenic lymphocytes between thirteen and fifteen weeks of gestation (Kay et al., 1970; Papiernik, 1970; August et al., 1971; Carr et al., 1973; Stites et al., 1974, 1975; Mumford et al., 1978; Hayward, 1981; Toivanen et al., 1981). PHA reactivity of fetal lymphocytes increases to that of adult peripheral blood T cells by about eighteen weeks of gestation (Stites et al., 1975; Hayward, 1981). T-cell responsiveness to the mitogen concanavalin A (con A) is not seen until thirteen to fourteen weeks of gestation in the thymus and eighteen weeks of gestation in the spleen (Pirofsky et al., 1973; Mumford et al., 1978; Leino et al., 1980; Toivanen et al., 1981). Neither PHA nor con A responsiveness is appreciably detected in fetal liver or bone marrow cells until at least eighteen weeks of gestation (Pirofsky et al., 1973; Leino et al., 1980; Toivanen et al., 1981).

The ability of T cells to recognize foreign MHC determinants in MLCs is not seen in the thymus until approximately thirteen weeks of gestation and in the peripheral blood and spleen for an additional one to two weeks (Carr et al., 1973; Pirofsky et al., 1973; Stites et al., 1974). Interestingly, MLC responsiveness has been demonstrated in $7\frac{1}{2}$ weeks' gestational fetal liver cultures (Carr et al., 1973). However, these results are not easily interpreted, since thymic development and T-cell differentiation have not yet occurred. The ability of cytotoxic T cells to kill allogeneic target cells is not demonstrated in CML assays using thymocytes until fifteen to twenty-two weeks of gestation and is not comparable to that of adult peripheral blood lymphocytes until birth (Granberg & Hirvonen, 1980; Rayfield et al., 1980; Toivanen et al., 1981). Indeed, many T lymphocytes in the newborn still have CML reactivity of about half normal levels (Granberg & Hirvonen, 1980).

In summary, the earliest indication of true T-cell function *in utero* is the PHA responsiveness of thymocytes from ten-week-old fetuses which pre-dates con A and MLC responsiveness of thymocytes by two to five weeks and CML reactivity by an additional few weeks. As well, immunocompetence of peripheral T lymphocytes appears approximately two or more weeks after thymocyte function is detected *in vitro*.

Acknowledgments

M. E. and M. J. C. were supported in part by grants from the National Institutes of Health P01-AI29512 and AI07395, The March of Dimes Birth Defects Foundation (6-221), Bank of America–Giannini Fellowship, and Merck–AFCR MD-PhD Postdoctoral Fellowship Award.

References

ABE, J. (1989) Immunocytochemical characterization of lymphocyte development in human embryonic and fetal livers. *Clinical Immunology & Immunopathology*, **51**, 13–21.

ACUTO, O. & REINHERZ, E. L. (1985) The human T-cell receptor. *New England Journal of Medicine*, **312**, 1100–11.

ADKINS, B., MUELLER, C., OKADA, C. Y., REICHERT, R. A., WEISSMAN, I. L. & SPRANGRUDE, G. L. (1987) Early events in T-cell maturation. *Annual Review of Immunology*, **5**, 325–65.

ALLEN, P. M., STRYDOM, D. J. & UNANUE, E. R. (1984) Processing of lysozyme by macrophages: Identification of the determinant recognized by two T cell hybridomas. *Proceedings of the National Academy of Sciences, USA*, **81**, 2489–93.

ALLISON, J. P. & LANIER, L. (1987) Structure, function, and serology of the T-cell antigen receptor complex. *Annual Review of Immunology*, **5**, 503–40.

ANTIN, J. H., EMERSON, S. G., MARTIN, P., GADOL, N. & ALT, K. A. (1986) Leu-1$^+$(CD5$^+$) B cells. A major lymphoid subpopulation in human fetal spleen: phenotypic and functional studies. *Journal of Immunology*, **136**, 505–10.

ASHWELL, J. D., CHEN, C. & SCHWARTZ, R. H. (1986) High frequency and nonrandom distributions of alloreactivity in T cell clones selected for recognition of foreign antigen in association with self class II molecules. *Journal of Immunology*, **136**, 389–95.

ASMA, G. E. M., PICHLER, W., SCHUIT, H. R. E., KNAPP, W. & HIJMANS, W. (1977) The development of lymphocytes with T- or B-membrane determinants in the human foetus. *Clinical & Experimental Immunology*, **29**, 278–85.

AUGUST, C. A., BERKEL, I., DRISCOLL, S. & MERLER, E. (1971) Onset of lymphocyte function in the developing human fetus. *Pediatric Research*, **5**, 539–47.

BALTIMORE, D. (1974) Is terminal deoxynucleotide transferase a somatic mutagen in lymphocytes. *Nature*, **248**, 409–11.

BANK, I., DePINHO, R. A., BRENNER, M. B., CASSIMERIS, J., ALT, F. W. & CHESS, L. (1986) A functional T3 molecule associated with a novel heterodimer on the surface of immature human thymocytes. *Nature*, **322**, 179–81.

BARRETT, D. J., STENMARK, S., WARA, D. W. & AMMANN, A. J. (1981) Helper cell function of human fetal thymocytes. *Cellular Immunology*, **59**, 17–25.

BEVAN, M. J. (1984) High determinant density may explain the phenomenon of alloreactivity. *Immunology Today*, **5**, 128–30.

BJORKMAN, P. J., SAPER, M. A., SAMRAOUI, B., BENNETT, W. S.,

STROMINGER, J. L. & WILEY, D. C. (1987) Structure of the human class I histocompatibility antigen, HLA-A2. *Nature*, **329**, 506–12.

BLUE, M. C., CRAIG, K. A., ANDERSON, P., BRANTON, K. R. & SCHLOSSMAN, S. F. (1988) Evidence for specific association between class I major histocompatibility antigens and the CD8 molecules of human suppressor/cytotoxic cells. *Cell*, **54**, 413–21.

BLUE, M. L., DALEY, J. F., LEVINE, H. & SCHLOSSMAN, S. F. (1985) Class II major histocompatibility complex molecules regulate the development of the T4$^+$T8$^-$ inducer phenotype of cultured human thymocytes. *Proceeding of the National Academy of Sciences, USA*, **82**, 8178–82.

BORST, J., ALEXANDER, S., ELDER, J. & TERHORST, C. (1983) The T3 complex on human T lymphocytes involves four structurally distinct glycoproteins. *Journal of Biological Chemistry*, **258**, 5135–41.

BRENNER, M. B., McLEAN, J., DIALYNAS, D. P., STROMINGER, J. L., SMITH, J. A., OWEN, F. L., SEIDMAN, J. G., IP, S., ROSE, F. & KRANGEL, M. S. (1986) Identification of a putative second T-cell receptor. *Nature*, **322**, 145–9.

BUCKLEY, R. H., DEES, S. C. & O'FALLON, W. M. (1968) Serum immunoglobulins: I. Levels in normal children and uncomplicated childhood allergy. *Pediatrics*, **41**, 600–11.

BURTON, D. R. (1985) Immunoglobulin G: Functional sites. *Molecular Immunology*, **22**, 161–206.

CAMPANA, D., JANOSSY, G., COUSTAN-SMITH, E., AMLOT, P. L., TIAN, W-T., IP, S. & WONG, L. (1989) The expression of T cell receptor-associated proteins during T cell ontogeny in man. *Journal of Immunology*, **142**, 57–66.

CAPRA, J. D. & KEHOE, J. M. (1975) Hypervariable regions, idiotypy and the antigen combining site. *Advances in Immunology*, **20**, 1–40.

CARR, M. C., STITES, D. P. & FUDENBERG, H. H. (1973) Dissociation of responses to phytohemagglutinin and adult allogeneic lymphocytes in human foetal lymphoid tissues. *Nature*, **24**, 279–81.

CEDERQUIST, L. L. & LITWIN, S. D. (1974) Production of α-1 and α-2 immunoglobulin heavy chains during fetal life. *Journal of Immunology*, **112**, 1605–8.

CHAN, A. & MAK, T. W. (1989) Genomic organization of the T cell receptor. *Cancer Detection Prevention*, **14**, 261–5.

CHAN, L., MacDERMOT, R. P. & SCHLOSSMAN, S. F. (1974) Immunologic functions of isolated human lymphocyte subpopulations. II. Antigen triggering of T and B cells *in vitro*. *Journal of Immunology*, **113**, 1122–7.

CLARK, E. A. & LEDBETTER, J. A. (1989) Leukocyte cell surface enzymology: CD45 (LCA,T200) is a protein tyrosine phosphatase. *Immunology Today*, **10**, 225–8.

COOPER, M. D. & BURROWS, P. D. (1989) B-cell differentiation. In: *Immunoglobulin Genes*, pp. 1–21. Eds. T. Honjo, F. W. Alt & T. H. Rabbitts. Academic Press, New York.

DAVIE, J. M. (1985) Antipolysaccharide immunity in man and animals. In: *Hemophilus Influenzae: Epidemiology, Immunology, and Prevention of Diseases*, pp. 129–34. Eds. S. H. Sell & P. F. Wright. Elsevier Biomedical, New York.

DENNING, S. A., KURTZBERG, J., LESLIE, D. S. & HAYNES, B. F.

(1989) Human postnatal CD4⁻ CD8⁻ CD3⁻ thymic T cell precursors differentiate *in vitro* into T cell receptor bearing cells. *Journal of Immunology*, **142**, 2988–97.

DOYLE, C. & STROMINGER, J. L. (1987) Interaction between CD4 and class II MHC molecules mediates cell adhesion. *Nature*, **330**, 256–9.

DUPONT, B., Ed. (1989*a*) Histocompatibility testing. In: *Immunobiology of HLA*, vol. 1, Springer-Verlag, New York.

DUPONT, B., Ed. (1989*b*) Immunogenetics and Histocompatibility. In: *Immunobiology of HLA*, vol. 2, Springer-Verlag, New York.

EDELMAN, G. M. & GALL, W. E. (1969) The antibody problem. *Annual Review of Biochemistry*, **38**, 415–66.

FLEISCHER, B. & WAGNER, H. (1986) Significance of T4 or T8 phenotype of human cytotoxic T-lymphocyte clones. *Current Topics in Microbiology & Immunology*, **126**, 101–9.

FORMAN, J. (1987) Determinants on major histocompatibility complex class I molecules recognized by cytotoxic T lymphocytes. *Advances in Immunology*, **41**, 135–79.

FOWLKES, B. J. & PARDOLL, D. M. (1989) Molecular and cellular events of T cell development. *Advances in Immunology*, **44**, 207–62.

FURLEY, A. J., MIZUTANI, S., WEILBAECHER, K., DHALIVAL, H. S., FORD, A. M., CHAN, L. C., MOLGAARD, H. V., TOYONAGA, B., MAK, T., VAN DER ELSEN, P., GOLD, D., TERHOST, C. & GREAVES, M. F. (1986) Developmentally regulated rearrangement and expression of genes encoding the T cell receptor–T3 complex. *Cell*, **46**, 75–87.

GADOL, N. & ALT, K. A. (1986) Phenotypic and functional characterization of human Leu1 (CD5) B cells. *Immunological Reviews*, **93**, 23–34.

GATHINGS, W. E., LAWTON, A. R. & COOPER, M. D. (1977) Immuno-fluorescent studies of the development of pre-B cells, B lymphocytes and immunoglobulin isotype diversity in humans. *European Journal of Immunology*, **7**, 804–10.

GITLIN, D. & BIASUCCI, A. (1969) Development of γG, γA, γM, B$_{ic}$/B$_{ia}$, C′I esterase inhibitor, caeruloplasmin, transferin, hemopexin, haptoglobin, fibrinogen, plasminogen, antitrypsin, orosomucoid, B lipoprotein, α2 macroglobin and pre-albumin in the human conceptus. *Journal of Clinical Investigation*, **48**, 1433–46.

GOLDMAN, A. S. & GOLDMAN, R. M. (1977) Primary immunodeficiencies in humoral immunity. *Pediatric Clinics of North America*, **24**, 277–91.

GRANBERG, C. & HIRVONEN, T. (1980) Cell-mediated lympholysis by fetal and neonatal lymphocytes in sheep and man. *Cellular Immunology*, **51**, 13–22.

HARDY, R. R. & HAYAKAWA, K. (1986) Development and physiology of LY-1 B and its human homolog, Leu-1B. *Immunological Reviews*, **93**, 53–79.

HAYNES, B. F., SCEARCE, R. M., LOBACH, D. F. & HENSLEY, L. C. (1984) Phenotypic characteristics and ontogeny of mesodermal-derived and endocrine epithelial components of the human thymic microenvironment. *Journal of Experimental Medicine*, **159**, 1149–68.

HAYNES, B. F., SINGER, K. H., DENNING, S. M. & MARTIN, M. E., (1988) Analysis of expression of CD2, CD3, and T cell antigen receptor molecules during early human fetal thymic development. *Journal of Immunology*, **141**, 3776–84.

HAYNES, B. F., DENNING, S. M., SINGER, K. H. & KURTZBERG, J.

(1989) Ontogeny of T-cell precursors. A model for the initial stages of human T-cell development. *Immunology Today*, **10**, 87–91.

HAYRY, P. & DEFENDI, V. (1970) Mixed lymphocyte cultures produce effector cells. Model *in vitro* for allograft rejection. *Science*, **168**, 133–5.

HAYWARD, A. R. (1981) Development of lymphocyte responses and interactions in the human fetus and newborn. *Immunological Reviews*, **57**, 39–60.

HIETER, P. A., HOLLIS, G. F., KORSEMEYER, S. J., WALDMAN, T. A. & LEDER, P. (1981) Clustered arrangement of immunoglobulin constant region genes in man. *Nature*, **294**, 536–40.

HILSCHMANN, N. & CRAIG, L. C. (1965) Amino acid sequence studies with Bence–Jones proteins. *Proceedings of the National Academy of Sciences, USA*, **53**, 1403–9.

HOKLAND, P., RITZ, J., SCHLOSSMAN, S. F. & NADLER, L. M. (1985) Orderly expression of B cell antigens during the in vitro differentiation of nonmalignant human pre-B cells. *Journal of Immunology*, **135**, 1746–51.

HONJO, T., SHIMIZU, A. & YAOITA, Y. (1989) Constant region genes of the immunoglobulin heavy chain and the molecular mechanisms of class switching. In: *Immunoglobulin Genes*, pp. 123–49. Eds. T. Honjo, F. W. Alt & T. H. Rabbitts. Academic Press, New York.

HUNIG, T. & BEVAN, M. J. (1981) Specificity of T-cell clones illustrates altered self hypothesis. *Nature*, **294**, 460–2.

ISHIZAKA, T. & ISHIZAKA, K. (1975) Biology of immunoglobulin E. Molecular basis of reaginic hypersensitivity. *Progress in Allergy*, **19**, 60–121.

JANEWAY, C. A., JONES, B. & HAYDAY, A. (1988) Specificity and function of T cells bearing γδ receptors. *Immunology Today*, **9**, 73–6.

JANOSSY, G., BOLLUM, F. J., BRADSTOCK, K. F., McMICHAEL, A., RAPSON, N. & GREAVES, M. F. (1979) Terminal transferase-positive human bone marrow cells exhibit the antigenic phenotype of common acute lymphoblastic leukemia. *Journal of Immunology*, **123**, 1525–9.

JELINEK, J. E. & LIPSKY, P. E. (1987) Regulation of human B lymphocyte activation, proliferation and differentiation. *Advances in Immunology*, **40**, 1–59.

KABELITZ, D. (1990) Do CD2 and CD3-TCR T-cell activation pathways function independently? *Immunology Today*, **11**, 44–7.

KAPPLER, J. W., ROEHM, N. & MARRACK, P. (1987) T cell tolerance by clonal elimination in the thymus. *Cell*, **49**, 273–280.

KAY, H. E. M., DOE, J. & HOCKLEY, A. (1970) Response of human foetal thymocytes to phytohaemagglutinin (PHA). *Immunology*, **18**, 393–6.

KINCADE, P. W. & PHILLIPS, R. A. (1985) B lymphocyte development. *Federation Proceedings*, **44**, 2874–80.

KODAIRA, M., KINASHI, T., UMEMURA, I., MATSUDA, F., NOMA, T., ONO, Y. & HONJO, T. (1986) Organization and evolution of variable region genes of the human immunoglobulin heavy chain. *Journal of Molecular Biology*, **190**, 529–41.

KORSMEYER, S. J., HEITER, P. A., SHARROW, S. O., GOLDMAN, C. K., LEDER, P. & WALDMANN, T. A. (1982) Normal human B cells display ordered light chain rearrangements and deletions. *Journal of Experimental Medicine*, **156**, 975–85.

KRONENBERG, M., SIU, G., HOOD, L. E. & SHASTRI, N. (1986) The molecular genetics of the T-cell antigen receptor and T-cell antigen recognition. *Annual Review of Immunology*, **4**, 529–91.

LANDRETH, K. S., KINCADE, P. W., LEE, G., GATHINGS, W. E. & FU, S. M. (1982) Enrichment of human marrow lymphocytes with monoclonal antibodies to murine antigens. *Proceedings of the National Academy of Sciences*, USA, **79**, 2370–4.

LANIER, L. L & WEISS, A. (1986) Presence of Ti (WT31) negative T lymphocytes in normal blood and thymus. *Nature*, **324**, 268–70.

LAWTON, A. R., SELF, S., ROYAL, J. A. & COOPER, M. D. (1972) Ontogeny of B lymphocytes in the human fetus. *Clinical Immunology & Immunopathology*, **1**, 84–93.

LeFRANC, M. P. (1988) The human T-cell rearranging gamma (TRG) genes and the gamma T-cell receptor. *Biochimie*, **70**, 901–8.

LEINO, A., HIRVONEN, T. & SOPPI, E. (1980) Ontogeny of phytohemagglutinin and concanavalin A responses in the human fetus: Effect of thymosin. *Clinical Immunology & Immunopathology*, **17**, 547–55.

MASON, D. W. (1986) Effector mechanisms in allograft rejection. *Annual Review of Immunology*, **4**, 119–45.

MASON, D. W., DALLMAN, M. J., ARTHUR, R. P. & MORRIS, P. J. (1984) Mechanisms of allograft rejection: The roles of cytotoxic T-cells and delayed-type hypersensitivity. *Immunological Reviews*, **77**, 167–84.

MATZINGER, P. & BEVAN, M. J. (1977) Why do so many lymphocytes respond to major histocompatibility antigens? *Cellular Immunology*, **29**, 1–5.

MEUER, S. C., ACUTO, O., HUSSEY, R. E., HODGDON, J.C., FITZGERALD, K. A., SCHLOSSMAN, S. F. & REINHERZ, E. L. (1983) Evidence for the T3-associated 90K heterodimer as the T-cell antigen receptor. *Nature*, **303**, 808–10.

MEUER, S. C., SCHLOSSMAN, S. F. & REINHERZ, E. L. (1982) Clonal analysis of human cytotoxic T lymphocytes: T4$^+$ and T8$^+$ effector T cells recognize products of different major histocompatibility regions. *Proceedings of the National Academy of Sciences, USA*, **79**, 4395–9.

MILER, I. (1983) The immunity of the human foetus and newborn infant. In: *Developments in Perinatal Medicine*, vol. 3, pp.12–59, Martinus Nijhoff Publishers, The Hague.

MORIMOTO, C., LETVIN, N. L., BOYD, A. W., HAGAN, M., BROWN, H. M., KORNACKI, M. & SCHLOSSMAN, S. F. (1985a) The isolation and characterization of the human helper inducer T cell subset. *Journal of Immunology*, **134**, 3762–9.

MORIMOTO, C., LETVIN, N. L., DISTASO, J. A., ALDRICH, W. R. & SCHLOSSMAN, S. F. (1985b) The isolation and characterization of the human suppressor inducer T cell subset. *Journal of Immunology*, **134**, 1508–15.

MUMFORD, D. M., SUNG, J. S., WALLIS, J. O. & KAUFMAN, R. H. (1978) The lymphocyte transformation response of fetal hemolymphatic tissue to mitogens and antigens. *Pediatric Research*, **12**, 171–5.

NATVIG, J. B. & KUNKEL, H. G. (1973) Human immunoglobulins: Classes, subclasses, genetic variants, and idiotypes. *Advances in Immunology*, **161**, 1–59.

NISONOFF, A., HOPPER, J. E. & SPRING, S. G. (1975) *The Antibody Molecule*. Academic Press, New York.

NORMENT, A., SALTER, R. D., PARHAM, P., ENGELHARD, V. H. &

LITTMAN, D. R. (1988) Cell–cell adhesion mediated by CD8 and MHC class I molecules. *Nature*, **336**, 79–81.

NOSSAL, G. J. V. (1983) Cellular mechanisms of immunologic tolerance. *Annual Review of Immunology*, **1**, 33–62.

OWEN, J. J. T. (1977) Ontogenesis of lymphocytes. In: *B and T Cells in Immune Recognition*, pp. 21–34. Eds. F. Loor & G. E. Roelants. John Wiley & Sons.

PAPIERNIK, M. (1970) Correlation of lymphocyte transformation and morphology in the human fetal thymus. *Blood*, **36**, 470–8.

PILARSKI, L. M. & DEANS, J. P. (1989) Selective expression of CD45 isoforms and of maturation antigens during human thymocyte differentiation: observations and hypothesis. *Immunological Letters*, **21**, 187–98.

PIROFSKY, B., DAVIES, G. H., RAMIREZ-MATEOS, J. C. & NEWTON, B. W. (1973) Cellular immune competence in the human fetus. *Cellular Immunology*, **6**, 324–8.

PRINDULL, G. (1974) Maturation of cellular and humoral immunity during human embryonic development. *Acta Paediatrica Scandinavica*, **63**, 607–15.

RATHBURN, G., BERMANN, J. F., YANCOPOULOS, G. & ALT, F. W. (1989) Organization and expression of the mammalian heavy-chain variable-region locus. In: *Immunoglobulin Genes*, pp. 76–90. Eds. T. Honjo, F. W. Alt & T. H. Rabbitts. Academic Press, New York.

RAULET, D. H. (1989) The structure, function, and molecular genetics of the γ/δ T cell receptor. *Annual Review of Immunology*, **7**, 175–207.

RAVETCH, J. V., SIEBENLIST, U., KORSEMEYER, S., WALDMAN, T. & LEDER, P. (1981) Structure of the human immunoglobulin μ locus: Characterization of embryonic and rearranged J and D genes. *Cell*, **27**, 583–91.

RAYFIELD, L. S., BRENT, L. & RODECK, C. H. (1980) Development of cell-mediated lympholysis in human foetal blood lymphocytes. *Clinical & Experimental Immunology*, **42**, 561–70.

REINHERZ, E. L. (1985) A molecular basis for thymic selection: Recognition of T11 induced thymocyte expansion by the T3-Ti antigen/MHC receptor pathway. *Immunology Today*, **6**, 75–9.

REINHERZ, E. L., MEUER, S.C. & SCHLOSSMAN, S. F. (1983) The delineation of antigen receptors on human T lymphocytes. *Immunology Today*, **4**, 5–8.

REINHERZ, E. & SCHLOSSMAN, S. F. (1980) The differentiation and function of human T lymphocytes. *Cell*, **19**, 821–7.

REIS, M. D., GRIESSER, H. & MAK, T. W. (1989) T cell receptor and immunoglobulin gene rearrangements in lymphoproliferative disorders. *Advances in Cancer Research*, **52**, 45–80.

ROSENTHAL, P., RIMM, I. J., UMIEL, T., GRIFFIN, J. D., OSATHA-NONDH, R., SCHLOSSMAN, S. F. & NADLER L. M. (1983) Ontogeny of human hematopoietic cells: Analysis utilizing monoclonal antibodies. *Journal of Immunology*, **31**, 232–7.

SAMELSON, L. E., HARFORD, J. B. & KLAUSNER, R. D. (1985) Identification of the components of the murine T cell antigen receptor complex. *Cell*, **43**, 223–31.

SEIDMAN, J. G. & LEDER, P. (1978) The arrangement and rearrangement of antibody genes. *Nature*, **276**, 790–5.

SHA, W. C., NELSON, C. A., NEWBERRY, R. D., KRANTZ, D. M.,

RUSSEL, J. H. & LOH, D. Y. (1988) Positive and negative selection of an antigen receptor on T cells in transgenic mice. *Nature*, **336**, 73–6.

SIEBENLIST, U., RAVETCH, J. V., KORSMEYER, S., WALDMANN, T. & LEDER, P. (1982) Human immunoglobulin D segments encoded in tandem multigenic families. *Nature*, **294**, 631–5.

SIVERSTEIN, A. M. & LUKES, R. J. (1962) Fetal responses to antigenic stimulus: 1. Plasmacellular and lymphoid reactions in the human fetus to intrauterine infection. *Laboratory Investigation*, **11**, 918–32.

SONDEL, P. M., CHEN, L., MacDERMOTT, R. P. & SCHLOSSMAN, S. F. (1975) Immunologic functions of isolated human lymphocyte subpopulations. III. Specific allogeneic lympholysis mediated by human T cells alone. *Journal of Immunology*, **114**, 982–7.

STITES, D. P., CALDWELL, J., CARR, M. C. & FUDENBERG, H. H. (1975) Ontogeny of immunity in humans. *Clinical Immunology & Immunopathology*, **4**, 519–27.

STITES, D. P., CARR, M. C. & FUDENBERG, H. H. (1974) Ontogeny of cellular immunity in the human fetus: Development of responses to phytohemagglutinin and to allogeneic cells. *Cellular Immunology*, **11**, 257–21.

STITES, D. & TERR, A. (eds.) (1991) *Basic and Clinical Immunology.* Appelton & Lange.

SWAIN, S. L. (1983) T cell subsets and the recognition of MHC class. *Immunological Reviews*, **74**, 129–42.

TEH, H. S., KISIELOW, P., SCOTT, B., KISHI, H., UEMATSU, Y., BLUTHMANN, H. & VON BOEHMER, H. (1988) Thymic major histocompatibility antigens and the α-β T cell receptor determine the CD4/CD8 phenotype of T cells. *Nature*, **335**, 229–35.

TOIVANEN, P., UKSILA, J., LEINO, A., LASSILA, O., HIRVONEN, T. & RUUSKANEN, O. (1981) Development of mitogen responding T cells and natural killer cells in the human fetus. *Immunological Review*, **57**, 89–105.

TOMASI, T. B. (1972) Secretory immunoglobulins. *New England Journal of Medicine*, **287**, 500–6.

TORIBIO, M. L., ALONSO, J. M., BARCENA, A., GUTIERREZ, J. C., de la HERA, A., MARCOS, M. A. R., MARQUEZ, C. & C. MARTINEZ-A, C. (1988) Human T-cell precursors; Involvement of the IL-2 pathway in the generation of mature T cells. *Immunological Reviews*, **104**, 55–79.

TOWNSEND, A. & BODMER, H. (1989) Antigen recognition by class I-restricted T lymphocytes. *Annual Review of Immunology*, **7**, 601–24.

UNANUE, E. R. (1984) Antigen-presenting function of the macrophage. *Annual Review of Immunology*, **2**, 395–428.

UNDERDOWN, B. J. & SCHIFF, J. M. (1986) Immunoglobulin A: Strategic defense initiative at the mucosal surface. *Annual Review of Immunology*, **4**, 389–417.

van FURTH, R., SCHUIT, H. R. E. & HIJMANS, W. (1965) The immunological development of the human foetus. *Journal of Experimental Medicine*, **122**, 1173–88.

von BOEHMER, H., KARJALAINEN, K., PELKONEN, J., BORGULYA, P. & RAMMENSEE, H.-G. (1988) The T-cell receptor for antigen in T-cell development and repertoire selection. *Immunological Reviews*, **101**, 21–37.

VOSSEN, J. M. (1975) Membrane associated immunoglobulin determinants

126

on bone marrow and blood lymphocytes in the paediatric age group and on fetal tissues. *Annals of the New York Academy of Sciences*, **254**, 262–79.

WANG, F., GREGORY, C. D., ROWE, M., RICKINSON, A. B., WANG, D., BIRKENBACH, M., KIKUTANI, H., KISHIMOTO, T. & KIEFF, E. (1987) Epstein–Barr virus nuclear antigen 2 specifically induces expression of the B cell activation antigen CD23. *Proceedings of the National Academy of Sciences, USA*, **84**, 3452–6.

WEISS, A. & IMBODEN, J. B. (1987) Cell surface molecules and early events involved in human T lymphocyte activation. *Advances in Immunology*, **41**, 1–38.

WHEELAHAN, J. & McKENZIE, I. F. C. (1987) The role of T4$^+$ and Ly2$^+$ cells in skin graft rejection in the mouse. *Transplantation*, **44**, 273–80.

WINKELHAKE, J. L. (1978) Immunoglobulin structure and effector functions. *Immunochemistry*, **15**, 695–714.

WU, L. Y. F., BLANCO, A., COOPER, M. D. & LAWTON, A. R. (1976) Ontogeny of B lymphocyte differentiation induced by pokeweed mitogen. *Clinical Immunology & Immunopathology*, **5**, 208–17.

YANCOPOULOS, G. D. & ALT, F. W. (1986) Regulation of the assembly and expression of variable region genes. *Annual Review of Immunology*, **4**, 339–68.

ZACHAU, H. G. (1989) Immunoglobulin light-chain genes of the K type in man and mouse. In: *Immunoglobulin Genes*, pp. 91–109. Eds. T. Honjo, F. W. Alt & T. H. Rabbitts. Academic Press, New York.

ZOLA, H. (1987) The surface antigens of human B lymphocytes. *Immunology Today*, **8**, 308–15.

ZUCKER-FRANKLIN, D., GREAVES, M. F., GROSSI, C. E. & MARMONT, A. M. (1981) *Atlas of Blood Cells, Function and Pathology*, 2nd ed., pp. 345–660. Lea & Febiger, Philadelphia.

CHAPTER 5

The procurement of human fetal tissues for clinical transplantation. Practice and problems

L. WONG

CONTENTS

THERE HAS BEEN A RECENT RENEWED INTEREST in the use of human fetal tissues for clinical transplantation. At present this use is small in comparison to use in research. However, provided that the ethical and moral concerns of society can be resolved, the potential for medical benefit is considerable.

The procurement of human fetal tissues for transplantation and research are essentially similar, except that, for the former, steps should be taken to ensure the safety of the tissues for the recipient. Only the principles of procurement can be covered in this general article which is largely based on fourteen years of the author's practical experience in acting as an intermediary in the procurement of and working with human fetal tissues. It must be emphasized that any views expressed are those of the author. The ethical and legal requirements discussed are those which are currently in force within the United Kingdom at the time of writing.

For the purposes of this article the definition of human fetal tissue transplantation is taken as the transplantation of tissues or cells from a human fetus into a human recipient for therapeutic purposes. Although pregnancy may be regarded as a form of naturally occurring embryo transplant, the intrauterine implantation of human embryos derived from in vitro fertilization techniques is not included under this definition. With the possible exceptions of human fetal donor thymus transplantation and adult donor bone marrow transplantation, the essential difference between adult organ and fetal tissue transplantation is that adult organ transplantation aims to replace a non-functional organ with a like but fully functional mature organ, whereas fetal tissue transplantation aims to transplant immature tissues or cells which have the potential to grow and mature within the host.

There is a lack of consistency in the definitions of embryo and fetus that are used in the embryological literature and those used in ethical and legal documents. However, since the use of fetal tissues in clinical transplantation in the United Kingdom comes within the remit of the recommendations of the Polkinghorne Report (1989), the definition of fetus used in this article is taken from that Report and covers the period of development from implantation until term.

Embryologists recognize at least two stages of development, an embryonic stage from fertilization until the end of the eighth week of gestation followed by a fetal stage ending at term. Therefore, the definition of fetus as used in the Polkinghorne Report covers a much longer period of development including that part of the embryonic stage following implantation in addition to the fetal stage. For the purposes of this article the definition of embryo when used in the context of the Human Fertilisation and Embryology Act (1990) will be used with the meaning as intended by that Act.

Reported uses of human fetal tissues

Clinical transplantation

The use of human fetal tissue in clinical transplantation has been limited and has met with varying degrees of success. In the majority of instances, work is still in the early stages of development, whereby variables influencing clinical outcome still remain to be determined. The most established example is that of human fetal thymus transplantation for the treatment of the severe form of the DiGeorge syndrome. The object here is one of replacement of a deficient thymus. The epithelium of the transplanted thymus then induces the differentiation of host stem cells into T cells. This has been the subject of a recent review (Buckley, 1988).

Fetal liver contains cells involved in early haemopoiesis and lymphopoiesis. Therefore, it has been used as a source of immature cells for reconstitution in a range of conditions that are characterized by defects in these cells lineages, e.g. immunodeficiency syndromes (Touraine *et al.*, 1987), aplastic anaemia and leukaemia (Lucarelli *et al.*, 1983). With the possible exception of severe combined immunodeficiency, only limited success has been achieved from such uses. In both fetal thymus and fetal liver transplantation an upper gestational age limit is set, the purpose being to minimize the risk of the simultaneous transplantation of mature T cells thought to be responsible for the graft versus host reaction.

Attempts have been made to treat inherited enzyme deficiencies, such as the inherited metabolic storage diseases, with fetal tissue transplantation. In this instance the object is to establish a population of fetal cells within the recipient which could then supply the deficient enzyme. Fetal liver cells have been used (Touraine *et al.*, 1987) as well as amniotic cells (Akle *et al.*, 1985), but because of insufficient data results have been difficult to assess.

Attempts have been made to treat insulin-dependent diabetes with human fetal pancreatic transplants. The object was to transplant fetal pancreatic islet cells, which would then multiply and develop into mature insulin secreting islets within the recipient thereby controlling the diabetes. There has been no long-term success (Stegall *et al.*, 1988) in spite of evidence from rodent xenograft models that such an approach should be feasible (Hullett *et al.*, 1987). However, work in this area is still at an early stage of development.

The treatment of Parkinson's disease by the transplantation of human fetal substantia nigra cell-rich mesencephalic tissue has been the most recent use of human fetal tissues in clinical transplantation. The objective in this instance is to transplant fetal substantia nigra cells of adequate growth and developmental potential such that not only would the deficient cells be replaced but also the transplanted cells would be capable of integrating into the brain of the recipient. Therefore, the gestational age of the transplanted fetal cells is likely to be of importance. The first objective evidence of engraftment has been reported recently (Lindvall *et al.*, 1990). However, this use of human fetal tissues is in the early stages of clinical evaluation. The medulla of the fetal adrenal gland has also been used to treat Parkinson's disease (Madrazo *et al.*, 1988), but long-term follow-up has not yet been reported.

The use of human fetal tissue in clinical transplantation is therefore still largely in the early stages of scientific development. The potential for such use is considerable, judging from preliminary work in animals.

However, in spite of this potential, the use of human fetal tissues in clinical transplantation has been explored only to a very limited extent. This has been largely a consequence of the ethical and moral concerns of society over the transplantation of tissues of human fetal origin and the illogical linkage of such usage with the issues of abortion.

Research and diagnostic virology

It is important to put the use of human fetal tissues in clinical transplantation into perspective. At present, the predominant use of human fetal tissues in the United Kingdom is in the area of research and diagnostic virology, and some examples in which the author has been involved as an intermediary in the procurement of fetal tissues are given in Table 5.1. Research use covers all the biological sciences. Its use in diagnostic virology involves virus isolation and identification, either in cell culture monolayers or organ cultures, and forms an essential part of health care without which such services would not be able to function effectively.

Ethical and legal considerations

The procurement and the specific uses of human fetal tissues in the United Kingdom are subject to legal and ethical considerations. Although obtaining fetal tissues and transplantation procedures are technically feasible, the actual use may not be ethically acceptable. Nowadays, ethics has become the major consideration. The ethical and legal constraints upon the use of human fetal tissue are in a constant state of change, which is a reflection of the pace of scientific advancement in this area and the consequent ethical and moral dilemmas thus generated.

At present the relevant ethical guidelines for the use of human fetal tissues within the United Kingdom are those contained within the Polkinghorne Report (1989). A prominent feature of this document is the principle of separation, which is designed to prevent the donor of fetal tissues from influencing the user and vice versa. It is recommended that, in practice, this is best achieved if fetal tissues are obtained through an independent third party. The clinical management of the mother should not be influenced by the potential use of the tissues. Consent for the use of the tissues should be obtained in a manner which does not indicate the specific use of the tissues to the mother. If the tissue or the mother are to be tested to ensure the safety of the tissues then consent must be obtained from the mother. Tissue must not be sent outside the United Kingdom. No financial inducements should be

Table 5.1. *Examples of projects in which human fetal tissues or cells are used*

Examples of projects	Examples of tissues or cells
Virology	
Clinical diagnostic virology using cell cultures for virus isolation and identification	Lung fibroblasts and kidney epithelial cells
Rapid identification of cytomegalovirus	Lung fibroblasts
Identification of JC virus	Brain spongioblasts
The effect of interferon-γ on rhinoviruses in organ culture	Nasal mucosa and trachea
Susceptibility of the brain to human immunodeficiency virus	Brain
Growth of parvovirus B19 in cells of erythroid lineage	Liver or bone marrow
HLA restriction in viral infected epithelial cell targets	Kidney
Bacteriology	
In vitro infection of Schwann cells with leprosy bacillus and histocompatibility antigen induction	Schwann cells from peripheral nerves
Susceptibility of cells in culture to bacterial toxins	Various tissues
Identification of *Clostridium difficile* toxin by effect on lung fibroblasts in culture	Lung fibroblasts
Effect of vaccines on the binding of *Bordetella pertussis* to ciliated respiratory epithelium	Trachea
Immunology	
Specificity evaluation of monoclonal antibodies	Various tissues
Oncofetal antigen isolation and specific antibody production	Pancreas, intestine, kidney, ovary and testis
Detection of autoimmune cytotoxic cell membrane antibodies to islet cells in diabetes mellitus	Pancreatic islet cells
Detection of the target cardiac cell in neonatal autoimmune heart block	Heart
Lymphocyte ontogeny. Development of T and B lymphocyte subpopulations. T-cell receptor ontogeny	Thymus, spleen, bone marrow and liver
Induction of the expression of HLA histocompatibility class II antigens in vitro as a possible pathogenic basis for cardiac rejection and diabetes mellitus	Heart and pancreatic islet cells
Lymphocyte epithelial interactions and differentiation in the thymus	Thymus
Detection of polymorphic T-cell histocompatibility antigens	Thymus
Acetylcholine receptors at the neuromuscular junction and the effect of myasthenia gravis sera on neuromusclar transmission	Muscle
Haematology	
Isolation of a possible human homologue of 'erythroid developmental agglutinin'	Muscle and bone marrow
Haemopoietic stem cell growth factors	Bone marrow, liver and spleen
Haemopoietic cell stromal interactions. Stromal colony stimulating growth factors	Bone marrow, spleen and liver

133

Table 5.1 (*cont.*)

Examples of projects	Examples of tissues or cells
Blood group substances ABO blood group expression and specific glycosyl transferase enzymes	Umbilical cord as source of fetal blood. Placenta
Molecular biology and genetics	
Production of cDNA libraries as an adjunct to finding specific gene probes in genetic disorders e.g. muscular dystrophy; Wilm's tumour; cystic fibrosis; and Frederick's ataxia	Muscle, brain, kidney, pancreas, spinal cord and dorsal root ganglia
Specific mRNA expression in different tissues during development using Northern blotting with specific probes or polymerase chain reaction amplification of cDNA using specific primers, e.g. the glucose-6-phosphate dehydrogenase gene; actin and myosin genes; T-cell receptor gamma gene; and cell adhesion molecule genes	Various tissues
mRNA isolation and translation to peptides for comparison between normal and Down's syndrome patients	Brain
In vitro gene transfection of cells in tissue culture	Skin fibroblasts
Aromatic DNA adducts and their role in carcinogenesis	Various tissues
Radiation damage to the DNA of cells in tissue culture induced by alpha particles	Lung fibroblasts
Anatomy and embryology	
Autonomic innervation of viscera	Intestine
Development of human cerebellum	Brain
Development of neurotransmitters in the brain	Brain
Development of cytokeratins and myoepithelial cells in human fetal salivary glands	Parotid and submandibular salivary glands
Development of the fetal prostate	Pelvis
Development of the fetal breast	Breast
Tissue culture and cell physiology	
Epithelial mesenchymal interactions	Skin
Growth factors and definition of the cell populations in human placenta	Placenta
Definition of nerve cells in culture using various markers	Brain and dorsal root ganglia
Adrenal cell culture and hormone production	Adrenal
Production of cell lines using retroviral vectors to insert growth promoting genes	Various tissues
Culture of dopamine producing cells of mesencephalic tissue	Brain
Development of cell adhesion molecules	Dorsal root ganglia and skin

involved. Ethical committees have the responsibility for vetting and monitoring specific project proposals and for ensuring that the fetal tissues have been procured and used in a manner which conform to ethical and legal requirements.

If fetal tissues are obtained from therapeutic abortions then these must be performed in accordance with the Abortion Act (1967) and the amendments to this Act contained within the Human Fertilisation and Embryology Act (1990). If the fetus has had a period of extrauterine viability prior to death then the Human Tissue Act (1961) must be observed. The Polkinghorne Report recommendations are concerned mainly with the postimplantation fetus and permit the use of fetal tissues from dead fetuses only, i.e. a fetus which is dead in the sense of a whole intact living organism. However, the Human Fertilisation and Embryology Act of 1990 is primarily concerned with the early stages of embryonic development and permits the use of live embryos under or equal to fourteen days postfertilization age but only under strictly controlled conditions as specified within the provisions of that Act. The Human Fertilisation and Embryology Act (1990) will also need to be observed if live fetal gametes, and embryos derived from manipulations upon these, are used. Although it is understood that the Human Organ Transplants Act (1989) was not intended to apply to the use of human fetal tissues in clinical transplantation, this could be subjected to clarification in the future.

It is not possible to deal with the practical implementation of the ethical and legal requirements of the use of human fetal tissues in this short chapter, and this would need to be dealt with separately.

Sources of human fetal tissues

Human fetal tissues become available as a consequence of spontaneous abortions, stillbirth or therapeutic abortions. Owing to the clinical circumstances in which *spontaneous abortion and stillbirth* occur, the tissues from these sources are generally of poor viability.

Methods of *therapeutic abortion* can be divided into surgical and medical. Medical methods are followed by surgical methods if the abortion is incomplete. For the purposes of this chapter the methods are discussed only in so far as they affect tissue viability and the ability to identify and therefore recover the tissues after evacuation. Technical details of the specific methods are described in text books of gynaecology (Burkman & King, 1984; Jeffcoate's Principles of Gynaecology, 1987) and the gynaecological literature (Castadot, 1986).

As a general principle, the viability of the tissue decreases with increasing length of time from the initiation of the procedure to the evacuation of the fetus. The method used is dependent upon current gynaecological practice and relates to the gestational age. In general, second trimester terminations are performed by medical induction; however, some centres extend use of surgical methods into the second trimester. First trimester terminations are performed by surgical methods but this trend may change in the future with the introduction of newer medical methods.

Surgical methods of therapeutic abortion

Hysterectomy and hysterotomy. These methods involve an intra-abdominal pelvic operation with either removal of the uterus with the fetus *in situ* (hysterectomy) or an incision into the uterus followed by removal of the fetus and membranes (hysterotomy). Both these methods produce an intact fetus and therefore all organs and tissues are potentially recoverable. Also as the interval between removal of the fetus and fetal death is brief, the tissues are of good viability. These methods of termination are now rarely used.

Cervical dilatation followed by surgical evacuation. These methods are dependent upon dilatation of the cervix with surgical dilators and/or laminaria tents followed by surgical evacuation of the fetal tissues with a curette, suction curette, syringe or forceps or a combination of these. These approaches are variously described as suction; vacuum aspiration; dilatation and curettage; dilatation and evacuation; and dilatation and extraction.

The time interval between the onset of fetal death and the evacuation of fetal tissues is brief, consequently the fetal tissues are of good viability. However, the extent of tissue disruption, and therefore the ability to identify and successfully recover the various tissues and organs, is very dependent upon the exact method used for evacuation.

Medical methods of therapeutic abortion

These methods involve the use of drugs such as oxytocin, the derivatives of prostaglandin, hyper-osmolar urea, hypertonic sodium chloride and more recently the antiprogestogens. In general, the principle behind these methods involves the induction of a form of 'labour'; the uterine contractions being finally responsible for the evacuation of the fetal tissues. Depending upon the drugs used, administration may be by various routes, e.g. intravenous infusion, intra-amniotic and intravaginal. A combination of drugs may be used, e.g. prostaglandins in combination with intra-amniotic urea. The drug protocols are designed to maximize efficacy of fetal evacuation with a minimum of drug side effects to the mother, e.g. pain and vomiting. The methods may also be supplemented by preliminary cervical dilatation with laminaria tents.

If medical methods fail to produce a complete abortion then surgical evacuation is the final method. Although these methods result in an intact fetus, tissue viability is in general inferior to that obtained with surgical methods. Viability is dependent upon a number of factors, i.e. the period of fetal hypoxia consequent upon the time between drug administration and fetal death, the time between fetal death and evacuation, and the effect of the drugs *per se* on the fetal tissues; for example, intra-amniotic hyper-osmolar urea and hypertonic sodium chloride are both very toxic to the fetal tissues.

In addition, there can be considerable variation in the viability of fetal tissues that are derived from medical inductions using the same method. This, in part, is due to variations in the technique used by individual gynaecologists. Therefore, fetal tissues should be evaluated for viability for a particular method as practised by a particular centre.

A more recent method of medical termination involves the use of the antiprogestogen RU486. This drug, which interferes with implantation, is then followed by a prostaglandin derivative to assist uterine evacuation (Cameron & Baird, 1988; Silvestre *et al.*, 1990). At present, this method has been confined to first trimester terminations, and recovery and viability of the fetal tissues has not yet been reported in the literature.

Dissection and identification of fetal organs and tissues

After uterine evacuation, the tissues should be maintained at 4 °C and dissected as soon as possible under sterile conditions using non-touch surgical technique. Recovered organs and tissues are then placed into appropriate sterile solutions in sterile containers.

The successful recovery of organs and tissues as a general principle depends upon the gestational age, the organ or tissue concerned, and the level of optical assistance used when undertaking the dissections. If the fetus is intact then the successful recovery of organs is largely a matter of dissection. In surgically disrupted fetal tissues, the degree of surgical disruption, and therefore the exact method of surgical termination used, is an important additional factor which determines successful recovery.

The majority of organs and tissues which are commonly used for research can be readily recovered from disrupted fetal tissues using naked eye dissection (Wong, 1988). Nevertheless, considerable difficulty can be experienced in the recovery of some organs and tissues from such disrupted tissues. Examples of the techniques used to locate some organs and tissues in disrupted fetal tissues are given below.

The *pancreas* is often found attached to other organs which can be readily identified. The location of these organs therefore facilitates the location of the pancreas. In their absence, it is difficult to identify pancreatic tissue with certainty.

If the stomach is identified then the body of the pancreas may be found attached to the posterior aspect. If intestinal tissue is identified then the head of the pancreas may be found partially encircled by the duodenum. If the spleen is located then the tail of the pancreas may be found attached to its root.

The *liver* can be identified as brown friable fragments of tissue. It can be confused at times with old blood clot which has taken on a brownish discolouration. However, in cases of uncertainty, examination of a wet preparation under microscopy is helpful.

Discrete lobes of the *thymus*, rather than entire glands, are usually found. The surface is smooth and lobulation can be discerned. At times, finding the thymus in disrupted fetal tissues of early gestational age can be facilitated if the sternum or anterior chest wall is found. The thymus may then be found often loosely attached to the posterior aspect of the upper sternum.

Midbrain tissue is required as a source of substantia nigra cells in the treatment of Parkinson's disease. The gestational age used by Lindvall has been reported in the literature as eight to ten weeks (Lindvall *et al.*, 1988, 1990). The fetal tissues available in this age range are disrupted surgically.

Brain tissue is very fragile, so that successful recovery is difficult, and very dependent on the extent of tissue disruption. If the cranium is still intact, a rare occurrence in disrupted fetal tissues, then location is straightforward. If the skull cap is dislocated, but the contents are still relatively intact then the midbrain may be located. Difficulty in the successful recovery of mesencephalic tissue from disrupted fetuses has led some Swedish workers to advocate a modification of the abortion technique (Seiger, 1988; Gustavii, 1989).

It must be emphasized at this point that any modification of abortion technique with a view to the potential use of fetal tissues is ethically unacceptable within the United Kingdom. Such a practice would be in direct contravention of the Polkinghorne Report (1989). Any modification should be done solely in the interest of the clinical management of the mother.

With the exception of the testes, which may be identified as discrete ovoid organs in second trimester disrupted fetal tissues, the location of the *gonads* depends mainly upon the identification of a relatively intact pelvis. The gonads are then identified by anatomical situation and structure.

Up to six weeks gestational age the gonad is developmentally indifferent. The identification of the gonad as ovary or testis on a gross anatomical basis is not possible, with confidence, until the second trimester. At this stage, it is also feasible to determine the sex from the external genitalia, thus providing confirmatory evidence as to the nature of the gonad. However, the nature of the gonad can be indirectly determined in younger fetuses if the genetic sex is determined by methods such as Y-body fluorescence.

The *adrenal* is readily identified as a pyramidal, brownish and soft structure either as a discrete organ or attached to the kidney in very young fetuses.

Bone marrow is recovered readily by irrigation of the marrow of long bones.

Assessing fetal tissue for clinical transplantation

Quantity of fetal tissue required

This has been established only for the transplantation of the fetal thymus in the DiGeorge syndrome where one thymus gland is sufficient. In the majority of instances, because of lack of data, the optimal amount of the tissue which is required remains to be determined. Although various estimated amounts form the basis of clinical transplantation protocols, such decisions are often influenced by the availability of tissue.

Evaluation of the viability of fetal tissues

Knowledge of the level of viability of the tissue transplanted is of crucial importance, since the subsequent clinical assessment of the success or failure of the transplant will assume adequate viability. Viability is a relative term and, therefore, is pitched at different levels. The level which is most relevant to fetal tissue transplantation is that the transplanted cells should be able to grow (multiply) or at least survive and function within the recipient.

The in vitro viability 'test' that best correlates with this level is that the cells to be transplanted should at least be able to grow (multiply) or survive and function in tissue culture. Therefore, a sample of the tissue to be transplanted should be evaluated for viability within tissue culture. If transplant tissue cannot be spared for this purpose because of shortage, then a number of other tissues should be taken from the same fetus and evaluated for viability within tissue culture. The viability of the tissue to be used for transplantation can then be evaluated indirectly by the ability of these other tissues to grow in tissue culture.

The relative viabilities of various tissues in culture have been determined in previous experiments. Although the results of such evaluation will not be available before transplantation, unless the tissue has been cryopreserved and used pending results, they will be required none-the-less in the event of graft failure in order to exclude inadequate tissue viability as a cause.

In the first instance, it must be decided which source of fetal tissues is most likely to result in tissues that are satisfactory for transplantation. The best practical guidance is that the fetal tissues obtained from a particular abortion procedure, as practised by a particular centre, should have been shown consistently to be successful within tissue culture in the past. Most of the author's practical experience comes from the use of fetal tissues derived from three categories of termination, i.e. hysterotomy, suction and a combination of intra-amniotic urea and prostaglandin (Wong, 1988).

Hysterotomy and suction terminations have been found to produce tissues of good and equivalent viability and are eminently suitable for tissue culture and therefore for transplantation. Combined intra-amniotic urea and prostaglandin terminations, generally but not invariably, result in tissues of poor viability. This is attributed mainly to the effects of urea. Although it may be possible to culture some tissues from some fetuses, this is unpredictable, therefore fetal tissues from this method of termination will not be suitable for transplantation. Some prostaglandin protocols, without intra-amniotic urea, have been found by some to produce tissue which is satisfactory for tissue culture. Therefore, tissue from such terminations should be satisfactory for transplantation.

Estimation of the gestational age of the fetus

The accurate estimation of fetal age is important where it is necessary that cells of the appropriate stage of differentiation are to be transplanted. One group of workers have chosen substantia nigra cell-rich tissue from fetuses of eight to ten weeks' gestational age for the treatment of Parkinson's disease (Lindvall *et al.*, 1988, 1990). This choice has been influenced by evidence that more mature cells may have lost the capacity to integrate into host brain tissues.

Another factor determining the gestational age of the tissue to be transplanted is the presence of mature T cells in fetal tissues of older gestational age. This factor influences the choice of fetal thymus used for the treatment of the DiGeorge syndrome where the upper gestational age limit is set at fourteen weeks (Buckley, 1988). In many instances the optimal gestational age of the tissue required for transplantation is unknown because of insufficient clinical data. Aging is important if such information is eventually to become available.

The estimation of fetal age from fetal measurements is standard practice. At present Tables 5.2, 5.3 and 5.4 are used by the author. The data for these tables have been derived from statistical analysis of cases by the author and will be presented in a separate article. Crown–rump length is used for intact fetuses, see Table 5.2. Either foot length or hand measurements are used for disrupted fetuses, see Tables 5.3 and 5.4 respectively.

Markers for following the chimeric state

Appropriate fetal tissues should be set aside to determine markers for following the chimeric state. Possible markers include sex; histocompatability antigens; blood group antigens; isoenzymes; and chromosome and DNA polymorphisms. Fetal tissue markers such as α-fetoprotein production in fetal liver transplants may also be of value as evidence of engraftment.

Measures to ensure the safety of the fetal tissues for the recipient

It is often not possible to do exhaustive testing to exclude all infective and genetic risk of the fetal tissues to the recipient. The amount of testing which is feasible is limited by the interval between obtaining the fetal tissue and the time of transplantation. If the tissues are preserved then the permissible duration of preservation becomes the limiting factor.

Rapid methods for diagnosis are being developed constantly for both viral infections (Richman *et al.*, 1984; Lee & Hallsworth, 1990) and genetic disorders (Reiss & Cooper, 1990), and testing that may not be feasible at present may become so in the future. In any event, testing protocols will need to be worked out and any risk which is consequent upon limited testing should be explained to the recipient and balanced against her or his clinical condition. Tests should not be excluded on the grounds that the results will not be available before transplantation as they may be of value in the subsequent clinical management of the recipient.

141

Table 5.2. *Equivalent menstrual age (weeks) vs crown–rump length (cm)*

Crown–rump length (cm)	Equivalent menstrual age (weeks)	Crown–rump length (cm)	Equivalent menstrual age (weeks)
1.5	9.0	5.5	11.8
1.6	9.1	6.0	12.2
1.7	9.1	6.5	12.5
1.8	9.2	7.0	12.9
1.9	9.3	7.5	13.2
2.0	9.4	8.0	13.6
2.1	9.4	8.5	13.9
2.2	9.5	9.0	14.3
2.3	9.6	9.5	14.6
2.4	9.6	10.0	15.0
2.5	9.7	10.5	15.3
2.6	9.8	11.0	15.7
2.7	9.8	11.5	16.0
2.8	9.9	12.0	16.4
2.9	10.0	12.5	16.7
3.0	10.1	13.0	17.1
3.1	10.1	13.5	17.5
3.2	10.2	14.0	17.8
3.3	10.3	14.5	18.2
3.4	10.3	15.0	18.5
3.5	10.4	15.5	18.9
3.6	10.5	16.0	19.2
3.7	10.6	16.5	19.6
3.8	10.6	17.0	19.9
3.9	10.7	17.5	20.3
4.0	10.8	18.0	20.6
4.1	10.8	18.5	21.0
4.2	10.9	19.0	21.3
4.3	11.0	19.5	21.7
4.4	11.0	20.0	22.0
4.5	11.1	20.5	22.4
4.6	11.2	21.0	22.7
4.7	11.3	21.5	23.1
4.8	11.3	22.0	23.4
4.9	11.4	22.5	23.8
5.0	11.5		

Notes:
(i) With the fetus in the seated position, the crown–rump length is taken as the perpendicular distance between the plane on which it is seated and the plane in contact with the top of the head. (ii) Gestational age is the equivalent menstrual age less two weeks. (Assuming midcycle ovulation in 4-week cycle.) (iii) Data in the table derived from the statistical analysis of 4260 cases.

Table 5.3. *Equivalent menstrual age (weeks) vs foot length (mm)*

Foot length (mm)	Equivalent menstrual age (weeks)	Foot length (mm)	Equivalent menstrual age (weeks)
2.0	9.5	26.5	16.7
2.5	9.7	27.0	16.8
3.0	9.9	27.5	16.9
3.5	10.1	28.0	17.0
4.0	10.3	28.5	17.1
4.5	10.4	29.0	17.2
5.0	10.6	29.5	17.3
5.5	10.8	30.0	17.4
6.0	11.0	30.5	17.6
6.5	11.1	31.0	17.7
7.0	11.3	31.5	17.8
7.5	11.5	32.0	17.9
8.0	11.6	32.5	18.0
8.5	11.8	33.0	18.1
9.0	12.0	33.5	18.2
9.5	12.1	34.0	18.3
10.0	12.3	34.5	18.4
10.5	12.4	35.0	18.5
11.0	12.6	35.5	18.6
11.5	12.7	36.0	18.7
12.0	12.9	36.5	18.8
12.5	13.0	37.0	18.9
13.0	13.2	37.5	19.1
13.5	13.3	38.0	19.2
14.0	13.5	38.5	19.3
14.5	13.6	39.0	19.4
15.0	13.8	39.5	19.5
15.5	13.9	40.0	19.6
16.0	14.0	40.5	19.7
16.5	14.2	41.0	19.8
17.0	14.3	41.5	19.9
17.5	14.4	42.0	20.0
18.0	14.6	42.5	20.1
18.5	14.7	43.0	20.2
19.0	14.8	43.5	20.3
19.5	15.0	44.0	20.4
20.0	15.1	44.5	20.5
20.5	15.2	45.0	20.6
21.0	15.3	45.5	20.7
21.5	15.5	46.0	20.8
22.0	15.6	46.5	20.9
22.5	15.7	47.0	21.0
23.0	15.8	47.5	21.1
23.5	15.9	48.0	21.2
24.0	16.1	48.5	21.3
24.5	16.2	49.0	21.4
25.0	16.3	49.5	21.5
25.5	16.4	50.0	21.6
26.0	16.5		

Notes:
(i) Foot length is taken as the distance between the heel and the tip of the big toe. (ii) Gestational age is the equivalent menstrual age less two weeks. (Assuming midcycle ovulation in 4-week cycle.) (iii) Data in the table derived from the statistical analysis of 5403 cases.

Table 5.4. *Equivalent menstrual age (weeks) vs wrist–index-finger length (mm)*

Wrist–index-finger length (mm)	Equivalent menstrual age (weeks)	Wrist–index-finger length (mm)	Equivalent menstrual age (weeks)
2.0	9.5	21.5	16.7
2.5	9.7	22.0	16.9
3.0	10.0	22.5	17.0
3.5	10.2	23.0	17.2
4.0	10.5	23.5	17.3
4.5	10.7	24.0	17.5
5.0	10.9	24.5	17.6
5.5	11.1	25.0	17.7
6.0	11.3	25.5	17.9
6.5	11.6	26.0	18.0
7.0	11.8	26.5	18.2
7.5	12.0	27.0	18.3
8.0	12.2	27.5	18.4
8.5	12.4	28.0	18.6
9.0	12.6	28.5	18.7
9.5	12.8	29.0	18.8
10.0	13.0	29.5	19.0
10.5	13.2	30.0	19.1
11.0	13.3	30.5	19.2
11.5	13.5	31.0	19.4
12.0	13.7	31.5	19.5
12.5	13.9	32.0	19.6
13.0	14.0	32.5	19.8
13.5	14.2	33.0	19.9
14.0	14.4	33.5	20.0
14.5	14.6	34.0	20.2
15.0	14.7	34.5	20.3
15.5	14.9	35.0	20.4
16.0	15.1	35.5	20.6
16.5	15.2	36.0	20.7
17.0	15.4	36.5	20.8
17.5	15.5	37.0	20.9
18.0	15.7	37.5	21.1
18.5	15.8	38.0	21.2
19.0	16.0	38.5	21.3
19.5	16.1	39.0	21.5
20.0	16.3	39.5	21.6
20.5	16.4	40.0	21.7
21.0	16.6		

Notes:

(i) Wrist–index-finger length is taken as the distance between the flexion crease at the wrist on flexion of the hand, to the tip of the extended index finger. (ii) Gestational age is the equivalent menstrual age less two weeks. (Assuming midcycle ovulation in 4-week cycle.) (iii) Data in the table derived from the statistical analysis of 829 cases.

Assessment and reduction of infective risk

There have been no reports of infection in recipients of fetal tissue transplantation which could have been unequivocally attributed to the donor as the ultimate source. Nevertheless, such reports have appeared in the case of adult organ transplantation (Clarke, 1987; Erice *et al.*, 1988). The risk of infection is therefore a real one requiring necessary precautions.

Assuming that the procedures following evacuation of the fetus from the uterus maintain sterility, the fetal tissues themselves may be infected by the mother as a result of intrauterine transmission of maternal infection, e.g. syphilis, toxoplasma, herpes simplex, vaccinia, cytomegalovirus, rubella, hepatitis B virus, human immunodeficiency virus (Lewis *et al.*, 1990; European Collaborative Study, 1991), varicella zoster (Alkalay *et al.*, 1987), parvovirus type B19 (Brown, 1989). The fetal tissues may also be contaminated by infected maternal fluids and secretions during evacuation of the fetus, this being the more common mode of transmission in the case of hepatitis B and herpes simplex. Therefore, it is advisable to test the mother as well as the fetal tissues themselves for evidence of infection. The screening for infection in pregnancy and the risk of transmission to the fetus has been the subject of a review by Klapper & Morris (1990).

Although it is not possible to prevent all infections being passed on to the recipient by the fetal tissues, a number of practical measures can be taken to minimize the risks. The approach is to evaluate infective risk at three levels: i.e. the mother, the fetal tissues and the recipient. Rational decisions can then be made whether to use the tissues and what tests for infection will be required.

The following procedures should be carried out to evaluate the risk of infection from the mother:

(i)   Fetal tissues from a termination which has been done because the mother had an infection during pregnancy, and which may be transmitted to the fetus, should be avoided. Examples include: rubella; cytomegalovirus; human immunodeficiency virus (HIV); hepatitis B; and toxoplasmosis

(ii) Fetal tissues from terminations in which the mother is a known carrier must be avoided, e.g. hepatitis B or HIV

(iii) Some active infections in the mother can be safely excluded in the fetus if she is known to have specific immunity, e.g. rubella

(iv) The mother's blood should be tested serologically for evidence of infection, and in particular for recent infection by the detection of class IgM specific antibodies. Blood may also be

145

examined using molecular techniques to detect specific DNA sequences of microorganisms. The range of microorganisms to be tested for should be decided for each transplantation protocol. However, because of the grave consequence to the recipient, some infections should always be tested for, e.g. syphilis, hepatitis B and HIV

The following procedures should be carried out to evaluate and reduce the risk of infection in the fetal tissues:

(i) Fetal tissues from spontaneous abortions will have a higher risk of being infected because of the circumstances in which this occurs, and are therefore best avoided

(ii) Fetal tissues may be tested by culturing representative tissue fragments for the identification of microorganisms. The possibility of the contamination of fetal tissues with vaginal commensals such as *Candida albicans* should be considered in such tests. The fetal tissues may also be tested using molecular techniques by searching for the specific DNA sequences of the microorganisms in the tissues. If fetal serum is available, this may be tested serologically for class IgM specific antibodies as evidence of recent infection

(iii) A mother may be incubating HIV at the time of termination and be serologically negative, but the fetal tissues are infected. Ideally, the fetal tissues should therefore tested for HIV using the polymerase chain reaction technique (Laure *et al.*, 1988; Loche & Mach, 1988; Ou *et al.*, 1988) if this possibility is to be excluded. The choice of placenta, as the tissue to be tested, might be appropriate in view of the suggested mode of intrauterine transmission (Lewis *et al.*, 1990). If the tissue is cryopreserved prior to use then the recommendations of the Expert Advisory Group on AIDS should be followed. These are that an HIV seronegative donor at the time of donation (the mother in the case of fetal tissues) should be retested after at least ninety days, and the tissue used only if the donor remains seronegative (Department of Health PL/CMO(90)2, 1990)

(iv) The risk of contamination of the fetal tissues can be reduced if the fetal tissues are washed in sterile solutions before transplantation. In practice, this simple measure has been very effective in reducing bacterial and fungal contamination in the tissue culture of tissues from disrupted fetuses

(v) The fetal tissues may be incubated and washed in antibiotics and antifungal solutions prior to transplantation. This simple

146

measure has also been very effective in reducing the incidence of bacterial and fungal infections in the routine use of disrupted fetuses for tissue culture

(vi)   The investigation of the in vitro treatment of fetal tissues with antiviral agents to reduce the risk of viral contamination might merit future investigation

The following procedures should be carried out to evaluate the risk of infection in the recipient:

(i)   The immunity of the recipient to specific infections should be assessed. For example, if the recipient is already a carrier of hepatitis B or HIV then the possibility of contamination of the donor fetal tissues with these viruses will not need to be rigorously excluded

(ii)   The possibility of active immunization before transplantation should be considered e.g. hepatitis B

(iii)   The general immune status of the recipient should be evaluated. For example, it should be decided if the recipient is immunodeficient or if immunosuppression is to be used in the transplantation protocol

(iv)   The prophylactic use of antimicrobials in the recipient should be considered

Assessment and reduction of risk of genetic abnormality

The clinical significance of transplanting genetically abnormal human fetal tissues into a human recipient is unknown. Nevertheless, the transplantation of a population of genetically abnormal cells which have the ability to grow and multiply in the host would be ethically unacceptable. Therefore the fetal tissues should be assessed for the risk of genetic abnormality and those at risk or shown to be abnormal should not be used.

The same conditions arise as described for the assessment of infective risk. Time is the limiting factor which determines the number of laboratory tests for genetic abnormality that can be done before transplantation. In addition to the tests, a number of factors which reduce the risk of transplanting genetically abnormal fetal tissue will need to be considered. The approach is to evaluate genetic risk in the fetal tissues at the level of the mother and the fetus. Then it can be decided rationally whether to use the tissues and what laboratory tests for genetic abnormality are required.

147

Fetal tissues from a mother known to have or to be a carrier of a genetic disease should not be used.

The following procedures should be carried out to evaluate and reduce genetic risk in the fetal tissues:

(i)   The incidence of karyotypic abnormality is estimated at 41.8% in spontaneous abortions and 2.24% in therapeutically induced abortions, these figures having been calculated from a review of several series (Wright, 1976). It is therefore advisable not to use fetal tissues from spontaneous abortions if karyotypic analyses cannot be performed before transplantation, a possible exception being where the spontaneous abortion has been shown to result from a gynaecological condition such as cervical incompetence

(ii) Fetuses showing evidence of anatomical abnormality should not be used, since a proportion of these will have genetic abnormalities

(iii) Where feasible, karyotypic and DNA analysis on fetal tissues for genetic abnormality should be performed before transplantation

Manipulations on fetal tissues before transplantation

Ideally, if the precise cells that are required for transplantation to treat a given condition are known then these cells could be isolated from the fetal tissues and transplanted to the recipient. This avoids the problem of contamination of the graft with cells which are not required for the transplant, e.g. cells of the immune system in particular, which could facilitate graft rejection or initiate a graft versus host reaction. Manipulations on fetal tissues before clinical transplantation have been done with these objectives in mind.

In general, fetal tissues are transplanted as tissue fragments (for example, fetal thymus) or as cell suspensions (for example fetal liver). A period of preliminary cell culture in vitro may have been used. An example of this is the culture of human fetal thymus for thymic epithelium and for the elimination of mature T cells prior to its use in the treatment of the DiGeorge syndrome (Thong et al., 1978). This preliminary culture achieved two purposes. Firstly, it allowed transplantation of those cells responsible for immunological reconstitution, i.e. thymic epithelium. Secondly, it eliminated mature T cells responsible for the graft versus host reaction.

A further example is the organ culture of fetal pancreas with a view to reducing the population of donor antigen presenting cells thought to contribute to graft rejection (Thomson et al., 1983).

Another approach has been to incorporate the fetal tissues into diffusion chambers as a transplant so that cells cannot pass out of the chamber whereas soluble factors can. This technique was used for transplants of fetal thymic tissue, in order to block the egress of lymphoid cells. This approach thus prevented the graft versus host reaction, but at the same time allowed the diffusion of thymic hormones thought to be responsible for immunological reconstitution (Steele *et al.*, 1972).

Maintenance of fetal tissues between donation and transplantation

As soon as possible after donation, the fetal tissues should be maintained at 4 °C. They are dissected to obtain the required tissues for grafting, which are then washed with a physiological solution to clear them of contaminating material such as red cells. Tissues for grafting are then cut into fragments or made into cell suspension, whichever is appropriate, and then maintained at 4 °C in a buffered tissue culture medium or an equivalent physiological solution containing nutrients. Antibiotics may be added as an extra safeguard against bacterial contamination.

Just as in adult organ transplantation, the time between donation and transplantation should be minimized in so far as logistics permit. In contrast to adult organ transplantation, where the viability of a large intact organ such as a kidney is to be maintained, fetal tissues to be transplanted comprise very much smaller tissue fragments or cell suspensions. The resulting shorter diffusion distances for nutrients and waste metabolic products make the maintenance of fetal tissues much easier.

There have been no studies on the relative survival of different types of fetal tissue maintained in suspension before transplantation. The extrapolation of evidence gained from fetal tissue culture following storage of tissue fragments in suspension indicates that relative survival declines from fibroblasts, epithelial cells to neuronal cells on the scale ranging from a few days to hours. However, as a compromise between feasible logistics and viability, and to reduce the risk of contamination, fetal tissues should be transplanted on the same day as donation; in the case of neuronal cells, this should be within hours.

Preservation of fetal tissues for clinical transplantation

The ability to preserve human fetal tissues such that they would be suitable for transplantation after prolonged storage would have many advantages. This would allow time to do quality control and

149

characterization on the tissues before transplantation, and so make it possible to ensure that the tissues to be transplanted are of adequate viability, free from infection and not genetically abnormal. Tissue with optimal markers for following the chimeric state in a particular recipient could be chosen, and histocompatibility matching would become feasible. Preservation would allow the pooling of tissues where a large amount of tissue is required. Tissue would be available when it is required clinically. The feasibility of the formation of a bank of preserved tissue has been indicated by a number of reports. For example, it has been shown that human fetal pancreas can be maintained in long-term organ culture (von Dorche *et al.*, 1987; Tuch & Turtle, 1987). The cryopreservation of both human fetal pancreas (Brown *et al.*, 1980; Kühn *et al.*, 1990) and substantia nigra cells (Redmond *et al.*, 1988) are possible (see Chapter 12, this volume).

Conclusions

The recently renewed interest in the use of human fetal tissue in clinical transplantation is an acknowledgement of the considerable potential benefit of this unique therapeutic approach. Although interest has been tempered by the ethical and moral concerns of society, these concerns have been addressed largely by the recent introduction of new ethical guidelines and legislation. Therapy using human fetal tissue transplantation is still in the early stages of scientific development. The introduction of cryopreservation techniques has made a reality of banks of characterized tissue, free from infection and genetic abnormality and suitable for clinical use.

References

AKLE, C., McCOLL, I., DEAN, M., ADINOLFI, M., BROWN, S., FERSOM, A. H. & MARSH, J. (1985) Transplantation of amniotic epithelial membranes in patients with mucopolysaccharidoses. *Experimental and Clinical Immunogenetics*, **2**, 43–8.

ALKALAY, A. L., POMERANCE, J. J. & RINION, D. L. (1987) Fetal varicella syndrome. *Journal of Paediatrics*, **111**, 320–23.

BROWN, J., KEMP, J. A., HURT, S. & CLARK, W. R. (1980) Cryopreservation of human fetal pancreas. *Diabetes*, **29**, 70–3.

BROWN, K. E. (1989) What threat is human parvovirus B19 to the fetus? A review. *British Journal of Obstetrics & Gynaecology*, **96**, 764–7.

BUCKLEY, R. H. (1988) Fetal thymus transplantation for the correction of congenital absence of the thymus (DiGeorge's Syndrome).In: *Report of the Human Fetal Tissue Transplantation Research Panel*, Vol. II, pp. D50–D57. Consultants to the Advisory Committee to the Director, National Institutes of Health.

BURKMAN, R. T. & KING, T. M. (1984) Second-trimester termination of pregnancy. In: *Obstetrics & Gynaecology, Part B: Gynaecology*, pp. 241–53. Eds. E. M. Symonds, & F. P. Zuspan. Marcel Dekker, Inc, New York.

CAMERON, I. T. & BAIRD, D. T. (1988) Early pregnancy termination: a comparison between vacuum aspiration and medical abortion using prostaglandin (16, 16 dimethyl-trans-delta$_2$-PGE$_1$ methyl ester) or the antiprogestogen RU 486. *British Journal of Obstetrics & Gynaecology*, **95**, 271–6.

CASTADOT, R. G. (1986) Pregnancy termination: techniques, risks, and complications and their management. *Fertility & Sterility*, **45**, 5–17.

CLARKE, J. A. (1987) HIV transmission and skin grafts. *Lancet*, **i**, 983.

DEPARTMENT OF HEALTH PL/CMO (90)2 (1990) HIV infection, tissue banks and organ donation. Health Publications Unit, Lancashire, UK.

ERICE, A., RHAME, F., SULLIVAN, C., DUNN, D., JACKSON, B. & BALFOUR, H. H., Jr. (1988) Human immunodeficiency virus (HIV) infection in organ transplant recipients (OTRS). *IV International Conference on AIDS*. Book 2, p. 363. Stockholm, June 12–16.

EUROPEAN COLLABORATIVE STUDY (1991) Children born to women with HIV-1 infection: natural history and risk of transmission. *Lancet*, **337**, 253–60.

GUSTAVII, B. (1989) Fetal brain transplantation for Parkinson's disease: technique for obtaining donor tissue. *Lancet*, **i**, 565.

HULLET, D. A., FALANY, J. L., LOVE, R. B., BURLINGHAM, W. J., PAN, M. & SOLLINGER, H. W. (1987) Human fetal pancreas – a potential source for transplantation. *Transplantation*, **43**, 18–22.

JEFFCOATE'S PRINCIPLES OF GYNAECOLOGY (1987) 5th Edition. *Sterilisation and termination of pregnancy*, pp. 617–32. Ed. V. R. Tindall. Butterworths Scientific Ltd, Guildford, UK.

KLAPPER, P. E. & MORRIS, D. J. (1990) Screening for viral and protozoal infections in pregnancy. A review. *British Journal of Obstetrics & Gynaecology*, **97**, 974–83.

KÜHN, F., WACHS, J. H., RÜCKERT, J., SETTMACHER, U., SCHULTZ, H. J., MATTHES, G., BOLLMANN, R., HAHN, H. J., RATZMANN, K. P. & WOLFF, H. (1990) Tissue bank of human fetal pancreas. *Transplantation Proceedings*, **22**, 683–4.

LAURE, F., ROUZIOUX, C., VEBER F., JACOMET, C., COURGNAUD, V., BLANCHE, S., BURGARD, M., GRISCELLI, C. & BRECHOT, C. (1988) Detection of HIV1 DNA in infants and children by means of the polymerase chain reaction. *Lancet* **ii**, 538–41.

LEE, P. C. & HALLSWORTH, P. (1990) Rapid viral diagnosis in perspective. *British Medical Journal*, **300**, 1413–18.

LEWIS, S. H., REYNOLDS-KOHLER, C., FOX, H. E. & NELSON, J. A. (1990) HIV-1 in trophoblastic and villous Hofbauer cells, and haematological precursors in eight-week fetuses. *Lancet*, **335**, 565–8.

LINDVALL, O., BRUNDIN, P., WIDNER, H., REHNCRONA, S., GUSTAVII, B., FRACKOWIAK, R., LEENDERS, K. L., SAWLE, G., ROTHWELL, J. C., MARSDEN, C. D. & BJÖRKLUND, A. (1990) Grafts of fetal dopamine neurons survive and improve motor function in Parkinson's disease. *Science*, **247**, 574–7.

LINDVALL, O., GUSTAVII, B., ÅSTEDT, B., LINDHOLM, T., REHNCRONA, S., BRUNDIN, P., WIDNER, H., BJORKLUND, A., LEENDERS, K. L., FRACKOWIAK, R., ROTHWELL, J. C., MARSDEN, C. D., JOHNELS, B.L., STEG, G., FREEDMAN, R., HOFFER, B. J., SIEGER, A., STRÖMBERG, I., BYGDEMAN, M. & OLSON, L. (1988) Fetal dopamine-rich mesencephalic grafts in Parkinson's disease. *Lancet*, **ii**, 1483–4.

LOCHE, M. & MACH, B. (1988) Identification of HIV-infected seronegative individuals by a direct diagnostic test based on hybridization to amplified viral DNA. *Lancet*, **ii**, 418–21.

LUCARELLI, G., IZZI, T., PORCELLINI, A., DELFINI, C., GALIMBERTI, M., POLCHI, P., MORETTI, L., MANNA, A. & SPARAVENTI, G. (1983) Fetal liver transplantation in aplastic anemia and acute leukaemia. In: *Recent Advances in Bone Marrow Transplantation*, pp. 865–874. Ed. Gale, R. P. Alan R. Liss, Inc, New York.

MADRAZO, I., LÉON, V., TORRES, C., AGUILERA, M. del C., VARELA, G., ALVAREZ, F., FRAGA, A., DRUKER-COLIN, R., OSTROSKY, F., SKUROVICH, M. & FRANCO, R. (1988) Transplantation of fetal substantia nigra and adrenal medulla to the caudate nucleus in two patients with Parkinson's disease. *New England Journal of Medicine*, **318**, 51.

OU, C.-Y., KWOK, S., MITCHELL, S. W., MACK, D. H., SNINSKY, J. J., KREBS, J. W., FEORINO, P., WARFIELD, D. & SCHOCHETMAN, G. (1988) DNA amplification for direct detection of HIV-1 in DNA of peripheral blood mononuclear cells. *Science*, **239**, 295–7.

POLKINGHORNE REPORT (1989) *Review of the Guidance on the Research Use of Fetuses and Fetal Material.* CM 762. HMSO, London.

REDMOND, D. E. Jr., NAFTOLIN, F., COLLIER, T. J., LERANTH, C., ROBBINS, R. J., SLADEK, C. D., ROTH, R. H. & SLADEK, J. R. Jr.

(1988) Cryopreservation, culture, and transplantation of human fetal mesencephalic tissue into monkeys. *Science*, **242**, 768–71.

REISS, J. & COOPER, D. N. (1990) Application of the polymerase chain reaction to the diagnosis of human genetic disease. *Human Genetics*, **85**, 1–8.

RICHMAN, D., SCHMIDT, N., PLOTKIN, S., YOIKEN, R., CHERENSKY, M., McINTOSH, K. & MATTHEIS, M. (1984) Summary of a workshop on new and useful methods in rapid viral diagnosis. *Journal of Infectious Diseases*, **150**, 941–51.

SEIGER, Å. (1988) Collection and use of aborted central nervous system material. *Fetal Therapy*, **3**, 8–13.

SILVESTRE, L., DUBOIS, C., RENAULT, M., REZVANI, Y., BALIEU, E.-E. & ULMANN, A. (1990) Voluntary interruption of pregnancy with mifepristone (RU 486) and a prostaglandin analogue. *New England Journal of Medicine*, **322**, 645–8.

STEELE, R. W., LIMAS, C., THURMAN, G. B., SCHUELEIN, M., BAUER, H. & BELLANTI, J. A. (1972) Familial thymic aplasia. Attempted reconstitution with fetal thymus in a Millipore diffusion chamber. *New England Journal of Medicine*, **287**, 787–91.

STEGALL, M. D., SUTHERLAND, D. E. R. & HARDY M. A. (1988) Registry report on clinical experience with islet transplantation. In: *Transplantation of the Endocrine Pancreas in Diabetes Mellitis*, pp. 224–33. Eds. Van Schilsgaarde & Hardy, M. A. Elsevier, Amsterdam.

THOMSON, N. M., HANCOCK, W. M., LAFFERTY, K. J., KRAFT, N. & AITKINS, R. C. (1983) Organ culture reduces Ia-positive cells present within the human fetal pancreas. *Transplantation Proceedings*, **15**, 1373–6.

THONG, Y. H., ROBERTSON, E. F., HENRY, G., RISCHBIETH, H. G., SMITH, G. J., BINNS, G. F., CHENEY, K. & POLLARD, A. C., (1978) Successful restoration of immunity in the DiGeroge syndrome with fetal thymic epithelial transplant. *Archives of the Diseases in Childhood*, **53**, 580–4.

TOURAINE, J. L., RONCAROLO, M. G., ROYO, C. & TOURAINE, F. (1987) Fetal tissue transplantation, bone marrow transplantation and prospective gene therapy in severe immunodeficiencies and enzyme deficiencies. *Thymus*, **10**, 75–87.

TUCH, B. E. & TURLE, J. R. (1987) Long-term organ culture of large numbers of human fetal pancreata: analysis of their insulin secretion. *Diabetic Medicine*, **4**, 116–21.

von DORCHE H. H., REIHER, H., HAHN, H.-J., FÄLT, K. & FALKMER, S. (1987) Tissue cultivation as a method for preservation of human fetal islet parenchyma – a correlated biochemical, immunohistochemical and morphometric investigation. *Diabetes Research*, **5**, 157–61.

WONG, L. (1988) Medical Research Council Tissue Bank. In: *Report of the Human Fetal Tissue Transplantation Research Panel*, Vol. II. pp. D267–D282. Consultants to the Advisory Committee to the Director, National Institutes of Health, USA.

WRIGHT, E. V. (1976) Chromosomes and human development. In: *The Biology of Human Fetal Growth*. Symposia of the Society for the Study of Human Biology, **15**, 237–52. Taylor and Francis, London.

CHAPTER 6

Transplantation of fetal haemopoietic and lymphopoietic cells in humans, with special reference to in utero transplantation

J.-L. TOURAINE

CONTENTS

THE TRANSPLANTATION of normal haemopoietic stem cells can cure a number of diseases in experimental animals as well as in humans. Stem cells, emerging from the yolk sac, migrate to the fetal liver and then to the bone marrow. In the latter two tissues, they develop in an appropriate microenvironment among a large variety of other cells. The bone marrow contains, in particular, T lymphocytes which developed in the thymus after this organ has been colonized by fetal liver or bone marrow prethymocytes and then returned back to the bone marrow or, to a lesser extent and only after the thirteenth week postfertilization, to the human fetal liver. Bone marrow transplantation (BMT) is a very effective treatment in many severe congenital disorders as well as in a number of inherited or acquired haematological diseases (Gatti *et al.*, 1968; Koning *et al.*, 1969; Thomas *et al.*, 1975; Bortin & Rimm, 1977; Touraine *et al.*, 1987).

Many patients have no HLA-identical donor available and the incompatible transplant is responsible for severe graft-versus-host disease (GvHD). Since GvHD is induced by the T lymphocytes which are present in the transplant and which react with host tissues (Grebe & Streilen, 1976; Korngold & Sprent, 1982), transplants from a donor who is not genotypically HLA-identical must be preceded by T cell depletion of the bone marrow. This manoeuvre reduces the incidence

155

of GvHD but is associated with an increased risk of graft failure, incomplete reconstitution, EBV-induced lymphomas, or leukaemia relapse (O'Reilly et al., 1983; Fischer et al., 1986). It is therefore of considerable interest that fetal liver stem cells can reconstitute the haemopoietic and lymphopoietic systems of experimental animals and humans without severe GvHD, even in cases of full donor–host incompatibility (Bortin & Saltzstein, 1969; Löwenberg, 1975; Touraine, 1983; Prümmer et al., 1985; Champlin et al., 1987; Touraine et al., 1987).

Since the pioneering work of Uphoff in 1958, much has been learned in the field of experimental and clinical fetal liver transplantation (FLT). Most of the studies have been carried out in mice (Löwenberg, 1975; Boersma, 1983). They have shown the effectiveness of fetal liver transplants in correcting the haematological and immunological consequences of lethal doses of irradiation (Uphoff, 1958; Löwenberg 1975; A. Aitouche & J.-L. Touraine, in preparation). Such an irradiation is the most frequent conditioning treatment given to mice in order to induce the take of allogeneic stem cells and invoke the immunological tolerance to the histoincompatible antigens expressed by these cells (A. Aitouche & J.-L. Touraine, in preparation). Following the establishment of a stable chimerism, full tolerance to tissues of the donor strain can be demonstrated. Fetal transplants can also cure the immunodeficiency of severe combined immunodeficiency (SCID) mice (Sanhadji et al., 1990), the leukaemia of AKR mice (Touraine et al., 1990), and improve significantly the neurological manifestations and the survival of mice which suffer from an inborn error of metabolism (IEM), the LSD mice (Veyron & Touraine, 1990). Addition of T cells from the same allogeneic donor can accelerate transplant take and a similar effect – without the associated risk of GvHD – appears to be obtainable using factors released by in vitro activated T lymphocytes (H. Plotnicky & J.-L. Touraine, in preparation). Fleischman et al. (1982) and Mintz (1985) have shown that haemopoietic stem cells from the fetal liver can induce reconstitution of erythroid cells in genetically anaemic murine fetuses when injected via the placental circulation. By using computerized statistical models the authors calculated that some animals must have been seeded by only a single donor stem cell which has been sufficient for reconstitution. Fetal tissue is also effective in reconstituting rats (Crouch, 1959; Kelemen et al., 1980) as well as larger and outbred animals: dogs (Löwenberg, 1975); horses (Perryman, 1980); sheep (Bunch et al., 1985); mini-pigs (Andreani et al., 1985); and monkey or sheep fetuses (Flake et al., 1986; Harrison et al., 1989).

The unique and remarkable properties of fetal stem cells, including their considerable capacities for proliferation and differentiation, their ability to become tolerant to host antigens, and to develop normally in the foreign host, have prompted the development of studies on human fetal liver transplantation. A reconstitution of good quality has been obtained in most patients treated, despite the lack of HLA-matching between donor and recipient (Touraine, 1983; Touraine *et al.*, 1987). Infants with SCID have received transplants of fetal liver, together with fetal thymus transplantation from the same allogeneic donor of less than 13 weeks postfertilization (Touraine, 1989; Touraine *et al.*, 1987). Patients with the most severe forms of DiGeorge syndrome have received fetal thymus transplants (J.-L. Touraine & M. G. Roncarolo, in preparation). Patients with severe aplastic anaemia and other haematological diseases can be treated by transplants of fetal liver in certain conditions (Gale, 1987; Kochupillai *et al.*, 1987*a, b*). The severity of inborn errors of metabolism can be improved by fetal liver transplants, and in patients with such diseases, the beneficial effect may result from transplantation of both stem cells and prehepatocytes (Touraine *et al.*, 1991*a*). More recently, fetal liver transplants *in utero* have been demonstrated to be feasible and effective when performed during the early stages of fetal development, immediately after prenatal diagnosis in the human fetus (Touraine 1990; Touraine *et al.*, 1989).

Ethical considerations when procuring fetal cells for transplantation

Fetal organ procurement was organized in accordance with the recommendations of the French National Committee for Bioethics (Touraine, 1985). A few hours following fetal death, the liver and the thymus were removed aseptically. Only fresh, not previously frozen, tissues and cells were used for transplantation.

The team responsible for organ procurement was fully distinct and independent from that involved in pregnancy termination. The ethical considerations were felt to be close to those associated with organ procurement from brain-dead cadavers. The ethics of abortion appeared to be a different matter, requiring its own distinct analysis. Whatever the law on abortion has been in any country, fetal cadavers have always been used to obtain tissue to participate in organ donation. The cause of abortion was not used as an ethical reason to refuse the donation of tissue, since it was considered that no direct association or 'complicity' existed between those inducing abortion and those removing the organs. Similarly, the surgeon who removes organs from a cadaver is not regarded as associated with the cause of death of this cadaver.

In the past, however, minority groups have suggested that the use of organs from voluntary abortions should be denied on the ground that such abortions were morally disputable. Their beliefs have not been supported by the various ethical committees that dealt with these matters. The committees believed that, in our present society, organ removal from a cadaver has no detrimental effect, including no adverse psychological effect on the donor's family, if there is no opposition to it. By contrast, the use of organs and cells removed after death, which are used for transplantation into a patient suffering from an otherwise lethal disease, has a greatly positive effect. Provided that strict conditions are followed, for example: lack of commercial use; lack of justification of abortion by the potential usefulness of the tissues; lack of opposition from parents; independence between teams; use for treatment of severe diseases only, etc., fetal tissue transplantation can thus be applied in the same conditions as organ transplantation (Touraine, 1985). It has even been stated that, in view of the very beneficial result of fetal tissue transplants and the absence of the drawbacks of organ removal from a dead body, it might be unethical to refuse this therapeutic possibility to patients who need it. To consider the human fetus as equivalent to a human being means that the fetus participates in the chain of solidarity between humans, exactly as if it was already a born individual. Recently, the in utero treatment of fetuses has become possible and it has followed the same ethical rules as applied to postnatal treatment. Helping a fetal patient means that transplantation can be undertaken when it is required. Solidarity means that organs can be removed from dead fetuses in order to treat live fetuses needing a transplantation.

Preparation of fetal cells for transplantation

The ages of fetal donors ranged from 7 weeks to 13 weeks postfertilization in transplants to immunodeficient patients and from 8 weeks to 22 weeks in transplants to patients with inborn errors of metabolism. The fetal thymus and liver were gently disrupted using a homogeneizer, and a single-cell suspension was thus prepared in RPMI-1640 medium supplemented with gentamycin.

The cells were counted and their viability was checked using the Trypan blue exclusion method. Those cell suspensions with insufficient viability, i.e. less than 70% when fetuses were below 13 weeks of age and less than 40% above this age, were discarded. The total number of living nucleated cells that were transplanted from an individual fetal liver varied greatly with the age of the fetal donor, and reached a mean of 8×10^8 cells. Thymuses which contained numerous thymocytes, i.e.

13 week-old thymuses, were irradiated with 4000 rads prior to their transplantation, together with syngeneic fetal liver cells, into patients with SCID.

Serological tests were performed on the maternal serum: antigens and antibodies for B hepatitis were assessed, and antibodies for CMV, HIV, C hepatitis, and HTLV 1 and 2 were measured. No tissue was used for transplantation when there was an identified risk of transmitting infectious disease, e.g. HIV infection, B or C hepatitis, septicaemia or other infections in the mother. The tissues were also discarded in cases of certain tumours or in cases of known chromosomal abnormalities. Bacteriological tests were performed on the cell suspension but the results were obtained after the transplant itself. These tests enabled the use of adequate antibiotics in cases of bacterial contamination. The cell suspension was then diluted in the appropriate volume of medium for intraperitoneal injection or intravenous infusion.

Postnatal fetal cell transplantation for severe immunodeficiency diseases or inborn errors of metabolism

Patients

In our Institute, the transplantation of fetal liver cells, in association with syngeneic thymic cells, was used to treat every SCID patient who had no HLA-identical donor available for a bone marrow transplantation. The first infant transplanted in this way was treated in 1976. Immunological reconstitution has been very successful, for the lethal disease has been completely cured, and the teenager is very healthy, living a fully normal life, without any sequelae or treatments. He is the oldest patient who has been cured of SCID thanks to fetal liver and thymus transplantation (FLTT).

Since then, 16 additional patients with SCID (including three with adenosine deaminase deficiency and two with bare lymphocyte syndrome (Touraine *et al.*, 1978; Touraine, 1981)) have also been treated by this method. Another patient with bare lymphocyte syndrome and 6 patients with complete and severe forms of the DiGeorge syndrome received a fetal thymus transplant between 1974 and 1990. Altogether, 24 patients with severe immunodeficiency diseases have been treated by fetal cell transplantation and twelve of them have been cured of their lethal disease (Figure 6.1). Following reconstitution, the clinical status has been very favorable and both the general condition and the immunological results have proven to be stable after the first years (Figure 6.1).

159

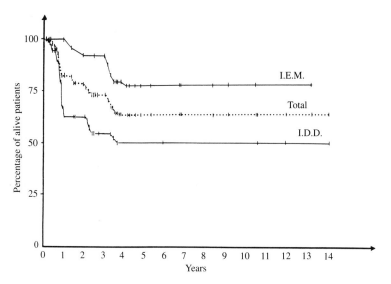

Figure 6.1. Survival of patients with severe immunodeficiency diseases (I.D.D.) or inborn errors of metabolism (I.E.M.), treated by fetal tissue transplantation. The global survival of all patients from these two groups is shown by the line 'Total'. (Reproduced from Touraine (1989) with the permission of *Bone Marrow Transplantation*.)

Proliferation of transplanted cells

Stem cells from fetal liver that were transplanted into these immunodeficient patients proliferated and differentiated in the allogeneic host, resulting in lymphocyte repopulation and immunological reconstitution. Because of their immaturity, stem cells that were confronted by allogeneic antigens acquired immunological tolerance to these antigens. No GvHD occurred initially because the stem cell suspension was devoid of any lymphocyte already engaged in T cell differentiation. Following the differentiation of some stem cells into T lymphocytes, none or only moderate and delayed GvHD was observed.

The immune reconstitution provided by fetal liver transplants can be enhanced by the simultaneous transplantation of thymus from the same donor (Bortin & Saltzstein, 1969; Pahwa *et al.*, 1977). This provides a syngeneic environment for T lymphocyte differentiation of transplanted stem cells. Such a fetal liver and thymus transplantation did not appear to result in an increased risk of GvHD (Bortin & Saltzstein, 1969), at least when the thymus was at an early stage of fetal development.

The number of transplants ranged from one to ten in each of these patients. Repeated transplants of fetal liver and thymus were performed to provide a larger number of stem cells in order to accelerate reconstitution. All patients with SCID were isolated in sterile 'bubbles' and decontaminated as much as possible prior to their transplantations. They were isolated for a prolonged period until a virtually complete reconstitution of cell-mediated immunity was obtained, no matter how long this process took, which could be between six months and $3\frac{1}{2}$ years. The adaptation of these young children to their limited environment has been remarkable and no significant psychological problem has been encountered, either during isolation or after their removal from the 'bubble'.

No attempt at HLA matching of donor and recipient was made. Graft take could be documented easily by identifying cells with an HLA phenotype different from that of the host. Several years after a successful transplant, the numbers of T lymphocytes, their subsets, the proliferative responses to mitogens, allogeneic cells and antigens, the helper T cell activities and the cytotoxic T cell responses were documented as being virtually normal. Immunoglobulin levels and antibody production following vaccination approached normal only after three or four years in most cases; immunoglobulins were of restricted heterogeneity initially then became normal.

Reconstitution of the recipient

Full reconstitution could develop despite a complete mismatch of HLA class I and class II antigens between donor and host. The separation of T and B lymphocyte populations, and the development of cell lines and clones from peripheral blood lymphocytes (PBL) of these patients, followed by HLA typing, showed that all T lymphocytes were of donor origin, while most B lymphocytes and monocytes were of host origin in the reconstituted and now chimeric SCID patients. Several experiments from our laboratory have demonstrated, repeatedly and beyond any doubt, that in such conditions, antigen presenting cells of the host type could effectively present tetanus toxoid antigens or Epstein–Barr virus antigens to the allogeneic T lymphocytes (Roncarolo *et al.*, 1986, 1988*a*; H. Plotnicky & J.-L. Touraine, in preparation). The antigenic peptide is, as usual, presented in the groove of an HLA molecule but, in this case, it is a different HLA molecule from that of the T lymphocyte itself. The study of numerous clones has shown that each T cell clone from these patients can recognize antigen in the context of one given allogeneic HLA determinant (Roncarolo *et al.*, 1986; Roncarolo *et al.*, 1988*a*, *b*).

Similarly, the in vivo defense against virus infections of various kinds has been normal and has not been hindered by the HLA mismatch between infected cells and cytotoxic T lymphocytes that are able to control the infection. Immunological tolerance was also very stable and there was no manifestation of autoimmunity in any of the treated

161

Figure 6.2. Two distinct
varieties of T lymphocytes
differentiating in the thymus,
one with 'Self + X' recognition
structures (left), the other with
'Allo + X' recognition
structures (right). TcR is T cell
receptor for antigen.

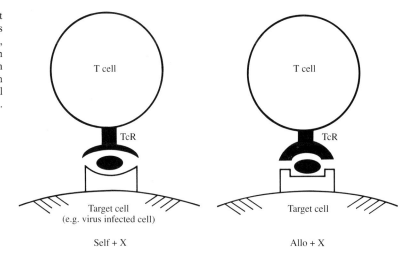

Figure 6.2. Two distinct varieties of T lymphocytes differentiating in the thymus, one with 'Self + X' recognition structures (left), the other with 'Allo + X' recognition structures (right). TcR is T cell receptor for antigen.

children, despite the presence of numerous T cell clones reactive against host antigens in the in vitro tests (Roncarolo *et al.*, 1988*b*; Spits *et al.*, 1990).

In contrast with predictions (Zinkernagel, 1978), T lymphocytes from these chimeric patients had no allogeneic restriction of their functions. This led us to postulate the 'Allo + X' hypothesis (Figure 6.2), according to which some T lymphocytes can develop a recognition for the X antigen in the context of allogeneic determinants instead of the previously known recognition for 'Self + X' (Touraine & Betuel, 1981; Touraine, 1983).

The ontogenic development of T lymphocytes with such recognition structures takes place primarily in the fetal thymus and might be envisioned schematically to occur as follows. A first degree of diversity develops with a variety of thymocytes which have a primary recognition structure for the histocompatibility antigens (possibly associated with a common peptide) (Figure 6.3). In normal circumstances, only those T cells with recognition for self-histocompatibility antigens are solicited, because the alloantigens are not encountered. These cells are induced to proliferate and to develop the full repertoire of antigen recognition in association with self recognition. In chimeric patients, a given set of other histocompatibility antigens is also presented continuously to T cells. Those T cells with recognition for the given alloantigens are then solicited, and they expand by proliferation and develop the gene rearrangement leading to the expression of the T cell receptor. Antigen recognition is then associated with alloantigen recognition. 'Self + X' and 'Allo + X' recognitions are supported by distinct T cells as shown by the analysis of T cell clones: each T cell clone is able to recognize the antigen presented by one histocompatibility determinant only. In chimeric patients, T cells that recognize antigen in the context of allo specificities are positively selected and are therefore found to be very numerous.

Clinical results

Half the patients with immunodeficiency disease had a very good result after fetal tissue transplantation. The causes of failure were mostly severe infections that were already apparent before transplantation: e.g. meningitis with neurologic consequences, resistant *Salmonella* infection, Bacille de Calmette et Guérin (BCG) infection, septicaemia associated with moderate and delayed GvHD. In addition, one child had haemorrhages with renal failure and one infant who had DiGeorge syndrome died of severe cardiopathy.

A variety of inborn errors of metabolism, without associated immunodeficiency, have been treated by fetal liver transplantation, in conjunction with a prolonged immunosuppressive therapy at moderate doses and comparable to those given in non-severe autoimmune diseases. No adverse effect of the treatment was observed. Thirty patients with inborn errors of metabolism had transplants and the diseases that were treated included those in the table below.

Diseases that were treated	No. of patients	Diseases that were treated	No. of patients
Gaucher	5	Hurler	2
Fabry	5	Metachromatic leucodystrophy	2
Familial amyloidosis	3	Adrenoleucodystrophy	1
Fucosidosis	2	Morquio B	1
Niemann Pick A	1	San Filippo B	1
Niemann Pick B	1	Hunter	1
Niemann Pick C	2	Gangliosidosis (GM 2)	1
Glycogenosis	2		

Most patients are in relatively good condition and display objective criteria of partial improvement (Touraine *et al.*, 1991*a*) (Figure 6.1). By comparison with children with immunodeficiency disease treated by fetal tissue transplantation, patients with inborn errors of metabolism were not cured completely by the fetal transplant but their disease was stabilized for some time after each transplant. Transplantation was repeated in order to maintain the clinical result but some patients with an already advanced deterioration, especially of the central nervous

Figure 6.3. Development and selection of a large variety of T lymphocytes with distinct recognition structures, during the differentiation process from the stem cell after migration to the thymus. In the figure, c.p. is 'common peptide'; auto Ag p is 'autoantigenic peptide'; p1 ... p4 are 'peptide 1 ... peptide 4'.

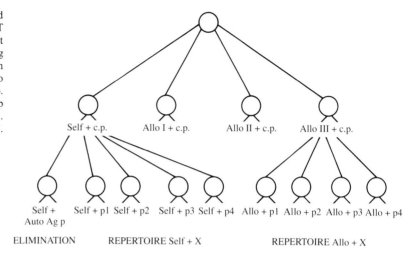

system, progressed eventually to a terminal condition. The serum levels of the defective enzymes were not increased dramatically, but the various substrates that were measured previously were decreased after fetal liver transplantation, and tissue deposits were stabilized. Donors selected for fetal liver transplantation in inborn errors of metabolism were relatively older than those chosen for the same treatment in severe combined immunodeficiency diseases. The respective part played by the stem cells and by the prehepatocytes in the partial improvement that was seen after transplantation is under investigation. The coculture of fetal cells with normal enzyme activities together with defective cells from the patients has shown how the latter benefit from the enzymes released by normal cells present in their vicinity. After transplantation, the viability of the fetal liver cells in the host could be monitored using the sequential measure of serum α-fetoprotein (AFP), and AFP levels rose sharply, then decreased progressively while the cells matured in one to two months.

In both immunodeficiency diseases and inborn errors of metabolism, fetal tissue transplantation has demonstrated beneficial effects. More precisely, 67% of the patients were either cured or improved significantly by the treatment and the survival curves showed a durable efficacy (Figure 6.1). However, almost one third of the patients did not enjoy a significant improvement as a result of fetal liver or thymus transplantation. In most cases, this lack of efficacy was due to either of two factors: (a) an insufficient graft take in patients with rejection capabilities; (b) late diagnosis of the initial disease and the presence of severe infection prior to transplantation. To overcome these two difficulties, we have recently developed in utero transplantation in fetuses with similar conditions that were diagnosed during pregnancy; we reasoned that the earlier the transplant was performed, the chances for graft take would be higher and the risks of infection would be lower.

Prenatal fetal liver transplantation for immunodeficiency diseases

Patients

The case reports of the first two patients treated by in utero fetal liver transplantation are summarized below. Both were fetuses with severe immunodeficiency disease that was diagnosed in mid-gestation. The first patient suffered from bare lymphocyte syndrome (BLS), a genetically-transmitted form of combined immunodeficiency due to a lack of expression of HLA antigens (Touraine 1981; Touraine *et al.*, 1978).

Infections, especially with opportunistic micro-organisms, are responsible for death of infants with BLS, unless they grow up isolated in a fully sterile atmosphere while they are successfully reconstituted with stem cell transplants (SCT). When carried out postnatally, however, such a stem cell transplant in the form of a transplant of either bone marrow or fetal liver is usually associated with graft failure due to the presence of allogeneic reactions in the host (i.e. persisting transplant immunity) and a high susceptibility to infections (i.e. defective immunity to infectious antigens).

This disease, which suggests that immune responses to allogeneic stimuli are acquired at an earlier ontogenic stage than immune responses to antigens, is therefore especially difficult to treat. In contrast with results in most cases of severe combined immunodeficiency disease, the transplantation of stem cells in these infants usually leads to graft rejection, unless a major conditioning regimen is administered prior to stem cell transplantation. Such a heavy chemotherapy is poorly tolerated by infants who are already infected. The prenatal diagnosis of bare lymphocyte syndrome can be performed by the HLA analysis of fetal blood lymphocytes (Durandy *et al.*, 1987) and pregnancy termination can be proposed if the parents wish, but at present the diagnosis is not performed before the sixteenth week postfertilization. Indeed, at this stage of fetal development fetoscopy and fetal blood drawing become possible, and HLA expression on normal lymphocytes is very significant (Royo *et al.*, 1987; Touraine *et al.*, 1989), so that the lack of HLA antigens cannot be attributed to a mere cell immaturity.

165

Case 1

Mrs T. had a first child who died of the bare lymphocyte syndrome before 2 years of age, despite an attempted stem cell transplant which did not result in stable graft take and immunological reconstitution. When she became pregnant again, she requested prenatal diagnosis. At 19 weeks postfertilization, a fetal blood sample (1.5 ml) was obtained by means of a direct umbilical cord puncture with a 20 G spinal needle, under ultrasound visualization (Daffos *et al.*, 1983; Berkowitz *et al.*, 1987). The placenta was posteriorly situated and the puncture of the umbilical vein was performed 2 cm ahead of the cord insertion on the placenta. The purity of the fetal blood sample was ascertained by means of Ii typing. Fetal blood lymphocytes were analysed for their expression of HLA antigens using fluorescent monoclonal antibodies and a cytofluorometer. The virtually complete lack of expression of both class I and class II HLA antigens at the cell surface, contrasting with findings in immunologically normal fetuses, led to the diagnosis of type III BLS. Three choices were offered to the parents:

(a) therapeutic abortion

(b) no treatment before birth and stem cell transplants after birth

(c) in utero stem cell transplant followed by a further postnatal stem cell transplant

She was informed that the latter treatment was unprecedented and that its results were therefore uncertain.

The parents decided to have the earliest possible transplant. In June 1988, at the twenty eighth week postfertilization, a second fetal blood puncture was performed under direct ultrasound visualization at the insertion of the umbilical vein on the placenta. Following the withdrawal of 5 ml fetal blood, a stem cell transplant was carried out by infusion into the umbilical vein of 7 ml culture medium containing a suspension of 16×10^6 fetal liver cells and fetal thymic epithelial cells (Touraine *et al.*, 1989). The technique for intravenous infusion was comparable to that used for intravascular intrauterine transfusions (Berkowitz *et al.*, 1987). Liver and thymic cells were obtained from two dead fetuses (aged 7 weeks and $7\frac{1}{2}$ weeks postfertilization). Over the months following the in utero transplant, no adverse effects were observed in the pregnant woman or in her baby, and the child (D. T.) was born normally in August 1988 (Table 6.1).

At birth, the diagnosis of bare lymphocyte syndrome was again confirmed but some cells with class I HLA antigens became progressively detectable. As shown in Figure 6.4, 10% of the lymphocytes had a normal expression of class I HLA antigens at the age of 1 month

Table 6.1. *Conditions and results of the first three fetal liver transplants carried out* in utero

Patients	Diseases	Ages of fetal patients[a]	Ages of fetal donors[a]	Date of transplant	Date of birth	Outcome
D.T.	BLS	28	7 & 7.5	30 Jun. 88	17 Aug. 88	Graft take (HLA) and immunological reconstitution
M.H.	SCID	26	7.5	8 Jun. 89	7 Aug. 89	Some graft take (Y chrom) and yet limited immunological reconstitution
M.R.	Thalassemia	12	9.5	10 Oct. 89	25 Mar. 90	Some graft take (Y chrom) and thalassemia still present

Note:
[a] Weeks postfertilization.
Source: Reproduced from Touraine *et al.* (1991*b*) with the permission of *Bone Marrow Transplantation.*

(Touraine *et al.*, 1989) and these cells were of donor origin, since their HLA specificities, of donor type, were not inherited from the child's parents. In particular, these cells expressed the HLA A9 specificity of donor origin, which made transplanted cells readily detectable in the initial test, both at birth and in subsequent tests. These results demonstrated the persisting engraftment of the fetal liver cells infused into the sick fetus. Based on past experience, graft take is known to be very difficult in BLS after birth, without heavy preconditioning. The engraftment was therefore attributed to the state of immaturity of the patient's immune system at the time of the transplant. Investigations carried out on the peripheral blood lymphocytes of the patient, at this same time, i.e., at the twenty eighth week postfertilization, indeed showed a more significant immaturity of T cells than is found in normal fetuses of identical age.

The expression of class II HLA antigens remained comparatively low at the surface of resting lymphocytes. This finding confirmed that B cell development does not occur as rapidly as T cell differentiation, following stem cell transplantation in immunodeficient patients (Touraine *et al.*, 1987).

As scheduled initially, the newborn was placed in a sterile bubble and, to accelerate reconstitution, he received seven additional transplants from nine fetal donors. This complementary treatment was carried out after the tests demonstrating an engraftment of the in utero transfused stem cells.

No engraftment of the cells that were infused after birth could be demonstrated, confirming the 'resistance' to transplantation in these patients. However, the number of cells deriving from the in utero transplant increased and was found to be 26% among peripheral blood

Figure 6.4. Cytofluorometric analysis of peripheral blood lymphocytes with W6/32 anti-HLA-ABC monoclonal antibody. A = normal cells; B = cells of the patient 1 month after birth (i.e. 3 months after fetal liver transplantation and before additional cell infusion). In B two populations of cells are identified, a larger one with HLA deficiency (patient's cells) and another, smaller, with normal HLA expression (donor-derived cells). (Reproduced from Touraine (1981) with the permission of *Lancet*.)

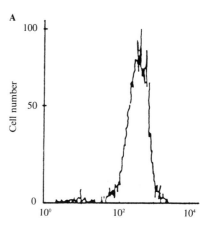

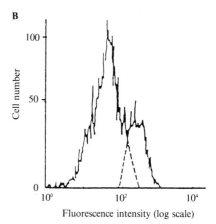

lymphocytes at 1 year. In parallel, T cell maturity and immunological reconstitution progressed. Although this reconstitution cannot yet be considered to be absolutely complete, the proliferative responses to antigens, including *Candida* antigens, cytomegalovirus (CMV) antigens, tetanus toxoid, etc., have occurred and progressed up to a normal degree. Immunoglobulin levels are still relatively low, a finding that is consistent with the previous observation of a slow reconstitution of humoral immunity following fetal liver transplantation (Touraine *et al.*, 1987).

Because of this T cell reconstitution from in utero transplanted cells and in view of the patient's good health, this infant was allowed to leave the isolator at the age of 16 months. The child's present condition is excellent. He has not developed any infection and he lives a normal life at home. He only receives immunoglobulins every month until he produces sufficient amounts of IgM and IgG.

After this first in utero fetal liver graft, and in view of the most encouraging results observed, a second fetus with immunodeficiency disease was treated prenatally in 1989.

Case 2

This second patient (M. H.) was a younger fetus with a complete form of severe combined immunodeficiency disease. He was treated with fetal liver in June 1989, at the age of 26 weeks postfertilization, after the prenatal diagnosis of severe immunodeficiency had been done. This revealed a complete lack of $CD2^+$, $CD3^+$, $CD4^+$, and $CD8^+$ lymphocytes in the peripheral blood of this fetus, while B cells were present, these findings being superimposable with those obtained in the first child of the family who also had severe combined immunodeficiency disease.

The transplant was carried out using the same conditions as in the first fetus who was treated in utero. It involved the intravenous infusion of 37×10^6 fetal liver cells through the umbilical vein of the fetal patient, under ultrasound control. The age of the donor was $7\frac{1}{2}$ weeks postfertilization; the age of the recipient at the time of the transplant was 26 weeks postfertilization. There were no side effects and the child was born normally in August 1989 (Table 6.1).

At birth, the female patient still had immunological manifestations of severe combined immunodeficiency disease. Therefore, she has been maintained in sterile isolation and has received additional infusions of fetal liver and thymus cells, with the aim to accelerate development of the in utero transplanted stem cells.

By amplification techniques, DNA fragments that are specific to the Y chromosome have been repeatedly demonstrated to be present in the DNA material prepared from the peripheral blood lymphocytes of this girl. Engraftment has been obtained, therefore, but the number of donor cells in this patient is considered to be still insufficient to sustain life in an unprotected environment. Isolation is prolonged until transplanted stem cells have proliferated further and have differentiated into T lymphocytes with adequate immune functions.

Prenatal fetal liver transplantation for thalassemia

The results obtained in immunodeficiency diseases prompted us to attempt in utero fetal liver transplants in fetal patients with severe non-immune haematological disorders. In such conditions, however, graft take may not be facilitated by immune incompetence of the fetal host, and we assumed that the grafting had to be carried out during the first trimester of pregnancy, at a time when normal fetuses have not yet developed cell-mediated immunity (Royo *et al.*, 1987).

Case 3

A pregnant woman with a family history of thalassemia solicited precocious prenatal diagnosis. By molecular biology techniques, the fetus was demonstrated to have β^0 thalassemia major. The mother refused abortion for religious reasons, and she asked for fetal liver transplantation *in utero*. She was informed of the uncertainty of results in such a disease.

The transplantation was carried out in a fetal patient (M. R.) whose age was 12 weeks postfertilization. The transplant consisted of the intraperitoneal injection of 3×10^8 viable fetal liver cells obtained from a fetus of $9\frac{1}{2}$ weeks postfertilization. There was no adverse effect in the mother nor in the recipient fetus. Birth occurred in March 1990 (Table 6.1). The site of puncture could hardly be seen on the abdominal skin of the newborn and ultrasound investigations demonstrated no modification of the abdominal wall.

Studies performed after birth showed presence of thalassemia. However, there were a few cells of donor origin: amplification techniques revealed Y chromosome-specific DNA fragments in the peripheral blood lymphocytes of this girl. In addition, haemoglobin A (HbA) was found to account for 0.9% of all haemoglobin (Table 6.2).

This infant received no further transplant and, one year after birth, was in very good general condition. Further investigations will follow the donor cells and determine whether they can proliferate to a larger degree and improve the thalassemic condition.

Conclusion

The efficacy of fetal liver transplantation in children and adults with a variety of diseases is most encouraging. In many cases, it already represents a valuable alternative to bone marrow transplantation, especially when there is no HLA-identical donor available. In the future, cultured stem cells from the fetal liver, administered together with appropriate factors, may offer a routine therapy to replace adequately any of the cell lineage of the haematopoietic or lymphopoietic system.

The most recent development of fetal liver transplantation, administered into human fetuses *in utero*, is described in detail herein. The feasibility and efficacy of grafting this tissue into fetuses, before the end of the first trimester in one case, gives results that are consistent with

Table 6.2. *Postnatal haematological data in the patient M. R.*

Girl with β^0 thalassemia who received fetal liver grafts during her fetal life.

Y chromosome (of donor origin): present		
HbA	=	0.9%
Hb	:	10 g/dl
MCH	:	23.8 pg
MCV	:	68.1 fl
WBC	:	14 000/μl

Note:
Hb is haemoglobin; MCH is haemoglobin per red cells; MCV is mean corpuscular volume; WBC are white blood cells.
Source: Reproduced from Touraine *et al.* (1991*b*) with the permission of *Bone Marrow Transplantation.*

experimental data in animals (Flake *et al.*, 1986; Harrison *et al.*, 1989). They confirm the model of induced tolerance described by Billingham *et al.* (1953), and demonstrate that the procedure can be effective in humans provided that transplantation is performed relatively younger in humans than in rodents (owing to the earlier development of the human immune system in the fetus). Stem cell engraftment is obtained consistently: it results in cure of inherited immunodeficiency and is likely to induce some improvement of other inborn errors of metabolism, such as thalassemia. To increase further the effectiveness of this procedure in the latter cases that do not involve immunodeficiency, it may be useful to increase the number of donor cells and to perform fetal liver transplantation in a fetal host who is even younger.

The main reasons for developing in utero grafts of fetal liver are the following:

(a) increased probability of graft take and chimerism, especially in diseases, such as bare lymphocyte syndrome in which a residual immunity can induce rejection, and even more so in diseases without immunodeficiency provided that it is performed in very young fetuses

(b) improved isolation at the time of the transplant, since the uterus is even better than a sterile bubble

(c) more optimal environment for fetal cell development when transplanted into the fetus rather than into the infant.

The earlier the transplant is performed the larger will be the chance of full and rapid development of the transplanted cells. Whether or not the use of additional therapy might be safe and beneficial for fetuses with normal immunity has not been investigated and will obviously have to be studied carefully in animal models before using with humans.

Fetal cell transplants can completely cure half the patients with severe congenital immunodeficiencies who are treated after birth (Touraine *et al.*, 1987). In utero transplants are likely to result in a higher rate of success, with a low incidence of rejection, even in difficult conditions e.g. bare lymphocyte syndrome or adenosine deaminase deficiency. At present in most cases, prenatal diagnosis of these conditions results in deciding to terminate the pregnancy. This new opportunity of in utero treatment may represent a more satisfying solution than abortion of the sick fetus. In inherited haematological diseases and in other inborn errors of metabolism it is also likely to offer a good therapeutic solution until gene therapy becomes more readily applicable and effective *in vivo*.

Acknowledgments

I am very grateful to F. Barbier, H. Bétuel, D. Frappaz, F. Freycon, L. Gebuhrer, E. Goillot, S. Laplace, N. Philippe, D. Raudrant, A. Rebaud, F. Rezzoug, M. G. Roncarolo, C. Royo, K. Sanhadji, G. Souillet, F. Touraine, C. Vullo and M. T. Zabot for their great contribution to patient care and to immunological studies.

Note added in proof. Since this chapter was written, the efficacy of in utero FLT has been further confirmed in the 3 patients: the first child is in very good health; the second infant has on-going immunological reconstitution and has left isolation to live normally at home; and the percentage of haemoglobin A has increased in peripheral blood of the third patient.

References

ANDREANI, M., DE BIAGI, M. CENTIS, F., MANNA, M., AGOSTI-
NELLI, F., FILIPETTI, A., GAUDENZI, G., MURETTO, P.,
GRIANTI, C., SOTTI, G., RIGON, A. & LUCARELLI, G. (1985) Fetal
liver transplantation in the mini-pig. In *Progress in Clinical and Biological
Research: Fetal Liver Transplantation*, pp. 205–17. Eds. R. P. Gale, J.-L.
Touraine & G. Lucarelli. Alan R. Liss, Inc., New York.

BERKOWITZ, R. L., CHITKARA, U., WILKINS, I., LYNCH, L. &
MEHALEK, K. E. (1987) Technical aspects of intravascular intrauterine
transfusions: Lessons learned from 33 procedures. *American Journal of
Obstetrics & Gynecology*, **157**, 4–9.

BOERSMA, W. J. A. (1983) Prothymocytes in mouse fetal liver. *Thymus*, **5**,
419–28.

BORTIN, M. M. & RIMM, A. A. (1977) Severe combined immunodeficiency
disease: Characterization of the disease and results of transplantation.
Journal of the American Medical Association, **238**, 591–600.

BORTIN, M. M. & SALTZSTEIN, E. C. (1969) Graft-versus-host inhibition:
Fetal liver and thymus cells to minimize secondary disease. *Science*, **164**,
316–18.

BILLINGHAM, R. E., BRENT, L. & MEDAWAR, P. B. (1953) Actively
acquired tolerance of foreign cells. *Nature*, **172**, 603–6.

BUNCH, C., WOOD, W. G. & KELLY, S. J. (1985) Fetal hemopoietic-cell
transplantation in sheep: An approach to the cellular control of hemoglobin
switching. In: *Progress in Clinical and Biological Research: Fetal Liver
Transplantation*, pp. 219–33. Eds. R. P. Gale, J.-L. Touraine & G. Lucarelli.
Alan R. Liss, Inc., New York.

CHAMPLIN, R. E., CAIN, G., STITZEL, K. & GALE, R. P. (1987) Sustained recovery of hematopoiesis and immunity following transplantation of
fetal liver cells in dogs. *Thymus*, **10**, 13–18.

CROUCH, B. G. (1959) Transplantation of fetal hemopoietic tissues into
irradiated mice and rats. In: *Proceedings of the Seventh Congress of the
European Society for Haematology*, p. 973, London.

DAFFOS, F., CAPELLA-PAVLOVSKY, M. & FORESTIER, F. (1983) A
new procedure for fetal blood sampling *in utero*. *American Journal of
Obstetrics & Gynecology*, **146**, 985–7.

DURANDY, A., CERF-BENSUSSAN, N., DUMEZ, Y. & GRISCELLI, C.
(1987) Prenatal diagnosis of severe combined immunodeficiency with
detective synthesis of HLA molecule. *Prenatal Diagnosis*, **7**, 27–31.

FISCHER, A., GRISCELLI, C., FRIEDRICH, W., KUBANECK, B.,
LEVINKSY, R., MORGAN, G., VOSSEN, J., WAGEMAKER, G. &
LANDAIS, P. (1986) Bone marrow transplantation for immunodeficien-
cies and osteopetrosis: European Survey, 1968–1985. *Lancet*, **ii**, 1080–3.

FLAKE, A. W., HARRISON, M. R., ADZICK, N. S. & ZANJANI, E. D.

(1986) Transplantation of fetal haemopoietic stem cells *in utero*: the creation of haemopoietic chimeras. *Science*, **233**, 776–8.

FLEISCHMAN, R. A., CLUSTER, R. P. & MINTZ, B. (1982) Totipotent hematopoietic stem cells: Normal self-renewal and differentiation after transplantation between mouse fetuses. *Cell*, **30**, 351–9.

GALE, R. P. (1987) Fetal liver transplantation in aplastic anemia and leukemia. *Thymus*, **10**, 89–94.

GATTI, R. A., ALLEN, H. D., MEUWISSEN, H. J., HONG, R. & GOOD, R. A. (1968) Immunological reconstitution in sex-linked lymphopenic immunological deficiency. *Lancet*, **ii**, 1366.

GREBE, S. C. & STREILEN, J. W. (1976) Graft-versus-host reactions: A review. *Advances in Immunology*, **22**, 119–221.

HARRISON, M. R., SLOTNICK, R. N., CROMBLEHOLME, T. M., GOLBUS, M. S., TARANTAL, A. F. & ZANJANI, E. D. (1989) In utero transplantation of fetal liver haemopoietic stem cells in monkeys. *Lancet*, **ii**, 1425–7.

KELEMEN, E., GULYA, E. & SZABO, L. (Hatvan) (1980) Xenogeneic transfer of fetal liver- and adult bone marrow-derived hemopoietic cells in rodents. In: *Fetal Liver Transplantation, Current Concepts and Future Directions*, pp. 168–74. Eds. G. Lucarelli, T. M. Fleidner & R. P. Gale. Excerpta Medica, Amsterdam.

KOCHUPILLAI, V., SHARMA, S., FRANCIS, S., NANU, A., MATHEW, S., BHATIA, P., DUA, H., KUMAR, L., AGGARWAL, S., SINGH, S., KUMAR, S., KARAK, A. & BHARGAVA, M. (1987a) Fetal liver infusion in aplastic anemia. *Thymus*, **10**, 95–102.

KOCHUPILLAI, V., SHARMA, S., FRANCIS, S., NANU, A., VERMA, I.C., DUA, H., KUMAR, L., AGGARWAL, S. & SINGH, S. (1987b) Fetal liver infusion in acute myelogenous leukæmia. *Thymus*, **10**, 117–24.

KONING, J. de, VAN BEKKUM, D. W., DICKE, A., DOOREN, L. J., van ROOD, J. J. & RADL, J. (1969) Transplantation of bone marrow cells and fetal thymus in an infant with lymphopenic immunological deficiency. *Lancet*, **i**, 1223–7.

KORNGOLD, R. & SPRENT, J. (1982) Features of T-cells causing H-2 restricted lethal graft-versus-host disease across minor histocompatibility barrier. *Journal of Experimental Medicine*, **155**, 182.

LOWENBERG, B. (1975) *Fetal liver cell transplantation*. Thesis. Erasmus University Rotterdam. Publication of the Radiobiological Institute of the Organisation for Health Research TNO, Rijswijk (ZH), The Netherlands.

MINTZ, B. (1985) Renewal and differentiation of totipotent hematopoietic stem cells of the mouse after transplantation into early fetuses. In: *Progress in Clinical and Biological Research: Fetal Liver Transplantation*, pp. 3–16. Eds. R. P. Gale, J.-L. Touraine & G. Lucarelli. Alan R. Liss, Inc., New York.

O'REILLY, R. J., KAPOOR, N., KIRKPATRICK, D., FLOMENBERG, N., POLLACK, M. S., DUPONT, B., GOOD, R. A. & REISNER, Y. (1983) Transplantation of hematopoietic cells for lethal congenital immunodeficiencies. In: *Primary Immunodeficiency Diseases, The March of Dimes Birth Defects Foundation*, pp. 129–37. Eds. R. J. Wedgwood, F. S. Rosen & N. W. Paul. Alan R. Liss, Inc., New York.

PAHWA, R., PAHWA, S., & GOOD, R. A., INCEFY, G. S. & O'REILLY, R. J. (1977) Rationale for combined use of fetal liver and thymus for immunological reconstitution in patients with variants of severe combined immunodeficiency. *Proceedings of the National Academy of Sciences, USA,* **74**, 3002–5.

PERRYMAN, L. E. (1980) Use of fetal tissues for immunoreconstitution in horses with severe combined immunodeficiency. In: *Fetal Liver Transplantation, Current Concepts and Future Directions,* pp. 183–97. Eds. G. Lucarelli, T. M. Fleidner & R. P. Gale. Excerpta Medica, Amsterdam.

PRÜMMER, O., RAGHAVARVACHAR, A., WERNER, C., CALVO, W., CARBONELL, F., STEINBACH, I. & FLIEDNER, T. M. (1985) Fetal liver transplantation in the dog. *Transplantation,* **39**, 349–55.

RONCAROLO, M. G., TOURAINE, J.-L. & BANCHEREAU, J. (1986) Cooperation between major histocompatibility complex mismatched mononuclear cells from a human chimera in the production of antigen-specific antibody. *Journal of Clinical Investigation,* **77**, 673–80.

RONCAROLO, M. G., YSSEL, H., TOURAINE, J.-L., BACCHETTA, R., GEBUHRER, L., DE VRIES, J. E. & SPITS, H. (1988a) Antigen recognition by MHC-incompatible cells of a human mismatched chimera. *Journal of Experimental Medicine,* **167**, 2139–52.

RONCAROLO, M. G., YSSEL, H., TOURAINE, J.-L., BETUEL, H. DE VRIES, J. E. & SPITS, H. (1988b) Autoreactive T cell clones specific for class I and class II HLA antigens isolated from a human chimera. *Journal of Experimental Medicine,* **167**, 1523–34.

ROYO, C., TOURAINE, J.-L. & DE BOUTEILLER, O. (1987) Ontogeny of T lymphocyte differentiation in the human fetus: Acquisition of phenotype and functions. *Thymus,* **10**, 57–73.

SANHADJI, K., NEGRIER, M. S. & TOURAINE, J.-L. (1990) Fetal liver cell transplantation in SCID mice. *Thymus,* **15**, 57–64.

SPITS, H., TOURAINE, J.-L., YSSEL, H., DE VRIES, J. E. & RONCAROLO, M. G. (1990) Presence of host-reactive and MHC-restricted T cells in a transplanted severe combined immunodeficient (SCID) patient suggest positive selection and absence of clonal deletion. *Immunological Reviews,* **116**, 101–16.

THOMAS, E. D., STOEB, R., CLIFT, R. A., FEFER, A., JOHNSON, F. L., NEIMAN, P. E., LERNER, K. G., GLUCKSBERG, H. & BUCKNER, C. D. (1975) Bone marrow transplantation. *New England Journal of Medicine,* **292**, 832–43 & 895–902.

TOURAINE, J.-L. (1981) The Bare Lymphocyte Syndrome: Report on the registry. *Lancet,* **i**, 319–21.

TOURAINE, J.-L. (1983) Bone marrow and fetal liver transplantation in immunodeficiencies and inborn errors of metabolism: Lack of significant restriction of T-cell function in long-term chimeras despite HLA-mismatch. *Immunological Reviews,* **71**, 103–21.

TOURAINE, J.-L. (1985) *Hors de la Bulle,* vol. 1. Flammarion, Paris.

TOURAINE, J.-L. (1989) New strategies in the treatment of immunological and other inherited diseases: Allogeneic stem cells transplantation. *Bone Marrow Transplantation,* **4**, (Supplement 4), 139–41.

TOURAINE, J.-L. (1990) In utero transplantation of stem cells in humans. *Nouvelle Revue Francaise d'Hématologie,* **32**, 441–4.

TOURAINE, J.-L. & BETUEL, H. (1981) Immunodeficiency diseases and expression of HLA antigens. *Human Immunology,* **2**, 147–53.

175

TOURAINE, J.-L., BETUEL, H., SOUILLET, G. & JEUNE, M. (1978) Combined immunodeficiency disease associated with absence of cell-surface HLA A and B antigens. *Journal of Pediatrics*, **93**, 47–51.

TOURAINE, J.-L., LAPLACE, S., REZZOUG, F., SANHADJI, K., GOILLOT, E., de BOUTEILLER, O., GARNIER, J.-L., POUTEIL-NOBLE, C., RAFFAELE, P., LIVROZET, J.-M., SAINT-MARC, T., VEYRON, P., ROYO, C., ZABOT, M.-T. & MAIRE, I. (1991*a*) Fetal liver transplantation in inborn errors of metabolism. *Journal of Inherited Metabolic Disease*, in press.

TOURAINE, J.-L., RAUDRANT, D., ROYO, C., REBAUD, A., RONCAROLO, M.G., SOUILLET, G., PHILIPPE, N., TOURAINE, F. & BETUEL, H. (1989) In utero transplantation of stem cells in the bare lymphocyte syndrome. *Lancet*, **i**, 1382.

TOURAINE, J.-L., RAUDRANT, D., VULLO, C., FRAPPAZ, D., FREYCON, F., REBAUD, A., BARBIER, F., RONCAROLO, M. G., GEBURHER, L., BETUEL, H. & ZABOT, M. T. (1991*b*) New developments in stem cell transplantation with special reference to the first in utero transplants in humans. *Bone Marrow Transplantation*, **7**, Supplement 3, 92–7.

TOURAINE, J.-L., RONCAROLO, M. G., ROYO, C. & TOURAINE, F. (1987) Fetal tissue transplantation, bone marrow transplantation and prospective gene therapy in severe immunodeficiencies and enzyme deficiencies. *Thymus*, **10**, 75–87.

TOURAINE, J.-L., ROYO, C. & GITTON, X. (1990) Are fetal liver cells able to amount a graft-versus-leukemia effect? *Experimental Hematology*, **18**, 657.

UPHOFF, D. E. (1958) Preclusion of secondary phase of irradiation syndrome by inoculation of fetal hematopoietic tissue following total-body X-irradiation. *Journal of the National Cancer Institute*, **20**, 625–32.

VEYRON, P. & TOURAINE, J.-L. (1990) Fetal liver cell transplantation: survival of affected grafted Balb/c LSD mice. *Transplantation Proceedings*, **22**, 2253–4.

ZINKERNAGEL, R. M. (1978) The thymus: Its influence on recognition of 'self-major-histocompatibility antigens' by T-cells and consequences for reconstitution of immunodeficiency. *Springer Seminars in Immunopathology*, **1**, 405.

CHAPTER 7

The biology of fetal brain tissue grafts:
from mouse to man

H. SAUER, S. B. DUNNETT and P. BRUNDIN

CONTENTS

NEURAL TRANSPLANTATION TO THE MAMMALIAN BRAIN is a field of long-standing interest to neuroscientists. Since the first reports on cortex or spinal cord grafting experiments around the turn of the century (Thompson, 1890; Shirres, 1905), the demonstration that immature brain tissue can survive (Dunn, 1917) and differentiate (Le Gros Clarke, 1940) in the adult host brain form milestones on the way to a more widespread application of neural grafting techniques since the early- and mid-seventies (Das & Altman, 1971). The finding that grafts of fetal ventral mesencephalic tissue, rich in dopamine (DA) neurons, can reverse lesion-induced functional deficits in an animal model of Parkinson's disease (Björklund & Stenevi, 1979; Perlow *et al.*, 1979) has led to increased interest in neural transplantation in a wide variety of animal models of neurodegenerative diseases and other forms of neuronal or neuroendocrine dysfunction. Neural transplants of fetal brain tissue have since been investigated in animal models of Huntington's chorea (Deckel *et al.*, 1983; Isacson *et al.*, 1986); Alzheimer's disease (Dunnett, 1990); hypogonadotropic hypogonadism (Krieger *et al.*, 1982; Gibson *et al.*, 1984); diabetes insipidus (Gash & Sladek, 1984); epilepsy (Barry *et al.*, 1987); demyelinating diseases (Lachapelle *et al.*, 1984); cerebellar ataxia (Sotelo & Alvarado-

Mallart, 1986); callosal agenesis (Smith *et al.*, 1987); spinal cord injury (Nygren *et al.*, 1977; Nornes *et al.*, 1983; Reier, 1985); cerebral ischemia and stroke (Mudrick *et al.*, 1988; Tønder *et al.*, 1989; Onifer & Low, 1990); cortical hypoplasia (Lee & Rabe, 1988, 1990); drug-induced prenatal brain damage (Yanai & Pick, 1988); and retinal degeneration (Turner & Blair, 1986).

The unique experimental situation created by grafting fetal brain tissue to the adult host brain has posed many fascinating questions. Which developmental characteristics does immature neural tissue display in a differentiated environment? How does the adult host brain react to the grafted immature tissue? Does this represent an unnatural situation where abnormal development and interaction occurs or may it allow for insights into the mechanisms governing neural differentiation, plasticity and regeneration? As has gradually emerged over the last fifteen years, the developmental potential of different fetal CNS tissues grafted to the adult brain is governed – at least in part – by several basic principles. In order to exemplify these principles, this review will concentrate on intracerebral grafts of fetal ventral midbrain tissue as a source of immature dopaminergic (DAergic) neurons in animal models of Parkinson's disease, which over the last years have led up to initial experimental clinical trials in patients.

Animal models of Parkinson's disease used in neural grafting research

The neuropathological hallmark of Parkinson's disease is a marked degeneration of DA neurons in the substantia nigra of the ventral midbrain and a concomitant decrease in DA content within the primary projection areas, i.e. the caudate nucleus and the putamen. This primary DA deficit leads to a well-defined neurological syndrome of rigidity, tremor, akinesia, and postural instability in man.

The first reliable animal model of Parkinson's disease was created by selectively destroying the DAergic neurons of the substantia nigra through intracerebral infusion of the catecholamine neurotoxin 6-hydroxydopamine (6-OHDA: Trantzer & Thoenen, 1967; Ungerstedt, 1968; Uretzky & Iversen, 1970). In rats, *bilateral* injections of 6-OHDA into the substantia nigra result in degeneration of the nigral DAergic cell populations and in a behavioral syndrome of profound akinesia, aphagia, adipsia, sensory inattention, and a hunched posture (Ungerstedt, 1971*b*; Marshall *et al.*, 1974; Marshall & Teitelbaum, 1977). *Unilateral* infusions of 6-OHDA into the mesotelencephalic DA projection, on the other hand, result in a marked imbalance of striatal DA content and a concomitant motor bias to the ipsilateral side

(Ungerstedt & Arbuthnott, 1970). Unilateral changes secondary to this DA depletion have been shown to occur in the host brain, such as DA receptor supersensitivity in the DA-depleted striatum (Ungerstedt, 1971*a*), and alterations of GABA receptor density in striatal output structures (Penney & Young, 1983; Pan *et al.*, 1985). The resulting behavioral changes include a curvature of the spine towards the side of the lesion; spontaneous motor asymmetry (i.e. a tendency to turn spontaneously towards the side of the lesion); drug-induced circling (towards the side of the lesion in response to challenge with DA-releasing drugs, such as amphetamine; or contralateral to the lesion in response to DA receptor-activating drugs, such as apomorphine or quinpirole); sensory inattention to stimuli applied from the side contralateral to the lesion; and an elevated threshold for initiating movements towards this side (Ungerstedt, 1971*a*, *b*). These behavioral asymmetries were found to be stable and quantifiable, and with a growing knowledge of DA pharmacology the 'rotating rat' model has been developed into a versatile and well-characterized tool in neuroscience and pharmacological research (see Pycock, 1980).

More recently, other animal models of Parkinson's disease have begun to be utilized in experiments with fetal nigral grafts. These studies involve, firstly, grafts into species other than the rat, including mice, cats and primates with unilateral 6-OHDA nigrostriatal lesions (Brundin *et al.*, 1986*a*; Trulson & Hosseini, 1987; Annett *et al.*, 1990). Secondly, the novel DA neurotoxin *N*-methyl-4-phenyl-1,2,3,6-tetrahydropyridine (MPTP) has been assessed following systemic administration in primates (Bakay *et al.*, 1985; Redmond *et al.*, 1986) and mice (Bohn *et al.*, 1987; Zuddas *et al.*, 1991); following intracarotid infusion to achieve unilateral denervation (Dubach *et al.*, 1988; Bankiewicz *et al.*, 1990); or following intracerebral administration of the neurotoxic metabolite MPP$^+$ in rats (Sirinatshingij *et al.*, 1990). Thirdly, the Weaver mutant mouse provides a model in which grafts can be assessed in a progressive neurodegenerative condition (Triarhou *et al.*, 1986, 1990) in contrast to the more acute nature of the lesions in the other models.

Factors governing the development of graft–host interactions

The developmental potential of fetal brain tissue transplants and donor age

All intracerebral grafting experiments conducted in mammals, irrespective of the type of neural tissue that is to be transplanted, share the common feature that the graft tissue has to be immature in order for it to survive transplantation to the host brain. The donor age limits

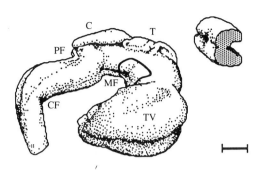

Figure 7.1. Drawing of a brain taken from a 25 mm crown–rump-length human fetus (approximately 8 weeks postconception). When preparing donor tissue for grafting to patients or animal models of Parkinson's disease, the ventral mesencephalon is microdissected from the brainstem of the aborted fetus with the help of fine watchmakers forceps and iridectomy scissors. Useful landmarks for dissection are the cervical (CF), pontine (PF), and mesencephalic flexures (MF), the developing cerebellum (C), the tectum (T) and the telencephalic vesicles (TV). The dissected piece contains the developing dopaminergic cell groups of the substantia nigra and the ventral tegmental area and has been demonstrated to survive well and yield functional effects when grafted to immunosuppressed experimental animals at a postconception age of up to 8 weeks. (The scale bar represents 1 mm.)

depend on: the specific type of tissue to be grafted; the technique used for transplantation; the graft location in the host brain; and the species from which the donor tissue is obtained. To give an example, fetal rat ventral mesencephalic tissue can survive grafting to the lateral ventricle as an undissociated tissue fragment up to embryonic day 18 (ED 18) (Simonds & Freed, 1990). When grafted to the anterior eye chamber, the upper age limit can be increased to postnatal day 1 (Seiger & Olson, 1977). When grafted as a dissociated cell suspension to the depth of the striatum, fetal rat ventral mesencephalic tissue survives well up to a donor age of ED 15–16 (Björklund *et al.*, 1980*a, b*; Brundin *et al.*, 1985, 1988*a*), although there is some suggestion that this upper age limit can be raised by pharmacological treatments that facilitate rapid vascularization of the newly grafted tissues (Finger & Dunnett, 1989). Ventral mesencephalic tissue *fragments* of the same age that are grafted to the striatal parenchyma, however, show only inferior survival (Stenevi *et al.*, 1976). Human fetal ventral mesencephalic tissue was found to have an upper donor age limit of 8–9 weeks postconception when grafted intrastriatally as a cell suspension into immunosuppressed rat hosts (Figure 7.1) (Brundin *et al.*, 1986*b*, 1988*b*).

Similar constraints apply also to other types of fetal brain tissue, such as *cerebellar* rat tissue which displays good Purkinje cell survival after suspension grafting only when taken from donor fetuses younger then ED 15. Other cerebellar neurons which have a more protracted neurogenesis, however, survive suspension grafting even when taken from early postnatal donors (Schmidt *et al.*, 1983*a*). Fetal *locus coeruleus* tissue rich in noradrenergic neurons, on the other hand, must be taken at a relatively early stage for suspension grafting to the hippocampus (ED 13–14), whereas the survival of rat *hippocampal* tissue fragments was found to be good even when grafted from donors between fetal day 20 and postnatal day 4 (Sørensen *et al.*, 1986). Equally, fragments of *tectal* tissue grafted to the midbrain of newborn rats display good survival when obtained from ED 15 and ED 18 but not ED 20 donor fetuses (Majda & Harvey, 1989); and intracerebral grafts of fetal rat *spinal cord* tissue survived well only when taken from donors younger than ED 16 (Reier *et al.*, 1983). Generally, the chances for good survival decrease when the graft tissue is dissected at a fetal stage that is past the period of neuronal proliferation and migration in the respective areas.

A second factor affecting the upper limit of donor age is imposed by the process of tissue preparation for each grafting technique. In particular, the dissociated cell suspension method involves a dissociation phase which, through axotomy and mechanical stress, further decreases the survival of graft tissue that was dissected in a state of axonal elongation. However, the advantage of being able to reach deep and circumscribed brain sites with suspension graft injections while causing minimal tissue trauma generally outweighs the stricter age limits required by the technique (Björklund *et al.*, 1980*b*).

A third factor possibly underlying donor age limitations may be partly related to the fact that more immature tissues can better endure prolonged periods of anoxia during the transplantation process.

The developmental potential of fetal brain tissue transplants and the graft location in the host brain

Fetal ventral mesencephalic DA neurons have been grafted to a number of structures in the adult host brain, including: the 6-OHDA-lesioned substantia nigra (Björklund *et al.*, 1983; Dunnett *et al.*, 1989); the striatum (cf. Stenevi *et al.*, 1976; Björklund *et al.*, 1980*a, b*; for review see Brundin & Björklund, 1987; Yurek & Sladek, 1990); the neocortex (Dunnett *et al.*, 1984; Herman *et al.*, 1986); the lateral hypothalamus (Björklund *et al.*, 1983); the septum (Herman *et al.*, 1986; Triarhou *et al.*, 1986); the tectum (Jaeger, 1985); the cerebellum (Ihara *et al.*, 1991); the lateral ventricle (apposed to the DA-depleted striatum; Perlow *et al.*, 1979; Freed *et al.*, 1980); and the choroidal fissure (apposed to the hippocampal formation; Björklund *et al.*, 1976; Stenevi *et al.*, 1976; Bischoff *et al.*, 1979).

When grafted to 'non-target' regions, such as the neocortex, the cerebellum and the lateral hypothalamus, grafts of dissociated fetal VM tissue generally display good survival. However, DA-rich fibres are primarily found within the transplant itself and display only very limited outgrowth into the surrounding non-target host brain tissue.

Fetal VM tissue placed in a cavity overlying (Björklund & Stenevi, 1979), or in the lateral ventricle adjacent to, the host striatum (Perlow *et al.*, 1979; Freed *et al.*, 1980) as well as dissociated grafts placed directly into the striatal parenchyma (Björklund *et al.*, 1980*b*; Doucet *et al.*, 1990) display a marked capacity to diffusely reinnervate and extend long axons through the DA-denervated host target, avoiding the fiber bundles of the internal capsule.

Equally, grafts of fetal VM tissue to the host septum show a reinnervation pattern reminiscent of the normal 'basket-like' DAergic innervation of the lateral septal nucleus (Herman *et al.*, 1986; Triarhou *et al.*, 1986).

When grafted to the 6-OHDA-lesioned substantia nigra, fetal ventral mesencephalic suspension grafts display essentially the same characteristics as grafts to 'non-target' regions of the host brain: they remain self-contained with no indication of DA fiber outgrowth along the medial forebrain bundle into the DA-denervated striatum (Björklund *et al.*, 1983; Dunnett *et al.*, 1989).

In contrast to the situation found in normal development, the grafted DA neurons must be placed within about 1 mm of the border of the striatum in order for their projections to be able to reach and reinnervate the striatum (see also Radel *et al.*, 1990). This restricted pattern of growth does not seem to reflect an intrinsic limitation of grafted DA neurons *per se*, since they display a marked capacity to extend long axons and reinnervate the host striatum through peripheral nerve 'bridge grafts' (Aguayo *et al.*, 1984; Gage *et al.*, 1985) or through tracks of dissociated fetal striatal tissue extending from VM grafts placed in the lesioned substantia nigra to the host striatum (Dunnett *et al.*, 1989). Moreover, Wictorin *et al.* (1990) have found that human telencephalic neurons xenografted to the excitotoxically lesioned striatum of immunosuppressed rats are capable of extending long axons through the host brain and reaching target areas that are beyond the reinnervation capacity of grafted rat striatal neurons. These and other grafting studies support the notion that there are mechanisms in the host brain that inhibit the outgrowth of syngeneic and allogeneic, but not necessarily xenogeneic, fetal CNS tissue grafts, and that the same mechanisms – possibly an active growth-inhibiting action of the host oligodendrocytes (Caroni & Schwab, 1988; for review see Schwab, 1990) – may be responsible for some aspects of the limited regenerative capacity of the damaged adult CNS.

Foster *et al.* (1985) produced further interesting evidence on the role of the target site in graft development. Mesencephalic serotonergic (5-HT) neurons, which normally project predominantly to the forebrain and only sparsely to the spinal cord, showed markedly decreased survival upon comparison with 'appropriate' intraspinal grafts derived from those medullary 5-HT-cell groups that normally innervate the spinal cord. Transplantation to the striatum – a target site predominantly for mesencephalic, but not for medullary, 5-HT-neurons – on the other hand demonstrates that the ability to reinnervate this target tissue is indeed restricted mostly to the 'appropriate' mesencephalic 5-HT neurons (Foster *et al.*, 1988). This finding, namely that fetal neurons producing the *same* neurotransmitter (but with *different* target preferences and dissected from different brain regions), do not display similar developmental characteristics when grafted to the same denervated target region (and are therefore not interchangeable in grafting experiments) is further supported by a series of studies in the cholinergic system.

Grafts rich in cholinergic neurons derived from the septal-diagonal band area were found to give rise to a markedly more extensive fiber outgrowth in their normal target area (the hippocampus) than identical transplants to the frontal cortex. Conversely, cholinergic grafts dissected from the nucleus basalis region, which normally projects predominantly to the neocortex, give rise to a markedly more extensive fiber outgrowth when implanted in the frontal cortex as compared to identical intrahippocampal grafts (Dunnett *et al.*, 1986*a*). 'Inappropriate' grafts of fetal *striatal* tissue rich in local cholinergic interneurons display only low survival rates when transplanted to the hippocampus (Gibbs *et al.*, 1986; Nilsson *et al.*, 1988); they form, however, normal synaptic connections. Cholinergic brainstem and spinal cord graft neurons survive better, but, on the other hand, show less fiber outgrowth and do *not* regularly form normal synaptic connections (Clarke *et al.*, 1990). In addition it was found that all types of 'inappropriate' intrahippocampal cholinergic grafts show different degrees of aberrant branching patterns within the layers of the host hippocampus (Nilsson *et al.*, 1988).

An interesting finding with respect to graft-derived reinnervation of 'non-target' areas is the denser than normal DA fiber ingrowth found in the hippocampus after grafting fragments of fetal ventral mesencephalic tissue to the choroidal fissure that is in close contact with the hippocampus (Björklund *et al.*, 1976; Stenevi *et al.*, 1976; Bischoff *et al.*, 1979). An abnormal hyperinnervation pattern from 'inappropriate' midbrain tissue was also found in a comparison of midbrain and medullary 5-HT neurons grafted to the 5-HT-denervated cerebellum of adult recipient rats (Ihara *et al.*, 1991).

These and many other studies highlight the importance of transplant location in the host brain as a determinant of graft development (see, for example, Figure 7.2). In summary, the wide range of phenomena that are encountered in graft experiments to 'target' and 'non-target' sites span from good survival and almost normal reinnervation patterns in appropriate graft locations to various degrees of impaired survival and/or development, abnormal growth characteristics and synapse formation in inappropriate graft sites.

It appears that these effects are to some degree interdependent, with,

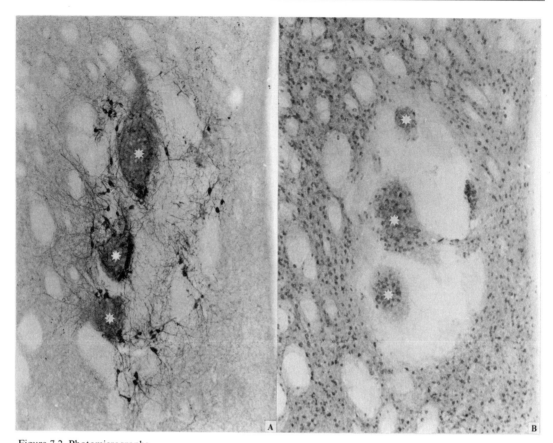

Figure 7.2. Photomicrographs of two adjacent sections through an intrastriatal rat-to-rat transplant of mixed fetal striatal and fetal ventral mesencephalic tissue. A is immunostained for the marker enzyme of catecholamine biosynthesis, tyrosine hydroxylase (TH); B is immunostained for the dopamine receptor-associated protein DARPP-32 as a marker for striatal tissue. Patches in the transplant (stars) represent striatal graft tissue. TH-immunoreactive cells can be seen within the graft. Although fetal striatal graft tissue is preferentially innervated by cografted mesencephalic dopamine neurons, the TH-cell number remains unaltered by addition of their fetal target tissue.

for example, poor graft survival reducing the density of fiber outgrowth and, conversely, contact to a target structure possibly influencing graft neuron survival. The findings discussed above suggest that both abnormal (e.g. distorted fiber lamination) and normal (e.g. formation of morphologically normal synapses) developmental features can occur independently in the same transplant. This implies that, far from following an 'all-or-nothing' pattern, different mechanisms in the host brain govern different aspects of neuronal development in a graded manner. This may have important implications for the potential application of neural growth factors in the treatment of neurodegenerative diseases.

The developmental potential of fetal brain tissue transplants and damage to the host brain

Numerous studies with grafts of different fetal brain tissues have demonstrated that the development of a transplant depends not only on its location within – and therefore on interaction with – an appropriate target tissue, but also on the cellular integrity of the host brain. Two distinct types of host brain damage have been found to influence several developmental parameters in fetal brain tissue grafts: *deafferentation* of the target structure as a result of a lesion in another brain area; and tissue damage of the target structure *itself*.

Injection of the neurotoxin 6-OHDA into the ascending dopaminergic projection from the ventral midbrain to the striatum results in a marked DA cell death in the substantia nigra from where this projection originates, with a corresponding DA loss in the striatal target area. Grafted fetal DA neurons from the ventral midbrain extend long axons through their *denervated* target structure and can form both a dense reinnervation pattern (Björklund *et al.*, 1983) and morphologically normal synapses (Freund *et al.*, 1985; Mahalik *et al.*, 1985; Clarke *et al.*, 1988). When grafted to the *non-denervated* striatum which still has an intact DAergic input, the degree of fiber outgrowth from grafted ventral mesencephalic DA cells as well as their cell body size was found to be decreased as compared to identical grafts into the DA denervated striatum (Schmidt *et al.*, 1981; Gage *et al.*, 1983; Doucet *et al.*, 1990).

Again, a supportive effect of target structure denervation on fetal brain tissue graft development has been described for other systems as well: when the hippocampal formation is cut off from its normal cholinergic afferents, several parameters of intrahippocampal graft survival and development are enhanced subsequently. Thus, grafts of fetal basal forebrain tissue rich in cholinergic neurons normally projecting to the hippocampus display enhanced growth, cell survival, cell body size, and choline acetyltransferase activity (the acetylcholine-producing enzyme) as compared to identical grafts to the non-denervated hippocampus (Gage & Björklund, 1986). Similarly, the recovery of partially lesioned host noradrenergic fibers originating in the locus coeruleus, or cholinergic fibers from the basal forebrain, as well as the survival of grafted sympathetic adrenergic neurons are all enhanced by hippocampal deafferentation (Björklund & Stenevi, 1981; Gage *et al.*, 1982, 1984). Removal of the hippocampal serotonin (5-HT) innervation results in the production of a humoral factor supporting the survival of grafted mesencephalic 5-HT neurons (Zhou *et al.*, 1987; Zhou & Azmitia, 1990).

Another interesting example of the importance of target structure damage comes from grafting experiments in an animal model of diabetes insipidus. Neurohypophysectomy in rats results in a marked proliferation of capillaries in the median eminence, whereas an anterior hypothalamic deafferentation leads to a lower density of capillaries. Grafting of fetal vasopressin-producing neurons revealed that a functional graft development occurred in neurohypophysectomized rats only, indicating that lesion-induced enrichment of the neurovascular target site plays a major role in this hypothalamic system (Marciano *et al.*, 1987).

It should also be noted in this context that intracranial grafts of fetal retina show a dense innervation pattern of the host tectum only after the normal visual inputs into this structure are eliminated by enucleation of the contralateral eye (McLoon & Lund, 1980), and that the specific reinnervation capacity of fetal entorhinal grafts placed in the adult hippocampus was found to be greatly enhanced by a preceding entorhinal deafferentation (Zhou *et al.*, 1989).

Several mechanisms have been proposed to govern the stimulatory effect of host brain lesions on transplant development and survival. Thus, it has been speculated that deafferentation of a given target structure in the host brain frees synaptic contacts which can then be occupied by graft neurons. A higher degree of graft–host interaction could in turn lend trophic support to the grafted cells and lead to increased survival rates. A possible model for trophic graft–host interaction involving the availability of sufficient target sites for neurons may exist in the chick embryo. Removal of a limb bud leads to a sharp increase in ontogenetic cell death of the spinal motoneurons, whereas an artificial *increase* in target structure availability through transplantation of an additional limb bud led to a *decrease* in ontogenetic cell death and thus to an abnormally high number of spinal motoneurons (Hollyday & Hamburger, 1976). Experimental evidence that the presence of, for example, unoccupied dendritic spines may play a direct role in governing graft survival and development is, however, scarce and not easy to interpret (Freed & Cannon-Spoor, 1988). Moreover, it is of interest in this context that deafferenting lesions have also been shown to induce or increase the secretion of diffusible trophic factors (Zhou *et al.*, 1987; Zhou & Azmitia, 1990), one of which, in the case of the deafferented hippocampus, is most likely identical to nerve growth factor (NGF) (cf. Gage & Björklund, 1987; see also Whittemore *et al.*, 1987).

Enhanced survival or development of intracerebral fetal brain tissue grafts has also been described in response to a tissue lesion at the graft site *itself*. Thus, grafts of fetal striatal tissue grow to a markedly larger size in the excitotoxically lesioned rat striatum than in the unlesioned striatum (Labandeira-Garcia *et al.*, 1991). The same also holds true for grafts of fetal nigral tissue, although the supranormal growth characteristics displayed in the excitotoxically lesioned striatum are not parallelled by increases in DA cell numbers (H. Sauer, unpublished observations). This increased growth capacity could possibly be an effect of additional growth space. However, the mechanism may be more complex than that, since wound fluids collected from focal brain lesions display a neurotrophic activity *in vitro* (Nieto-Sampedro *et al.*, 1982) and the survival of fetal striatal tissue grafts can be enhanced by the addition of such wound fluids (Nieto-Sampedro *et al.*, 1984). These results are supported also by other studies which demonstrate trophic activity at the site of focal brain wounds (Manthorpe *et al.*, 1983; Nieto-Sampedro *et al.*, 1984; Whittemore *et al.*, 1985; Heacock *et al.*, 1986; Finkelstein *et al.*, 1988).

Whereas the above studies discuss the effects of *externally* induced brain damage on the fate of neural grafts, Sotelo and colleagues have investigated the effects of a genetic progressive neurodegenerative disorder in the host. When fetal cerebellar tissue is grafted to the Purkinje cell deficient mutant mouse cerebellum, the transplanted cells display a remarkable capacity to migrate to their appropriate location and specifically to replace the lost host Purkinje neurons (Sotelo & Alvarado-Mallart, 1986, 1987). In contrast, grafts of fetal cerebellar anlage placed in the cerebellum of normal mice display abnormal development and interconnectivity and only occasional migration of Purkinje cells into the surrounding host brain tissue (Kawamura *et al.*, 1987; Sotelo & Alvarado-Mallart, 1988).

If lesions in the host brain can have a trophic effect on grafts of immature brain tissue, the inverse situation – a trophic effect of the grafted cells on the lesioned host brain – would also seem to be conceivable. Indeed, this has been demonstrated in several instances. Thus, grafts of fetal hypothalamic tissue have been shown specifically to protect neurons in the supraoptic nucleus from retrograde degeneration after neurohypophysectomy (Marciano *et al.*, 1989). Fetal occipital cortex grafts in neonatal rats were found similarly to ameliorate the degenerative effects of occipital cortex ablations on relay neurons in the dorsal lateral geniculate nucleus (Haun & Cunningham, 1984), and a protection from thalamic atrophy by fetal cortical grafts was also reported after frontal cortex lesions (Sørensen *et al.*, 1989). The degeneration of axotomized rubrospinal neurons is ameliorated by fetal spinal cord grafts (Bregman & Reier, 1986) and fetal cortical grafts were found to protect cholinergic basal forebrain projection neurons from excitotoxin-induced retrograde degeneration (Sofroniew *et al.*, 1986).

In summary, the following mechanisms are likely to be involved in the regulation of trophic graft–host interactions:

(i)   induction or increase of factors promoting neuronal survival and/or neurite outgrowth after deafferentation

(ii)   activation and mobilization of glial cells

(iii)   appearance of trophic activity at the site of focal brain lesions

(iv)   availability of appropriate target sites for graft or host neurons

(v)   changes of vasculature in response to injury

Far from being exclusive for a neural grafting situation, all these mechanisms are likely to play a role also in injury repair after brain lesions. They are, however, more clearly demonstrable with neural grafting techniques. Firstly, grafts of fetal neural tissue can be expected to react in a more plastic way to trophic stimuli by virtue of their immaturity. Secondly, by placing the neuronal population of interest at the actual site of injury/deafferentation it is possible to circumvent restrictions imposed on regenerating neurons by the adult brain environment – such as rapid glial scar formation or neurite outgrowth-inhibition. The neural transplantation approach has thus, by exposing the unfavorable features of the adult brain with respect to regeneration, unmasked the powerful trophic mechanisms active after brain lesions and provided fascinating insight into the intricate trophic interdependence of different brain systems.

The survival and development of fetal brain tissue transplants and immunological characteristics of both host brain and donor tissue

It has been known for a long time that allogeneic and xenogeneic grafts implanted into the brain exhibit a prolonged survival compared with transplantation into other sites in the body and that the general rules set up for graft rejection in the periphery do not seem to apply to the brain. As a result of these findings, the brain has been described as an immunologically privileged transplantation site (Medawar, 1948; Scheinberg *et al.*, 1964; Barker & Billingham, 1977; Widner & Brundin, 1988). This special immunological status of the brain, however, does not imply that survival of incompatible intracerebral grafts is permanent, nor does it mean that immune reactions cannot take place in the brain. The precise reason or reasons why the brain is immunologically privileged remain an enigma but, since the immunologically privileged status of the brain is of primary interest in the context of intracerebral neural grafting, it is worth mentioning briefly some of the proposed underlying mechanisms.

Lack of lymphatic drainage. Previously, it was believed that the brain completely lacked lymphatic drainage and, therefore, that the access of graft antigens to lymphatic tissue would be limited. Indeed, there are no classic lymph vessels in the brain but studies in rats indicate that antigens implanted in the brain can drain to deep cervical lymph nodes (Widner & Brundin, 1988), possibly through the perivascular and extracellular spaces to the cribiform lamina, and eventually to the lymphatics of the nasal mucosa (Bradbury & Westrop, 1983; Widner *et al.*, 1987; Bradbury, 1990; Cserr *et al.*, 1990).

Lack of antigen-presenting cells. It has previously been proposed that the brain lacks, or has very few, accessory cells that are capable of presenting antigens. However, cerebral endothelium, astrocytes and microglia have been proposed to possess this capacity (Fontana *et al.*, 1984; McCarron *et al.*, 1985; Traugott *et al.*, 1985; Wekerle *et al.*, 1986; Frei *et al.*, 1987; King & Katz, 1990; Poltorak & Freed, 1990).

Blocked effector mechanisms. It has been suggested that antigens implanted in the brain are drained primarily via the blood rather than by the less well-developed lymphatic system and thereby first reach lymphocytes in the spleen. Under these conditions it would seem possible that the spleen induces a state of unresponsiveness by producing antibodies that bind to transplantation antigens on the grafted cells and 'hide' them from the effector cells of the immune system ('enhancing antibodies': Kaplan & Streilein, 1974). Alternatively the spleen has been suggested to promote activity of a specific class of T lymphocytes that suppress immune responses (Streilein & Niederkorn, 1985). In the brain, however, this phenomenon has not been demonstrated, although splenectomy can indeed lower graft survival in the anterior chamber of the eye, another site exhibiting a degree of immunological privilege (Kaplan & Streilein, 1974).

The blood–brain barrier as an immunological barrier. The existence of a blood–brain barrier has been suggested to constitute an obstacle for lymphocyte traffic into the brain. Nevertheless, more recent evidence points to activated lymphocytes being able to pass an intact blood–brain barrier; moreover, there is also prolonged survival of grafted tissues that do not form a barrier, such as skin, when grafted to the brain (Stewart *et al.*, 1984; Head & Griffin, 1985).

Low immunogenicity of graft tissue. Unlike skin, for example, brain tissue normally expresses very low levels of, or no, major histocompatibility complex (MHC) antigens. This means that in grafting brain tissue one is implanting cells of low immunogenicity, which potentially could escape rejection by failing to identify themselves as foreign to the host immune system. However, experiments have shown that certain inductive signals can cause high expression of MHC antigens on brain tissue (Lampson & Fischer, 1984; Wong *et al.*, 1984; for a review see Lampson, 1987). Moreover, when implanted into the brain, cells in grafted neural tissue have been found to start expressing MHC antigens, possibly as a result of the inflammatory response that the surgical trauma evokes (Mason *et al.*, 1986; Nicholas *et al.*, 1987; Date *et al.*, 1988; Pollack *et al.*, 1990).

Presumably as a result of the mechanisms listed above, interspecies grafts of fetal brain tissue have indeed been shown to survive for prolonged times without immunosuppression (Björklund *et al.*, 1982; Daniloff *et al.*, 1984, 1985*a*, *b*; Inoue *et al.*, 1985; Vinogradova *et al.*, 1985; Kamo *et al.*, 1986, 1987; Finsen *et al.*, 1988). However, xenograft survival observed in these studies was not consistent in all specimens, and by now it is well established that good and consistent survival can best be obtained by continuous immunosuppressive treatment with cyclosporin A (CyA: Brundin *et al.*, 1985; Inoue *et al.*, 1985; Finsen *et al.*, 1988).

The chronically CyA-treated rat was used subsequently as a host for intracerebral grafts of human fetal mesencephalic tissue (Brundin *et al.*, 1986*b*, 1988*b*; Strömberg *et al.*, 1986, 1989; Clarke *et al.*, 1988; Sauer & Brundin, 1991) and it was shown that these animals could maintain their human xenografts for at least twenty-one weeks, whereas there was no survival of xenografted human DA neurons in non-immunosuppressed rats (Brundin *et al.*, 1988*b*).

Since an intact blood–brain barrier has been implicated in the maintenance of xenograft survival, an interesting observation was that the leakage of Evans Blue from cerebral blood vessels into the brain parenchyma subsided within twelve days after implantation of dissociated xenogeneic neural tissue (Brundin *et al.*, 1989). Thus, immunosuppression during and beyond the time it takes for the graft and surrounding host brain to acquire a blood–brain barrier does not in itself guarantee survival of xenografted tissue, which is consistent with the finding that activated lymphocytes are capable of crossing an intact blood–brain barrier (Wekerle *et al.*, 1986). In this context, it should be noted that intracerebral grafts of incompatible tissue that does *not* normally form a blood–brain barrier – such as skin – equally display prolonged survival (Stewart *et al.*, 1984; Head & Griffin, 1985). In summary, these findings indicate that the blood–brain barrier by itself does not seem to be the sole crucial factor governing the immunological privilege of the brain.

Both the observation that intracerebral xenografts are rejected eventually under normal conditions and the clear protective effect of CyA treatment suggest that the host immune system is indeed activated by intracerebral xenografts. A humoral antibody response was found in rat recipients of xenografted mouse (Lund *et al.*, 1987; Brundin *et al.*,

1989) and human (Brundin *et al.*, 1988*b*) fetal mesencephalic tissue. It is noteworthy that there was no measurable difference in the antibody response between animals with surviving and rejected grafts. It should be noted that although a humoral antibody response against MHC antigens indicates that these antigens are expressed in the grafts and that the afferent arc of the immune system (from the brain to the lymphatic tissue) is operative, the antibodies as such are not thought to play an important role in graft rejection, which is considered a cell-mediated process (Mason & Morris, 1986).

The finding that human fetal brain tissue can be immunogenic is of special relevance to the clinical situation, since grafts from a fetus to a patient with Parkinson's disease will necessarily be genetically incompatible. However, in the clinical situation the grafts will be *allogeneic*. Previous studies have shown that there is prolonged survival of allogeneic neural tissue grafts in different CNS sites (Zalewski *et al.*, 1978; Low *et al.*, 1983; Vinogradova *et al.*, 1985; Mason *et al.*, 1986; Sladek *et al.*, 1986; Bankiewicz *et al.*, 1987, 1990; Lund *et al.*, 1987; Date *et al.*, 1988; Fine *et al.*, 1988), but that in certain cases grafts incompatible at both major (MHC) and minor transplantation antigens are rejected (Mason *et al.*, 1986; Lund *et al.*, 1987; Nicholas *et al.*, 1987; Date *et al.*, 1988).

When allogeneic dissociated DA neurons are grafted between different inbred strains of mice there is good survival of the allografts in all the groups after six to seven weeks, quite comparable to syngeneic grafts, regardless of whether the donor and host differed at major or minor transplantation antigens, or both. Invariably, allogeneic *skin* grafts, between the same donor–host combinations, however, were rapidly rejected. Despite an apparently unimpaired allograft survival, a cellular response against the intracerebral grafts was demonstrated in some recipients, indicating that they were immunized (Widner *et al.*, 1989).

It is still too early to say whether a certain immunogenetical difference between donor and host is particularly favorable or unfavorable for allograft survival in the striatum. The presence of a cellular immunization response in the hosts points to the need for circumspection, since the hosts are primed for a rejection process and may be more likely to reject their grafts rapidly under certain conditions. This could account for the apparently more inconsistent survival of allografts, as compared to syngeneic grafts, and it is important in this context to note a study by Lawrence *et al.* (1990), who recently demonstrated that allogeneic grafts that are placed in the hippocampus may be invariably rejected. Furthermore, recent results from our own work with sequential intracerebral grafts of allogeneic fetal ventral mesencephalic tissue indicate that an immunization of the host occurs following the first transplant, and that this host response may result in impaired survival of a second intracerebral graft implanted fifteen weeks later. Moreover, challenging allograft recipients with an allogeneic skin graft can equally result in markedly decreased graft survival (Widner & Brundin, 1990).

In summary, there is need for caution, since the conclusions that can be drawn so far do *not* necessarily imply that allograft survival is *permanent*. Therefore, the observations that intracerebral allografts can immunize the host and that human fetal brain tissue can be immunogenic can be taken in support of the use of immunosuppression in clinical trials of neural grafting. Grafting without immunosuppression would leave a major factor of uncertainty, and the possible failure of a graft would be difficult to interpret.

Functional effects of grafting fetal brain tissue: lessons learned in the dopaminergic system

Long before all the parameters and conditions that govern the integration of transplanted fetal tissues into the host brain were identified, there was speculation about whether grafted neural tissues could influence the functional capacities of the host animal. Indeed, such philosophical speculations led Greene & Arnold (1945) to remark quizzically that guinea pigs bearing intracerebral grafts of human glioma tissues showed evidence of 'a marked increase in libido'. However, the behavioral consequences of neural transplants were first investigated systematically in the 6-OHDA lesion model of parkinsonism, and nigral grafts have been well studied under a wide variety of conditions.

The first demonstrations that nigral grafts can exert a functional influence on host behavior came with the demonstration of reversal of amphetamine- and apomorphine-induced rotation (Perlow *et al.*, 1979; Björklund & Stenevi, 1979; Freed *et al.*, 1980; Björklund *et al.*, 1980*a*). Although drug-induced rotation may be a rather artificial behavior, bearing little apparent relevance to human psychopathology, the power of these tests is that they are entirely objective, simple to quantify, and the rate of turning correlates highly with *post mortem* indices of the extent of the lesions (Hefti *et al.*, 1980; Dunnett *et al.*, 1987). Similarly, the degree of compensation of an initial high level of lesion-induced rotation after grafting provides an indicator that the extent of DAergic fiber ingrowth from the nigral grafts, whether measured anatomically or biochemically, has reached above a certain threshold level (Björklund *et al.*, 1980*a, b*; Schmidt *et al.*, 1983*b*;

Dunnett *et al.*, 1987; Brundin *et al.*, 1988*a*; Sauer & Brundin, 1991). Consequently, rotation provides a simple and non-invasive means of screening animals and determining *in vivo* the survival and integration of their individual grafts.

Recovery is not only observed in drug-dependent tests such as rotation. Embryonic nigral tissues have been found to be the most effective tissues for transplantation in dopamine-depleted animals, and they can yield amelioration or full recovery on many of the symptoms induced by 6-OHDA lesions in rats (and indeed also in other neurogenetic models in rodents and MPTP models in primates). This includes: spontaneous rotation and motor biases; contralateral sensory neglect; impairments in learning assessed by conditioned rotation and self-stimulation in rats with unilateral lesions; and the akinesia and bilateral neglect in rats with bilateral lesions (Dunnett *et al.*, 1981*a*, *b*, *c*, 1983*a*, *b*, 1986*b*; Fray *et al.*, 1983). Alternative non-embryonic dopamine-secreting tissues, such as adrenal medulla, carotid ganglion, neuroblastoma or transfected cell lines, have been considered as alternatives to embryonic mesencephalon for intracerebral transplantation. However, none of these alternatives has proved to be as effective functionally as the embryonic tissue, and, therefore, they are beyond the scope of the present book.

Nevertheless, even under optimal transplantation procedures currently available, recovery is not complete. In particular, there remain a few classes of behavioral impairment induced by dopaminergic denervation that have proved resistant to all attempts at dopamine cell transplantation tried so far: the profound aphagia and adipsia following bilateral nigrostriatal lesions; deficits in skilled contralateral paw use following unilateral nigrostriatal lesions; and impairments in hoarding behavior following ventral mesencephalic lesions (Dunnett *et al.*, 1983*b*, 1987; Herman *et al.*, 1986). A likely reason for this failure relates to the ectopic location of the grafts in the terminal striatum. Therefore, although the grafts can reinnervate their targets, and receive some limited afferent input from the host brain, they remain disconnected from the bulk of the normal afferent inputs received by the substantia nigra. However, nigral grafts implanted directly back into the nigra are without any detectable functional effect whatsoever, owing to their disconnection from appropriate targets (Dunnett *et al.*, 1983*a*). It is plausible that functions that are resistant to ectopic grafts will be restored only if the essential nigrostriatal circuitry itself can be reconstructed. This provides the rationale for the bridge grafting procedures currently under investigation (Aguayo *et al.*, 1984; Gage *et al.*, 1985; Dunnett *et al.*, 1989), in which embryonic nigra grafts are implanted in a homotopic nigral location, where they may be expected to attract more of the appropriate host inputs, in combination with a tissue bridge that will provide a substrate to stimulate and direct the growth of dopamine axons to reach and reinnervate the distant neostriatal targets. Although such surgical combinations now appear feasible (Dunnett *et al.*, 1989), they have not yet been developed to the stage of sufficient reliability to be taken to full functional assessment.

Clinical studies with grafts of fetal dopamine neurons in Parkinson's disease

After the first report on neural grafting trials involving human patients in 1905 (Shirres, 1905) it took eighty years before another report on clinical intracerebral transplantation appeared in the scientific literature (Backlund *et al.*, 1985). Since then, there have been numerous attempts to ameliorate parkinsonian symptoms by autografting catecholamine producing adrenal medulla. In general, non-neuronal catecholamine producing grafts have proven to be less effective in animal experiments and have yielded variable results in clinical studies (cf. W. J. Freed *et al.*, 1991). However, since these chromaffin cells are not of fetal origin they fall outside the scope of this book and will not be discussed further.

By the end of 1990, over 100 patients with Parkinson's disease had received grafts of fetal DA neurons at one of several centers worldwide. Several of these studies are still under way and therefore not yet available in the literature. The following account describes results from some of the centers that have been most active in the field and have so far reported their results either at meetings or in scientific journals.

In Mexico, mesencephalic tissue from 12 to 14-week-old spontaneously aborted fetuses has been implanted unilaterally in the head of the caudate nucleus with a transcallosal open surgical approach to 4 immunosuppressed patients (Madrazo *et al.*, 1990). The investigators have reported results 19–32 months postsurgery and describe an initial improvement occurring between 4 and 8 weeks after the operation. This improvement was maintained over three to four months after which a further decrease in symptoms was noted. The neurological improvement was bilateral and manifested in terms of a reduction in the time spent in 'off' (defined as a period with poor effect of L-dopa medication), reduction in rigidity, bradykinesia, postural imbalance and gait disturbances. Tremor was not affected.

In Cuba, over 30 immunosuppressed patients have received unilateral grafts using a modification of the Mexican technique, but with younger donor tissue that was derived from elective abortions (6–12 weeks postconception: Molina *et al.*, 1991). The patients, some of whom have been followed for twenty-four months, display a marked improvement of over 50% compared to preimplantation on three clinical rating scales. Moreover, the time spent in off was reduced and in 28 of the 30 patients the L-dopa dose was lowered. The clinical improvement was most pronounced contralaterally to the implant and seemed to develop gradually over the first six months following surgery, whereafter it remained stable.

Other groups have utilized a stereotaxic approach. In Birmingham, UK, at least 36 non-immunosuppressed patients have received unilateral grafts in either the caudate nucleus or the putamen (Hitchcock et al., 1990, 1991). Relatively large volumes (0.4–2 ml) of dissociated tissue from one aborted fetus aged 12–20 weeks have been implanted in each patient. So far, only results from the first set of 12 patients (grafted in the caudate) are available. Of these patients, nine have been followed for up to two years and four of these show sustained improvement in clinical rating.

From Yale University, USA (E. Redmond, personal communication, June 1990), 7 patients have been reported so far. They have received stereotaxic implants of 9 to 12-week-old fetal mesencephalon either unilaterally or bilaterally. The fetal donor tissue had been stored at liquid nitrogen temperature prior to grafting. One of the Yale patients died four months after grafting owing to aspiration pneumonia. At autopsy, there was survival of some graft tissue, but signs of surviving dopamine neurons were limited to one immunohistochemically stained cell found adjacent to the graft (Redmond et al., 1989). Clinical data on the other patients are still undergoing analysis.

In Denver, Colorado, USA, 2 patients have been given stereotaxic implants of tissue from one 6 to 8-week-old fetus each (C. R. Freed et al., 1990, 1991). So far, follow-ups at five months and fifteen months have been reported. The implant was distributed unilaterally over 10 to 12 sites in the striatum (both caudate and putamen). In one patient, the donor tissue was matched with regard to MHC class I antigens. The first patient was immunosuppressed, the second was not. In addition to regular clinical rating of symptoms in the hospital, the patients themselves conduct daily computer assisted movement analysis at home. The first patient has displayed a small functional effect with a reduction of motor symptomatology in drug-free phases; whereas the second patient has shown no motor effects. Analysis of the graft survival with positron emission tomography (PET), using radioactive fluorodopa as a label for cerebral dopamine systems, has been inconclusive (Freed et al., 1990).

In Sweden, 6 immunosuppressed patients have received unilateral or bilateral stereotaxic implants of dissociated mesencephalic tissue from

3–4 fetuses aged 6 to 8-weeks postconception. Grafts were placed in the putamen only (Lindvall *et al.*, 1990) or both the putamen and the caudate nucleus (Lindvall *et al.*, 1989). To date, clinical evaluation of four of the patients has been compiled. In summary, the first two patients displayed minor functional effects of no real therapeutic value (Lindvall *et al.*, 1989). Prior to surgery on the second two patients, some technical improvements were made in the procedure, e.g. a thinner implantation instrument was developed. Both these patients, who have received three unilateral implants in the putamen only, display improvements of a clearly therapeutic magnitude (Lindvall *et al.*, 1990, 1991). Antiparkinson medication is effective over greater proportions of the day and when the patients are off medication their rigidity and akinesia are clearly reduced as compared to pregraft testing. The effects are partly bilateral but most pronounced on the side of the body contralateral to the implants. PET has shown that both patients have a marked increase in flurodopa uptake compared with the level before grafting, which is indicative of the grafts surviving and containing dopamine neurons which can take up dopa. In certain restricted areas of the grafted putamen the levels of fluorodopa uptake approach those of normal subjects (Sawle *et al.*, 1991).

Conclusions

In the studies mentioned above, patient selection criteria, the antiparkinson medication, methods for clinical evaluation, the age of donor tissue and its preparation for implantation, the surgical techniques and the sites selected for implantation differ between groups in several or all points, which makes it difficult to compare results directly. For this reason it is at present impossible to say whether, in the future, the transplantation approach may represent a therapeutic alternative to conventional antiparkinson medication. It should be pointed out that this methodological diversity, although it may at first obscure the clinical feasibility of neural grafting, could turn out to be at least partly advantageous in the end by possibly providing answers to several issues that are unresolved at present.

Answers to some of the more technical questions may be found through animal experiments, such as optimization of donor tissue preparation for neural grafting; the development of safe storage techniques for donor tissue; the size of the implantation instrument; the role of immunosuppression, etc. However, there remain a number of clinical issues that probably cannot be approached with the animal models available currently, such as: are less severely affected patients more likely to benefit from a neural graft than patients who are severely incapacitated by the disease? Which of the symptoms of Parkinson's disease are most likely to be alleviated by a neural graft? Which bearing will an intracerebral graft have on the effectiveness of conventional antiparkinson medication and vice versa? Will the therapeutic graft effects fade with the normal progression of the disease or will the clinical symptoms remain stable after grafting?

Therefore, judging by both the preliminary clinical data so far available and the diversity of technical approaches, clinical neural grafting can be considered to be in an exploratory phase at present and it is likely that some or most of the questions mentioned above will be answered in the future.

There are, however, some important differences between the clinical studies that deserve special mention. Firstly, the choice of donor tissue is probably crucial. Animal studies suggest that if the dissociated tissue technique is used, the donor fetus should be no older than 8 weeks postconception (Carnegie stage 22) (Brundin *et al.*, 1986*b*, 1988*b*; Brundin, 1991). At best, older tissue has yielded only very poor survival when xenografted to immunosuppressed rats if dissociated prior to implantation, but may fare better if grafted in the form of solid pieces. Thus, one faces the question of selecting the optimal technique for a given donor tissue, and animal studies may in the future be helpful in developing an array of methods for preparation and implantation of donor tissues of different ages.

Secondly, it emerged from the ongoing clinical trials that a safe method for pregraft tissue storage would be most helpful in ensuring biological safety, immunological matching, and availability of the donor tissue on the day of surgery. However, animal studies suggest that pregraft cryopreservation of the donor tissue at temperatures below freezing may markedly reduce graft survival (Chanaud & Das, 1987; Collier *et al.*, 1988; Sauer *et al.*, 1992). Further experiments will show whether or nor this procedure is hazardous for the graft tissue.

Thirdly, the type of grafting technique constitutes an important variable, since it has been speculated that the open surgical technique may be more prone to induce a putative trophic host response (with concomitant collateral sprouting of residual host dopaminergic neurons) than the less traumatic stereotaxic surgery.

Lastly, one theory implies that transplanted dopamine cells might be effective owing to a diffuse release of dopamine into surrounding tissue rather than by restoring the precise nigro-striatal circuitry. This point is unclear, since transplanted dopamine neurons: form both 'correct' and 'incorrect' synaptic connections, as shown ultrastructurally; respond electrophysiologically to stimulation of the host brain, thus receiving regulatory host afferents; regulate dopamine release in response to medication. On the other hand, the clinical value of long-lived drugs that are active on dopamine receptors is well established, but long-term treatment with therapeutically relevant doses can cause undesirable side-effects, perhaps by modifying receptor sensitivity or the rates of dopamine synthesis. This is shown by the psychotic manifestations of long-term treatment with amphetamines or the tardive dyskinesias associated with treatments using dopamine antagonists.

Initial studies have shown that it is valuable to be able to assess graft survival with non-invasive techniques. So far, the PET technique would seem to provide the most useful method to monitor survival of grafted human dopamine neurons. With this tool it may be possible to correlate improvement in clinical performance with the size and precise location of the grafts, thus allowing for an optimization of the clinical grafting technique. However, it should be stressed that, as yet, neural grafting constitutes an experimental procedure only and, although we have come a long way from the rotating rodent to the parkinsonian patient, a great deal of research, development and constant re-evaluation remains before, if ever, it can provide a therapy for Parkinson's disease.

Acknowledgments

Work conducted in the laboratories in which the authors are active is supported by the following foundations and institutions:
the German Research Foundation (grant DFG/Oe 95 4-1/2); the German Parkinson Foundation (dPV e.V.); the Friedrich-Baur-Foundation; the German Federal Ministry of Research and Technology (BMFT 01 KL 9001); the Parkinson's Disease Society (UK); the British Medical Research Council; the Mental Health Foundation; the Swedish Medical Research Council (grant 04X-8666); the Neurologiskt Handikappades Riksförbund; the American Parkinson's Disease Association.

H. S. is supported by the Boehringer Ingelheim Foundation for Biomedical Research. P. B. is supported by 'Telefondirektör H. T. Cedergrens Uppfostringsfond.'

References

AGUAYO, A. J., BJÖRKLUND, A., STENEVI, U. & CARLSTEDT, T. (1984) Fetal mesencephalic neurons survive and extend long axons across peripheral nervous system grafts inserted in the adult rat striatum. *Neuroscience Letters*, **45**, 53–8.

ANNETT, L. E., DUNNETT, S. B., MARTEL, F. L., ROGERS, D. C., RIDLEY, R. M., BAKER, H. F. & MARSDEN, C. D. (1990) A functional assessment of embryonic dopaminergic grafts in the marmoset. *Progress in Brain Research*, **82**, 535–42.

AZMITIA, E. & BJÖRKLUND, A. (eds.) (1987) Cell and Tissue Transplantation Into the Adult Brain. *Annals of the New York Academy of Sciences*, **495**, 1–813.

BACKLUND, E.-O., GRANBERG, P.-O., HAMBERGER, B., KNUTSSON, E., MÅRTENSSON, A., SEDVALL, G., SEIGER, Å. & OLSON, L. (1985) Transplantation of adrenal medullary tissue to striatum in parkinsonism. First clinical trials. *Journal of Neurosurgery*, **621**, 169–73.

BAKAY, R. A. E., FIANDACA, M. S., BARROW, D. L., SCHIFF, A. & COLLINS, D. C. (1985) Preliminary report on the use of fetal tissue transplantation to correct MPTP-induced parkinsonian-like syndrome in primates. *Applied Neurophysiology*, **48**, 358–61.

BANKIEWICZ, K. S., JACOBOWITZ, D. M., PLUNKETT, R. J., OLDFIELD, E. H. & KOPIN, I. J. (1987) Injury induced sprouting into the caudate nucleus, after solid tissue implantation in MPTP-induced parkinsonian monkeys. *Society for Neuroscience Abstracts*, **46**, 16.

BANKIEWICZ, K. S., PLUNKETT, R. J., JACOBOWITZ, D. M., PORRINO, L., diPORZIO, U., LONDON, W. T., KOPIN, I. J. & OLDFIELD, E. H. (1990) The effect of fetal mesencephalon implants on primate MPTP-induced parkinsonism. *Journal of Neurosurgery*, **72**, 231–44.

BARKER, C. F. & BILLINGHAM, R. E. (1977) Immunologically privileged sites. *Advances in Immunology*, **25**, 1–54.

BARRY, D. I., KIKVADZE, I., BRUNDIN, P., BOLWIG, T. G., BJÖRKLUND, A. & LINDVALL, O. (1987) Grafted noradrenergic neurons suppress seizure development in kindling-induced epilepsy. *Proceedings of the National Academy of Sciences, USA*, **84**, 8712–15.

BISCHOFF, S., SCATTON, B. & KORF, J. (1979) Dopamine metabolism, spiperone binding and adenylate cyclase activity in the adult rat hippocampus after ingrowth from dopaminergic neurons from embryonic implants. *Brain Research*, **179**, 77–84.

BJÖRKLUND, A., DUNNETT, S. B., STENEVI, U., LEWIS, M. E. & IVERSEN, S. D. (1980a) Reinnervation of the denervated striatum by substantia nigra transplants: Functional consequences as revealed by pharmacological and sensorimotor testing. *Brain Research*, **199**, 307–33.

BJÖRKLUND, A., SCHMIDT, R. H. & STENEVI, U. (1980b) Functional reinnervation of neostriatum in the adult rat by use of intraparenchymal grafting of dissociated cell suspensions from the substantia nigra. *Cell and Tissue Research*, **212**, 39–45.

BJÖRKLUND, A. & STENEVI, U. (1979) Reconstruction of the nigrostriatal dopamine pathway by intracerebral nigral transplants, *Brain Research*, **177**, 555–60.

BJÖRKLUND, A. & STENEVI, U. (1981) In vivo evidence for a hippocampal adrenergic neurotrophic factor specifically released on septal deafferentation. *Brain Research*, **229**, 403–428.

BJÖRKLUND, A., STENEVI, U., DUNNETT, S. B. & GAGE, F. H. (1982) Cross-species neural grafting in a rat model of Parkinson's disease, *Nature*, **298**, 652–4.

BJÖRKLUND, A., STENEVI, U., SCHMIDT, R. H., DUNNETT, S. B. & GAGE, F. H. (1983) Intracerebral grafting of neuronal cell suspensions II. Survival and growth of nigral cell suspensions implanted in different brain sites. *Acta Physiologica Scandinavica*, Supplement, **522**, 9–18.

BJÖRKLUND, A., STENEVI, U. & SVENDGAARD, N.-A. (1976) Growth of transplanted monoaminergic neurones into the adult hippocampus along the perforant path. *Nature*, **262**, 787–90.

BOHN, M. J., CUPIT, L., MARCIANO, F. & GASH, D. M. (1987) Adrenal medulla grafts enhance recovery of striatal dopaminergic fibers. *Science*, **237**, 913–16.

BRADBURY, M. W. (1990) Overview of passage routes of interstitial fluid into the lymphatics: history and current concepts. In: *Pathophysiology of The Blood–Brain Barrier, Long Term Consequences of Barrier Dysfunction in The Brain*, pp. 403–12. Eds. B. B. Johansson, C. Owman & H. Widner, Elsevier, Amsterdam.

BRADBURY, M. W. & WESTROP, R. J. (1983) Factors influencing exit of substances from cerebrospinal fluid into deep cervical lymph of the rabbit. *Journal of Physiology*, **339**, 519–34.

BREGMAN, B. S. & REIER, P. J. (1986) Neural tissue transplants rescue axotomized rubrospinal cells from retrograde death. *Journal of Comparative Neurology*, 86–95.

BRUNDIN, P. (1991) Dissection, preparation and implantation of human embryonic brain tissue. In: *A Practical Approach to Neural Transplantation.* Ed. S. B. Dunnett. Oxford University Press, Oxford, in press.

BRUNDIN, P., BARBIN, G., STRECKER, R. E., ISACSON, O., PROCHIANTZ, A. & BJÖRKLUND, A. (1988a) Survival and function of dissociated rat dopamine neurones grafted at different developmental stages or after being cultured *in vitro*. *Developmental Brain Research*, **39**, 233–43.

BRUNDIN, P. & BJÖRKLUND, A. (1987) Survival, growth and function of dopaminergic neurons grafted to the brain. In: *Progress in Brain Research*, **71**, pp. 293–308. Eds. F. J. Seil, E. Herbert & B. M. Carlson. Elsevier, Amsterdam.

BRUNDIN, P., ISACSON, O. & BJÖRKLUND, A. (1985) Monitoring of cell viability in suspension of embryonic CNS tissue and its use as a criterion for intracerebral graft survival. *Brain Research*, **331**, 251–9.

BRUNDIN, P., ISACSON, O., GAGE, F. H., PROCHIANTZ, A. & BJÖRKLUND, A. (1986a) The rotating 6-hydroxydopamine-lesioned mouse as a model for assessing functional effects of neuronal grafting. *Brain Research*, **366**, 346–9.

BRUNDIN, P., NILSSON, O. G., STRECKER, R. E., LINDVALL, O. &

BJÖRKLUND. A. (1986b) Behavioral effects of human fetal dopamine neurons grafted in a rat model of Parkinson's disease. *Experimental Brain Research*, **65**, 235–40.

BRUNDIN, P., STRECKER, R. E., WIDNER, H., CLARKE, D. J., NILSSON, O. G., ÅSTEDT, B., LINDVALL, O. & BJÖRKLUND, A. (1988b) Human fetal dopamine neurons grafted in a rat model of Parkinson's disease: Immunolgical aspects, spontaneous and drug-induced behaviour, and dopamine release, *Experimental Brain Research*, **70**, 192–208.

BRUNDIN, P., WIDNER, H., NILSSON, O. G., STRECKER, R. E. & BJÖRKLUND, A. (1989) Intracerebral xenografts of dopamine neurons: the role of immunosuppression and the blood–brain barrier. *Experimental Brain Research*, **75**, 195–207.

CARONI, P. & SCHWAB, M. E. (1988) Two membrane protein fractions from rat central myelin with inhibitory properties for neurite growth and fibroblast spreading. *Journal of Cell Biology*, **106**, 1281–8.

CHANAUD, C. M. & DAS, G. D. (1987) Growth of neural transplants in rats: Effects of initial volume, growth potential, and fresh vs. frozen tissues, *Neuroscience Letters*, **80**, 127–33.

CLARKE, D. J., BRUNDIN, P., STRECKER, R. E., NILSSON, O. G., BJÖRKLUND, A. & LINDVALL, O. (1988) Human fetal dopamine neurons grafted in a rat model of Parkinson's Disease: Ultrastructural evidence for synapse formation using tyrosine hydroxylase immunocyto-chemistry. *Experimental Brain Research*, **73**, 115–26.

CLARKE, D. J., NILSSON, O. G., BRUNDIN, P. & BJÖRKLUND, A. (1990) Synaptic connections formed by grafts of different types of cholinergic neurons in the host hippocampus. *Experimental Neurology*, **107**, 11–22.

COLLIER, T. J., SLADEK, C. D., GALLAGHER, M. J., BLANCHARD, B. C., DALEY, B. F., FOSTER, P. N., REDMOND, D. E., ROTH, R. H. & SLADEK, J. R., Jr. (1988) Cryopreservation of fetal rat and non-human primate mesencephalic neurons: viability in culture and neural transplantation. In: *Transplantation in the Mammalian CNS, Progress in Brain Research*, **78**, 631–6. Eds. D. M. Gash & J. R. Sladek, Jr. Elsevier, Amsterdam.

CSERR, H. F., HARLING-BREG, C., ICHIMURA, Y. T., KNOPF, P. M. & YAMADA, S. (1990) Drainage of cerebral extracellular fluids into cervical lymph: an afferent limb in brain/immune system interactions. In: *Pathophysiology of the Blood-Brain Barrier, Long Term Consequences of Barrier Dysfunction in the Brain*, pp. 413–20. Eds. B. B. Johansson, C. Owman & H. Widner. Elsevier, Amsterdam.

DANILOFF, J. K., BODONY R. P. & WELLS J. (1985a) Cross-species neural transplants: embryonic septal nuclei to the hippocamal formation of adult rats. *Experimental Brain Research*, **59**, 73–82.

DANILOFF, J. K., LOW, W. C., BODONY, R. P. & WELLS, J. (1985b) Cross-species embryonic septal transplants: restoration of conditioned learning behavior, *Brain Research*, **346**, 176–180.

DANILOFF, J. K., WELLS, J. & ELLIS, J. (1984) Cross-species septal transplants: Recovery of choline acetyl transferase activity. *Brain Research*, **324**, 151–4.

DAS, G. D. & ALTMAN, J. (1971) Transplanted precursors of nerve cells: their fate in the cerebellums of young rats. *Science*, **173**, 637–8.

DATE, I., KAWAMURA, K. & NAKASHIMA, H. (1988) Histological signs of immune reactions against allogeneic solid neural grafts in the mouse cerebellum depend on the MHC locus. *Experimental Brain Research*, **73**, 15–22.

DECKEL, A. W., ROBINSON, R. G., COYLE, J. T. & SANBERG, P. R. (1983) Reversal of long-term locomotor abnormalities in the kainic acid model of Huntington's disease by day 18 fetal striatal implants. *European Journal of Pharmacology*, **93**, 287–8.

DOUCET, G., BRUNDIN, P., DESCARRIERES, L. & BJÖRKLUND, A. (1990) Effect of prior dopamine denervation on survival and fiber outgrowth from intrastriatal ventral mesencephalic grafts. *European Journal of Neuroscience*, **2**, 279–90.

DUBACH, M., SCHMIDT, R. H., MARTIN, R., GERMAN, D. C. & BOWDEN, D. M. (1988) Transplant improves hemiparkinsonian syndrome in nonhuman primate: intracerebral injection, rotometry, tyrosine hydroxylase immunohistochemistry. *Progress in Brain Research*, **78**, 491–6.

DUNN, E. H. (1917) Primary and secondary findings in a series of attempts to transplant cerebral cortex to the albino rat. *Journal of Comparative Neurology*, **27**, 565–82.

DUNNETT, S. B. (1990) Neural transplantation in animal models of dementia. *European Journal of Neuroscience*, **2**, 567–87.

DUNNETT, S. B., BJÖRKLUND, A., SCHMIDT, R. H., STENEVI, U. & IVERSEN, S. D. (1983a) Intracerebral grafting of neuronal cell suspensions. IV. Behavioural recovery in rats with unilateral implants of nigral cell suspensions in different forebrain sites. *Acta Physiologica Scandinavica*, Supplement, **522**, 29–37.

DUNNETT, S. B., BJÖRKLUND, A., SCHMIDT, R. H., STENEVI, U. & IVERSEN, S. D. (1983b) Intracerebral grafting of neuronal cell suspensions. V. Behavioural recovery in rats with bilateral 6-OHDA lesions following implantation of nigral cell suspensions. *Acta Physiologica Scandinavica*, Supplement, **522**, 39–47.

DUNNETT, S. B., BJÖRKLUND, A., STENEVI, U. & IVERSEN, S. D. (1981a) Behavioural recovery following transplantation of substantia nigra in rats subjected to 6-OHDA lesions of the nigrostriatal pathway. I. Unilateral lesions. *Brain Research*, **215**, 147–61.

DUNNETT, S. B., BJÖRKLUND, A., STENEVI, U. & IVERSEN, S. D. (1981b) Grafts of embryonic substantia nigra reinnervating the ventrolateral striatum ameliorate sensorimotor impairments and akinesia in rats with 6-OHDA lesions of the nigrostriatal pathway. *Brain Research*, **229**, 209–17.

DUNNETT, S. B., BJÖRKLUND, A., STENEVI, U. & IVERSEN, S. D. (1981c) Behavioural recovery following transplantation of substantia nigra in rats subjected to 6-OHDA lesions of the nigrostriatal pathway. II. Bilateral lesions. *Brain Research*, **229**, 457–70.

DUNNETT, S. B., BUNCH, S. T., GAGE, F. H. & BJÖRKLUND, A. (1984) Dopamine-rich transplants in rats with 6-OHDA lesions of the ventral tegmental area: Effects on spontaneous and drug-induced locomotor activity. *Behavioural Brain Research*, **13**, 71–82.

DUNNETT, S. B., ROGERS, D. C. & RICHARDS, S.-J. (1989) Nigrostriatal reconstruction after 6-OHDA-lesions in rats: Combination of dopamine-rich nigral grafts and nigrostriatal 'bridge' grafts. *Experimental Brain Research*, **75**, 523–35.

DUNNETT, S. B., WHISHAW, I. Q., BUNCH, S. T. & FINE, A. (1986a) Acetylcholine-rich neuronal grafts in the forebrain of rats; Effects of environmental enrichment, neonatal noradrenaline depletion, host transplantation site and regional source of embryonic donor cells on graft size and acetylcholinestrase-positive fibre outgrowth, *Brain Research*, **378**, 357–73.

DUNNETT, S. B., WHISHAW, I. Q., JONES, G. H. & ISACSON, O. (1986b) Effects of dopamine-rich grafts on conditioned rotation in rats with unilateral 6-OHDA lesions. *Neuroscience Letters*, **68**, 127–33.

DUNNETT, S. B., WHISHAW I. Q., ROGERS D. C. & JONES, G. H. (1987) Dopamine rich grafts ameliorate whole body motor asymmetry and sensory neglect but not independent limb use in rats with 6-hydroxydopamine lesions. *Brain Research*, **415**, 63–87.

FINE, A., HUNT, S. P., OERTEL, W. H., NOMOTO, M., CHONG, P. N., BOND, A., WATERS, C., TEMLETT, J. A., ANNETT, L., DUNNETT, S. B., JENNER, P. & MARSDEN, C. O. (1988) Transplantation of embryonic marmoset dopaminergic neurons to the corpus striatum of marmosets rendered parkinsonian by 1-methyl-4-phenyl-1,2,3,6-tetrahydropyridine. In: *Transplantation in the Mammalian CNS. Progress in Brain Research*, **82**, 723–8. Eds. S. B. Dunnett & S.-J. Richards. Elsevier, Amsterdam.

FINGER, S. & DUNNETT, S. B. (1989) Nimodipine enhances growth and vascularization of neural grafts. *Experimental Neurology*, **104**, 1–9.

FINKELSTEIN, S. P., APOSTOLIDES, P. J., CADAY, C. G., PROSSER, J., PHILIPS, M. F. & KLAGSBRUN, M. (1988) Increased basic fibroblast growth factor (bFGF) immunoreactivity at the site of focal brain wounds. *Brain Research*, **460**, 253–9.

FINSEN, B., POULSEN, P. H. & ZIMMER, J. (1988) Xenografting of fetal mouse hippocampal tissue to the brain of adult rats. Effect of cyclosporin A treatment. *Experimental Brain Research*, **70**, 117–33.

FONTANA, A., FIERZ, W. & WEKERLE, H. (1984) Astrocytes present myelin basic protein to encephalitogenic T-cell lines, *Nature*, **307**, 273–6.

FOSTER, G. A., SCHULTZBERG, M., GAGE, F. H., BJÖRKLUND, A., HÖKFELT, T., CUELLO, A. C., VERHOFSTAD, A. A. J., VISSER, T. J. & EMSON, P. C. (1988) Transmitter expression and morphological development of embryonic medullary and mesencephalic raphé neurones after transplantation to the adult rat central nervous system. III. Grafts to the striatum. *Experimental Brain Research*, **70**, 242–55.

FOSTER, G. A., SCHULTZBERG, M., GAGE, F. H., BJÖRKLUND, A., HÖKFELT, T., NORNES, H., CUELLO, A. C., VERHOFSTAD, A. A. J. & VISSER, T. J. (1985) Transmitter expression and morphological development of embryonic medullary and mesencephalic raphé neurones after transplantation to the adult rat central nervous system. I. Grafts to the spinal cord. *Experimental Brain Research*, **60**, 427–44.

FRAY, P. J., DUNNETT, S. B., IVERSEN, S. D., BJÖRKLUND, A. & STENEVI, U. (1983) Nigral transplants reinnervating the dopamine-depleted neostriatum can sustain intracranial self-stimulation. *Science*, **219**, 416–19.

FREED, C. R., BREEZE, R. E., ROSENBERG, N. L., SCHNECK, S. A., SCHROTER, G., LAFFERTY, K., TALMAGE, D. W., BARRETT, J. N., WELLS, T., MAZZIOTTA, J. C., HUANG, S. C., EIDELBERG, D. & ROTTENBERG, D. A. (1991) Fetal neural transplants for Parkinson's disease: results at 15 months. In: *Intracerebral Transplantation in Movement*

Disorders, 69–78. Eds. O. Lindvall, A. Björklund & H. Widner. Elsevier Science Publishers, Amsterdam.

FREED, C. R., BREEZE, R. E., ROSENBERGH, N. L., SCHNECK, S. A., WELLS, T., BARRETT, J. N., GRAFTON, S. T., HUANG, S. C., EIDELBERG, D. & ROTTENBERG, D. A. (1990) Transplantation of human fetal dopamine cells for Parkinson's disease. Results at 1 year. *Archives of Neurology*, **10**, 1268–75.

FREED, W. J. & CANNON-SPOOR, H. E. (1988) Cortical lesions increase reinnervation of the dorsal striatum by substantia nigra grafts. *Brain Research*, **446**, 133–43.

FREED, W. J., PERLOW, M. J., KAROUM, F., SEIGER, Å., OLSON, L., HOFFER, B. J. & WYATT, R. J. (1980) Restoration of dopamine function by grafting of fetal rat substantia nigra to the caudate nucleus. Long-term behavioral, biochemical and histochemical studies. *Annals of Neurology*, **8**, 510–19.

FREED, W. J., POLTORAK, M. & BECKER, J. B. (1991) Intracerebral adrenal medulla grafts: A review. *Experimental Neurology*, **110**, 137–66.

FREI, K., SIEPL, C., GROSCURTH, P., BODMER, S., SCHWERDEL, C. & FONTANA, A. (1987) Antigen presentation and tumor cytotoxicity by γ-interferon treated microglial cells, *European Journal of Immunology*, **17**, 1271–8.

FREUND, T. F., BOLAM, J. P., BJÖRKLUND, A., STENEVI, U., DUNNETT, S. B., POWELL, J. F. & SMITH, A. D. (1985) Efferent synaptic connections of grafted dopaminergic neurons reinnervating the host neostriatum: A tyrosine hydroxylase immunocytochemical study. *Journal of Neuroscience*, **5**, 603–16.

GAGE, F. H. & BJÖRKLUND, A. (1986) Enhanced graft survival in the hippocampus following selective denervation. *Neuroscience* **17**, 89–98.

GAGE, F. H. & BJÖRKLUND, A. (1987) Denervation-induced enhancement of graft survival and growth: A trophic hypothesis. *Annals of the New York Academy of Sciences*, **495**, 378–95.

GAGE, F. H., BJÖRKLUND, A. & STENEVI, U. (1982) Reinnervation of the partially deafferented hippocampus by compensatory collateral sprouting from spared cholinergic and noradrenergic afferents. *Brain Research*, **268**, 27–37.

GAGE, F. H., BJÖRKLUND, A. & STENEVI, U. (1984) Denervation induces a neuronal survival factor in adult rat hippocampus. *Nature*, **308**, 637–9.

GAGE, F. H., BJÖRKLUND, A., STENEVI, U. & DUNNETT, S. B. (1983) Intracerebral grafting of neuronal cell suspensions VIII. Survival and growth of implants of nigral and septal cell suspensions in intact brains of aged rats. *Acta Physiologica Scandinavica*, Supplement, **522**, 67–75.

GAGE, F. H., STENEVI, U., CARSTEDT, T., FOSTER, G., BJÖRKLUND, A. & AGUAYO, A. J. (1985) Anatomical and functional consequences of grafting mesencephalic neurons into a peripheral nerve 'bridge' connected to the denervated striatum. *Experimental Brain Research*, **60**, 584–9.

GASH, D. M. & SLADEK, J. R., Jr. (1984) Functional and non-functional transplants: studies with grafted hypothalamic and preoptic neurons. *Trends in Neurosciences*, **7**, 391–4.

GIBBS, R. B., ANDERSON, K. & COTMAN, C. W. (1986) Factors affecting innervation in the CNS: Comparison of three cholinergic cell types transplanted to the hippocampus of adult rats, *Brain Research*, **383**, 362–6.

GIBSON, M. J., CHARLTON, H. M., PERLOW, M. J., ZIMMERMAN, E. A., DAVIES, T. F. & KRIEGER, D. T. (1984) Preoptic area brain grafts in hypogonadal (hpg) female mice abolish effects of congenital hypothalamic gonadotropin-releasing hormone (GnRH) deficiency. *Endocrinology*, **114**, 1938–40.

GREENE, H. S. N. & ARNOLD, H. (1945) The homologous and heterologous transplantation of brain and brain tumours. *Journal of Neurosurgery*, **3**, 315–31.

HAUN, F. & CUNNINGHAM, T. J. (1984) Cortical transplants reveal CNS trophic interactions *in situ*. *Brain Research*, **15**, 290–4.

HEACOCK, A. M., SCHONFELD, A. R. & KATZMAN, R. (1986) Hippocampal neurotrophic factor: Characterization and response to denervation. *Brain Research*, **363**, 299–306.

HEAD, J. R. & GRIFFIN, S. T. (1985) Functional capacity of solid tissue transplants in the brain: evidence for immunological privilege. *Proceedings of the Royal Society, London, B*, **224**, 375–87.

HEFTI, F., MELAMED, E., SAHAKIAN, B. J. & WURTMAN, R. J. (1980) Circling behavior in rats with partial unilateral nigro-striatal lesions: Effects of amphetamine, apomorphine and DOPA. *Pharmacology, Biochemistry & Behavior*, **12**, 185–8.

HERMAN, J.-P., CHOULLI, K., GEFFARD, M., NADAUD, D., TAGH-ZOUTI, K. & LE MOAL, M. (1986) Reinnervation of the nucleus accumbens and frontal cortex of the rat by dopaminergic grafts and effects on hoarding behavior. *Brain Research*, **372**, 210–16.

HITCHCOCK, E. R., HENDERSON, B. T. H., KENNY, B. G. CLOUGH, C. G. HUGHES, R. C. & DETTA, A. (1991) Stereotactic implantation of fetal mesencephalon. In: *Intracerebral Transplantation in Movement Disorders, Experimental Basis and Clinical Experiences*, pp. 79–86. Eds. O. Lindvall, A. Björklund & H. Widner. Elsevier Science Publishers, Amsterdam.

HITCHCOCK, E. R., KENNY, B. G., CLOUGH, C. G., HUGHES, R. C., HENDERSON, B. T. H. & DETTA, A. (1990) Stereotactic implantation of foetal mesencephalon (STIM): the UK/experience. In: *Neural Transplantation. From Molecular Basis to Clinical Application. Progress in Brain Research*, **82**, pp. 328–33, Eds. S. B. Dunnett & S.-J. Richards. Elsevier, Amsterdam.

HOLLYDAY, M. & HAMBURGER, V. (1976) Reduction of the naturally occurring motor neuron loss by enlargement of the periphery, *Journal of Comparative Neurology*, **170**, 311–19.

IHARA, N., UEDA, S., TANABE, T. & SANO, Y. (1991) Transplantation of fetal medullary and raphé tissues into the cerebellum of denervated adult rats – an immunohistochemical study. *Brain Research*, 39–43.

INOUE, H. K. S., YOSHIDA, K. OHTANI, M., TOYA, S. & TSUKADA, Y. (1985) Cyclosporin A enhances the survivability of mouse cerebral cortex grafted into the third ventricle of rat brain. *Neuroscience Letters*, **54**, 85–90.

ISACSON, O., DUNNETT, S. B. & BJÖRKLUND, A. (1986) Graft-induced behavioral recovery in an animal model of Huntington's disease. *Proceedings of the National Academy of Sciences, USA*, **83**, 2728–32.

JAEGER, C. B. (1985) Cytoarchitectonics of substantia nigra grafts: a light and electron microscopic study of immunocytochemically identified dopa-minergic neurons and fibrous astrocytes. *Journal of Comparative Neurology*, **231**, 121–35.

KAMO, H., KIM, S. U., McGEER, P. L, ARAKI, M., TOMIMOTO, H. & KIMURA, H. (1987) Transplantation of cultured human spinal cord cells into the rat motor cortex: use of *Phaseolus vulgaris* leucoagglutinin as a cell marker. *Neuroscience Letters*, **76**, 163–7.

KAMO, H., KIM, S. U., McGEER, P. L. & SHIN, D. H. (1986) Functional recovery in a rat model of Parkinson's disease following transplantation of cultured human sympathetic neurons. *Brain Research*, **397**, 372–6.

KAPLAN, H. J. & STREILEIN, J. W. (1974) Do immunologically privileged sites require a functional spleen? *Nature*, **251**, 553–4.

KAWAMURA, K., NANAMI, T., KIKUCHI, Y. & SUZUKI, M. (1987) Cerebellar anlage transplanted into mature cerebellum. In: *Cell and Tissue Transplantation Into the Adult Brain. Annals of the New York Academy of Sciences*, **495**, pp. 726–9. Eds. E. Azmitia & A. Björklund. New York.

KING, P. D. & KATZ, D. R. (1990) Mechanisms of dendritic cell function. *Immunology Today*, **11**, 206–11.

KRIEGER, D. T., PERLOW, M. J., GIBSON, M. J., DAVIES, T. F., ZIMMERMAN, E. A., FERIN, M. & CHARLTON, H. M. (1982) Brain grafts reverse hypogonadism of gonadotropin-releasing hormone deficiency. *Nature*, **298**, 468–71.

LABANDEIRA-GARCIA, J. L., WICTORIN, K., CUNNINGHAM, E. T., Jr. & BJÖRKLUND, A. (1991) Development of intrastriatal striatal grafts and their afferent innervation from the host. *Neuroscience*, in press.

LACHAPELLE, F., GUMPEL, M., BAULAC, M., JAQUE, C., DUC, P. & BAUMANN, N. (1984) Transplantation of CNS fragments in the brain of shiverer mutant mice: Extensive myelination by implanted oligodendro-cytes. Immunocytochemical studies. *Developmental Neuroscience*, **6**, 325–34.

LAMPSON, L. A. (1987) Molecular bases of the immune response to neural antigens. *Trends in Neurosciences*, **10**, 211–16.

LAMPSON, L. A. & FISCHER, C. A. (1984) Weak HLA and β2-microglobu-lin expression of neuronal cell lines can be modulated by interferon, *Proceedings of the National Academy of Sciences, USA*, **81**, 6476–80.

LAWRENCE, J. M., MORRIS, R. J., WILSON, D. J. & RAISMAN, G. (1990) Mechanisms of allograft rejection in the rat brain, *Neuroscience*, **37**, 431–62.

LEE, M. H. & RABE, A. (1988) Neocortical transplants in the microencepha-lic rat brain: Morphology and behavior. *Brain Research Bulletin*, **21**, 813–224.

LEE, M. H. & RABE, A. (1990) Functional consequences of neocortical transplants in rats with a congenital brain defect: Electrophysiology and behavior. *Progress in Brain Research*, **82**, 359–66.

LE GROS CLARK, W. E. (1940) Neuronal differentiation in implanted foetal cortical tissue. *Journal of Neurology & Psychiatry*, **3**, 263–84.

LINDVALL, O., BRUNDIN, P., WIDNER, H., REHNCRONA, S., GUS-TAVII, B., FRACKOWIAK, R. LEENDERS, K. L., SAWE, G., ROTH-WELL, J. C., MARDSEN, C. D. & BJÖRKLUND, A. (1990) Grafts of fetal dopamine neurons survive and improve motor function in Parkinson's disease, *Science*, **242**, 574–7.

LINDVALL, O., REHNCRONA, S., BRUNDIN, P., GUSTAVII, B.,

ÅSTEDT, B., WIDNER, H., LINDHOLM, T., BJÖRKLUND, A., LEENDERS, K. L., ROTHWELL, J. C., FRACKOWIAK, R., MARSDEN, C. D., JOHNELS, B., STEG, G., FREEDMAN, R., HOFFER, B. J., SEIGER, Å., BYGDEMAN, M., STRÖMBERG, I. & OLSON, L. (1989) Human fetal dopamine neurons grafted into the striatum in two patients with severe Parkinson's disease. A detailed account of methodology and a 6-month follow-up, *Archives of Neurology*, **46**, 615–31.

LINDVALL, O., WIDNER, H., REHNCRONA, S., BRUNDIN, P., ODIN, P., GUSTAVII, B., FRACKOWIAK, R., LEENDERS, K. L., SAWLE, G., ROTHWELL, J. C., BJÖRKLUND, A. & MARSDEN, C. D. (1991) Transplantation of fetal dopamine neurons in Parkinson's disease: 1-year clinical and neurophysiological observations in two patients with putaminal implants. *Annals of Neurology*, in press.

LOW, W. C., LEWIS, P. R. & BUNCH, S. T. (1983) Embryonic neural transplants across a major histocompatibility barrier: survival and specificity of innervation. *Brain Research*, **262**, 328–33.

LUND, R. D., RAO, K., HANKIN, M. H., KUNZ, H. W. & GILL, T. J. (1987) Transplantation of retina and visual cortex to rat brains of different ages. Maturation, connection patterns, and immunological consequences, *Annals of the New York Academy of Sciences*, **495**, 227–41.

MADRAZO, I., FRANCO-BOURLAND, R., OSTROSKY-SOLIS, F., AGUILERA, M., CUEVAS, C., ZAMORANO, C., MORELOS, A., MAGALLON, E. & GUIZAR-SAHAGUN, G. (1990) Fetal homotransplants (ventral mesencephalon and adrenal tissue) to the striatum of parkinsonian subjects. *Archives of Neurology*, **47**, 1281–5.

MAHALIK, T. J., FINGER, T. E., STRÖMBERG, I. & OLSON, L. (1985) Substantia nigra transplants into denervated striatum of the rat: Ultrastructure of graft and host interconnections. *Journal of Comparative Neurology*, **240**, 60–70.

MAJDA, B. T. & HARVEY, A. R. (1989) Tectal tissue grafted to the midbrain of newborn rats: Effects of donor age on the survival, growth and connectivity of transplants. *Journal of Neural Transplantation*, **1**, 95–103.

MANTHORPE, M., NIETO-SAMPEDRO, M., SKAPER, S. D., LEWIS, E. R., BARBIN, G., LONGO, F. M., COTMAN, C. W. & VARON, S. (1983) Neuronotrophic activity in brain wounds of the developing rat. Correlation with implant survival in the wound cavity. *Brain Research*, **267**, 47–56.

MARCIANO, F. F., WIEGAND, S. J. & GASH, D. M. (1987) The role of target–graft interactions in the functional development of transplanted vasopressin neurons. *Annals of the New York Academy of Sciences*, **495**, 760–3.

MARCIANO, F. F., WIEGAND, S. J., SLADEK, J. R., Jr. & GASH, D. M. (1989) Fetal hypothalamic transplants promote survival and functional regeneration of axotomized adult supraoptic magnocellular neurons. *Brain Research*, **483**, 135–42.

MARSHALL, J. F., RICHARDSON, J. S. & TEITELBAUM, P. (1974) Nigrostriatal bundle damage and the lateral hypothalamic syndrome. *Journal of Comparative Physiology and Psychology*, **807**, 808–30.

MARSHALL, J. F. & TEITELBAUM, P. (1977) New considerations in the neuropsychology of motivated behavior. In: *Handbook of Psychopharmacology*, 7, pp. 201–29. Eds. L. L. Iversen, S. D. Iversen & S. H. Snyder. Plenum

Press, New York.

MASON, D. W., CHARLTON, H. M., JONES, A. J., LAVY, C. B., PUKLAVEC, M. & SIMMONDS, S. J. (1986) The fate of allogeneic and xenogeneic neuronal tissue transplanted into the third ventricle of rodents. *Neuroscience*, **19**, 685–94.

MASON, D. W. & MORRIS, P. J. (1986) Effector mechanisms in allograft rejection. *Annual Reviews in Immunology*, **4**, 119–45.

McCARRON, R. M., KEMPSKI, O., SPATZ, M. & McFARLIN, D. (1985) Presentation of myelin basic protein by murine cerebral vascular endothelial cells. *Journal of Immunology*, **134**, 3100–3.

McLOON, S. C. & LUND, R. D. (1980) Specific connections of retina transplanted to rat brain. *Experimental Brain Research*, **40**, 273–82.

MEDAWAR, P. B. (1948) Immunity to homologous grafted skin: III. The fate of skin homografts transplanted to the brain, to subcutaneous tissue, and to the anterior chamber of the eye. *British Journal of Experimental Pathology*, **29**, 58–69.

MOLINA, H., QUINONES, R., ALVAREZ, L., GALARRAGA, J., PIEDRA, J., SUAREZ, C., RACHID, M., GARCIA, J. C., PERRY, T. L., SANTANA, A., CARMENATE, H., MACIAS, R., TORRES, O., ROJAS, M. J., CORDOVA, F. & MUNOZ, J. L. (1991) Transplantation of human fetal mesencephalic tissue in caudate nucleus as treatment for Parkinson's disease. The Cuban experience. In: *Intracerebral Transplantation in Movement Disorders, Experimental Basis and Clinical Experiences*, pp. 99–110. Eds. O. Lindvall, A. Björklund & H. Widner. Elsevier Science Publishers, Amsterdam.

MUDRICK, L. A., LEUNG, P. P.-H., BAIMBRIDGE, K. G. & MILLER, J. J. (1988) Neuronal transplants used in the repair of acute ischemic injury in the central nervous system. *Progress in Brain Research*, **78**, 87–93.

NICHOLAS, M. K., ANTEL, J. P., STEFANSSON, K. & ARNASON, B. D. W. (1987) Rejection of fetal neocortical neural transplants by H-2 incompatible mice. *Journal of Immunology*, **139**, 2275–83.

NIETO-SAMPEDRO, M., LEWIS, E. R., COTMAN, C. W., MANTHORPE, M., SKAPER, S. D., BARBIN, G., LONGO, F. M. & VARON, S. (1982) Brain injury causes a time-dependent increase in neurotrophic activity at the lesion site. *Science*, **217**, 860–1.

NIETO-SAMPEDRO, M., WHITTEMORE, S. R., NEEDELS, D. L., LARSON, J. & COTMAN, C. W. (1984) The survival of brain transplants is enhanced by extracts from injured brain. *Proceedings of the National Academy of Sciences, USA*, **81**, 6250–54.

NILSSON, O. G., CLARKE, D. J., BRUNDIN, P. & BJÖRKLUND, A. (1988) Comparison of growth and reinnervation properties of cholinergic neurons from different brain regions grafted to the hippocampus. *Journal of Comparative Neurology*, **268**, 204–22.

NORNES, H., BJÖRKLUND, A. & STENEVI, U. (1983) Reinnervation of the denervated adult spinal chord of rats by intraspinal transplants of embryonic brain stem neurons. *Cell and Tissue Research*, **230**, 15–35.

NYGREN, L-G., OLSON, L. & SEIGER, Å. (1977) Monoaminergic reinnervation of the transected spinal cord by homologous fetal brain grafts. *Brain Research*, **129**, 227–35.

ONIFER, S. M. & LOW, W. C. (1990) Spatial memory deficit resulting from ischaemia-induced damage to the hippocampus is ameliorated by intrahippocampal transplants of fetal hippocampal neurons. *Progress in Brain Research*, **82**, 359–66.

PAN, H. S., PENNEY, J. B. & YOUNG, A. B. (1985) Gamma-aminobutyric acid and benzodiazepine receptor changes induced by unilateral 6-hydroxy-dopamine lesions of the medial forebrain bundle. *Journal of Neurochemistry*, **45**, 1396–404.

PENNEY, J. B. & YOUNG, A. B. (1983) Speculations on the functional anatomy of basal ganglia disorders. *Annual Reviews in Neuroscience*, **6**, 73–94.

PERLOW, M. J., FREED, W. J., HOFFER, B. J., SEIGER, Å., OLSON, L. & WYATT, R. J. (1979) Brain grafts reduce motor abnormalities produced by destruction of nigrostriatal dopamine system. *Science*, **204**, 643–7.

POLLACK, I. F., LUND, R. D. & RAO, K. (1990) MHC expression in spontaneous and induced rejection of intracerebral neural xenografts. *Progress in Brain Research*, **82**, 129–40.

POLTORAK, M. & FREED, W. J. (1990) Immunological reactions induced by intracerebral transplantation: Evidence that host microglia but not astroglia are the antigen-presenting cells. *Experimental Neurology*, **103**, 222–3.

PYCOCK, C. J. (1980) Turning behaviour in animals. *Neuroscience*, **5**, 461–514.

RADEL, J. D., HANKIN, M. H. & LUND, R. D. (1990) Proximity as a factor in the innervation of host brain regions by retinal transplants. *Journal of Comparative Neurology*, **300**, 211–29.

REDMOND, D. E., SLADEK, J. R., ROTH, R. H., COLLIER, T. J., ELSWORTH, J. D., DEUTCH, A. Y. & HABER, S. (1986) Fetal neuronal grafts in monkeys given methylphenyltetrahydropyridine. *Lancet*, **i**, 1125–7.

REDMOND, D. E. Jr., SPENCER, D., NAFTOLIN, F., LERANTH, C., ROBBINS, R. J., VOLLMER, T. L., ROTH, R. H., BUNNEY, B. S. & KIM, J. H. (1989) Cyropreserved human fetal neural tissue remains viable 4 months after transplantation into human caudate nucleus. *Society for Neuroscience Abstracts*, **15**, 123.

REIER, P. J. (1985) Neural tissue grafts and repair of the injured spinal chord. *Neuropathology & Applied Neurobiology*, **11**, 81–104.

REIER, P. J., PERLOW, M. J. & GUTH, L. (1983) Development of embryonic spinal cord transplants in the rat. *Developmental Brain Research*, **10**, 201–19.

SAUER, H. & BRUNDIN, P. (1991) Effects of cool storage on survival and function of intrastriatal ventral mesencephalic grafts. *Restorative Neurology and Neuroscience*, **2**, 123–35.

SAUER, H., FRODL, E. M., KUPSCH, A., ten BRUGGENCATE, G. & OERTEL, W. H. (1992) Cryopreservation, survival and function of intras-triatal fetal mesencephalic grafts in a rat model of Parkinson's disease. *Experimental Brain Research*, in press.

SAWLE, B. V., BLOOMFIELD, P. M., BJÖRKLUND, A., BROOKS, D. J., BRUNDIN, P., LEENDERS, K. L., LINDVALL, O., MARSDEN, C. D., REHNCRONA, S., WIDNER, H. & FRACKOWIAK, R. S. J. (1991) Transplantation of fetal dopamine neurons in Parkinson's disease: positron emission tomography [^{18}F]-6-L-flurodopa studies in two patients with putaminal implants. *Annals of Neurology*, in press.

SCHEINBERG, L. C., EDELMAN, F. L. & LEVY, A. W. (1964) Is the brain an immunologically privileged site? I. Studies based on intracerebral tumor transplantation and isotransplantation to sensitized hosts. *Archives in Neurology*, **11**, 248–64.

SCHMIDT, R. H., BJÖRKLUND, A. & STENEVI, U. (1981) Intracerebral grafting of dissociated CNS tissue suspensions: A new approach for neuronal transplantation to deep brain sites. *Brain Research*, **218**, 347–56.

SCHMIDT, R. H., BJÖRKLUND, A., STENEVI, U. & DUNNETT, S. B. (1983*a*) Intracerebral grafting of dissociated CNS tissue suspensions. In: *Nerve, Organ and Tissue Regeneration: Research Perspectives*, pp. 325–327. Ed. F. J. Seil. Academic Press, New York.

SCHMIDT, R. H., BJÖRKLUND, A., STENEVI, U., DUNNETT, S. B. & GAGE, F. H. (1983*b*) Intracerebral grafting of neuronal cell suspensions. III. Activity of intrastriatal nigral suspension implants as assessed by measurements of dopamine synthesis and metabolism. *Acta Physiologica Scandinavica*, Supplement **522**, 19–28.

SCHWAB, M. E. (1990) Myelin-associated inhibitors of neurite growth and regeneration in the CNS. *Trends in Neurosciences*, **13**, 452–6.

SEIGER, Å & OLSON, L. (1977) Quantification of fiber growth in transplanted central monoamine neurons, *Cell and Tissue Research*, **179**, 285–316.

SHIRRES, D. A. (1905) Regeneration of the axones of the spinal neurones in man. *Montreal Medical Journal*, **34**, 239–49.

SIMONDS, G. R. & FREED, W. J. (1990) Effects of intraventricular substantia nigra allografts as a function of donor age. *Brain Research*, **530**, 12–19.

SIRINATSHINGIJ, D. J. S., DUNNETT, S. B., NORTHROP, A. J. & MORRIS, B. J. (1990) Experimental hemiparkinsonism in the rat following chronic unilateral infusion of MPP$^+$ into the nigrostriatal dopamine pathway – III. Reversal by embryonic nigral dopamine grafts. *Neuroscience*, **37**, 757–66.

SLADEK, J. R., Jr, COLLIER, T. J., HABER, S. N., ROTH, R. H. & REDMOND, D. E., Jr. (1986) Survival and growth of fetal catecholamine neurons grafted into the primate brain. *Brain Research Bulletin*, **1**, 809–18.

SMITH, G. M., MILLER, R. H. & SILVER, J. S. (1987) Astrocyte transplantation induces callosal regeneration in postnatal acallosal mice. *Annals of the New York Academy of Sciences*, **495**, 185–205.

SOFRONIEW, M. V., ISACSON, O. & BJÖRKLUND, A. (1986) Cortical grafts prevent atrophy of cholinergic basal nucleus neurons induced by excitotoxic cortical damage. *Brain Research*, **378**, 409–15.

SØRENSEN, T., JENSEN, S., MØLLER, A. & ZIMMER, J. (1986) Intracephalic transplants of freeze-stored rat hippocampal tissue. *Journal of Comparative Neurology*, **252**, 468–82.

SØRENSEN, J. C., ZIMMER, J. & CASTRO, A. J. (1989) Fetal cortical transplants reduce the thalamic atrophy induced by frontal cortical lesions in newborn rats. *Neuroscience Letters*, **98**, 33–8.

SOTELO, C. & ALVARADO-MALLART, R. M. (1986) Growth and differentiation of cerebellar suspensions transplanted into the adult cerebellum of mice with heredo-degenerative ataxia. *Proceedings of the National Academy of Sciences, USA*, **83**, 1135–9.

SOTELO, C. & ALVARADO-MALLART, R. M. (1987) Embryonic and adult neurons interact to allow Purkinje cell replacement in mutant cerebellum. *Nature*, **327**, 421–3.

SOTELO, C. & ALVARADO-MALLART, R. M. (1988) Integration of grafted Purkinje cells into the host cerebellar circuitry in Purkinje cell degeneration mutant mouse. In: *Transplantation Into the Mammalian CNS. Progress in Brain Research*, **78**. pp. 141–53. Eds. D. M. Gash & J. R. Sladek, Jr. Elsevier, Amsterdam.

STENEVI, U., BJÖRKLUND, A. & SVENDGAARD, N.-A. (1976) Transplantation of central and peripheral monoamine neurons to the adult rat brain: techniques and conditions for survival. *Brain Research*, **114**, 1–20.

STEWART, P. A., CLEMENTS, L. G. & WILEY, M. J. (1984) Revascularization of skin transplanted to the brain: source of the graft endothelium. *Microvascular Research*, **28**, 113–24.

STREILEIN, J. W. & NIEDERKORN, J. Y. (1985) Characterization of the suppressor cell(s) responsible for anterior chamber-associated immune deviation (ACAID) induced in BALB/c mice by P815 cells. *Journal of Immunology*, **134**, 1381–7.

STRÖMBERG, I., ALMQUIST, P., BYGDEMAN, M., FINGER, T., GERHART, G., GRANHOLM, A.-C., MAHALIK, T. J., SEIGER, Å., HOFFER, B. & OLSON, L. (1989) Human mesencephalic tissue grafted to dopamine-denervated striatum of athymic rats: Light and electron microscopical histochemistry and in vivo chronoamperometric studies. *Journal of Neuroscience*, **9**, 614–24.

STRÖMBERG, I., BYGDEMAN, M., GOLDSTEIN, M., SEIGER, Å. & OLSON, L. (1986) Human fetal substantia nigra grafted to the dopamine denervated striatum of immunosuppressed rats: evidence for functional reinnervation. *Neuroscience Letters*, **71**, 271–6.

THOMPSON, W. G. (1890) Successful brain grafting. *New York Medical Journal*, **5**, 701–2.

TØNDER, N., SØRENSEN, T., ZIMMER, J., JØRGENSEN, M. B., JOHANSEN, F. F. & DIEMER, N. H. (1989) Neural grafting to ischemic lesions of the adult rat hippocampus. *Experimental Brain Research*, **74**, 512–26.

TRANTZER, J. P. & THOENEN, H. (1967) Ultramorphologische Veränderungen der sympathischen Nervenendigungen der Katze nach Vorbehandlung mit 5- und 6-Hydroxy-Dopamin. *Naunyn-Schmiedebergs Archives of Experimental Pathology and Pharmacology*, **257**, 343–4.

TRAUGOTT, U., SCHEINBERG, L. & RAINE, C. (1985) On the presence of Ia-positive endothelial cells and astrocytes in multiple sclerosis lesions and its relevance to antigen presentation. *Journal of Neuroimmunology*, **8**, 1–14.

TRIARHOU, L. C., LOW, W. C. & GHETTI, B. (1986) Transplantation of ventral mesencephalic anlagen to hosts with genetic nigrostriatal dopamine deficiency. *Proceedings of the National Academy of Sciences, USA*, **83**, 8789–93.

TRIARHOU, L. C., LOW, W. C. & GHETTI, B. (1990) Dopamine neuron grafting to the Weaver mouse neostriatum. *Progress in Brain Research*, **82**, 187–93.

TRULSON, M. E. & HOSSEINI, A. (1987) Dopamine neuron transplants: electrophysiological unit activity of intrastriatal nigral grafts in freely moving cats. *Life Sciences*, **40**, 2097–102.

TURNER, J. E. & BLAIR, J. R. (1986) Newborn rat retinal cells transplanted into a retinal lesion site in adult host eyes. *Developmental Brain Research*, **26**, 91–104.

UNGERSTEDT, U. (1968) 6-Hydroxydopamine induced degeneration of central monoamine neurons. *European Journal of Pharmacology*, **5**, 107–10.

UNGERSTEDT, U. (1971a) Post-synaptic supersensitivity after 6-hydroxydopamine induced degeneration of the nigro-striatal dopamine system. *Acta Physiologica Scandinavica*, Supplement, **367**, 49–68.

UNGERSTEDT, U. (1971b) Aphagia and adipsia after 6-hydroxydopamine induced degeneration of the nigro-striatal dopamine system. *Acta Physiologica Scandinavica*, Supplement, **367**, 95–122.

UNGERSTEDT, U. & ARBUTHNOTT, G. W. (1970) Quantitative recording of rotational behavior in rats after 6-hydroxydopamine lesions of the nigrostriatal dopamine system. *Brain Research*, **24**, 485–93.

URETSKY, N. J. & IVERSEN, L. L. (1970) Effects of 6-hydroxydopamine on catecholamine containing neurones in the rat brain. *Journal of Neurochemistry*, **17**, 269–78.

VINOGRADOVA, O. S., BRAGIN, A. G. & KITCHIGINA, V. F. (1985) Spontaneous and evoked activity of neurons in intrabrain allo- and xenografts of the hippocampus and septum. In: *Neural Grafting in the Mammalian CNS*, pp. 409–42. Eds. A. Björklund & U. Stenevi. Elsevier, Amsterdam.

WEKERLE, H., LININGTON, C., LASSMANN, H. & MEYERMAN, R. (1986) Cellular immune reactivity within the CNS. *Trends in Neurosciences*, **6**, 271–7.

WHITTEMORE, S. R., LARKFORS, L., EBENDAL, T., HOLETS, V. R., ERICSSON, A. & PERSSON, H. (1987) Increased beta-Nerve Growth Factor messenger RNA and protein levels in neonatal rat hippocampus following specific cholinergic lesions. *Journal of Neuroscience*, **7**, 244–51.

WHITTEMORE, S. R., NIETO-SAMPEDRO, M., NEEDELS, D. M. & COTMAN, C. W. (1985) Neuronotrophic factors for mammalian brain neurons: Injury induction in neonatal, adult and aged brain. *Developmental Brain Research*, **20**, 169–78.

WICTORIN, K., BRUNDIN, P., GUSTAVII, B., LINDVALL, O. & BJÖRKLUND, A. (1990) Reformation of long axon pathways in adult rat central nervous system by human forebrain neurons. *Nature*, **347**, 556–8.

WIDNER, H. & BRUNDIN, P. (1988) Immunological aspects of grafting in the mammalian central nervous system: a review and speculative synthesis. *Brain Research Reviews*, **13**, 287–324.

WIDNER, H. & BRUNDIN, P. (1990) Long-term survival, immunogenicity and functional effects of single and sequential intracerebral allogeneic fetal neuronal grafts in rats. In: *Immunological Basis for Intracerebral Reconstructive Transplantations*, pp. 123–35. Ed. H. Widner. Academic Thesis, Lund.

WIDNER, H., BRUNDIN, P., BJÖRKLUND, A. & MÖLLER, E. (1989) Survival and immunogenicity of dissociated allogeneic fetal neural dopamine-rich grafts when implanted into the brains of adult mice, *Experimental Brain Research*, **76**, 187–97.

WIDNER, H., JÖNSSON, B.-A., HALLSTADIUS, L., WINGÅRDH, K., STRAND, S. E. & JOHANSSON, B. B. (1987) Scintigraphic method to quantify the passage from brain parenchyma to the deep cervical lymph nodes in the rat. *European Journal of Nuclear Medicine*, **13**, 456–61.

WONG, G. H., BARTLETT, P. F., CLARK-LEWIS, I., BATTYE, F. & SCHRADER, J. W. (1984) Inducible expression of H-2 and Ia antigens on brain cells. *Nature*, **310**, 688–91.

YANAI, J. & PICK, C. G. (1988) Neuron transplantation reverses phenobar-bital-induced behavioral birth defects in mice. *International Journal of Developmental Neuroscience*, **6**, 409–16.

YUREK, D. M. & SLADEK, J. R., Jr. (1990) Dopamine cell replacement: Parkinson's Disease. *Annual Reviews in Neuroscience*, **13**, 415–40.

ZALEWSKI, A. A., GOSHGARIAN, H. G. & SILVERS, W. K. (1978) The fate of neurons and neurilemmal cells in the spinal cord of normal and immunologically tolerant rats. *Experimental Neurology*, **59**, 322–30.

ZHOU, F. C., AUERBACH, S. & AZMITIA, E. (1987) Denervation of serotonergic fibers in the hippocampus induced a trophic factor which enhances the maturation of transplanted serotoneric neurons but not norepinephrine neurons. *Journal of Neuroscience Research*, **17**, 235–46.

ZHOU, F. C. & AZMITIA, E. C. (1990) Neurotrophic factor for serotonergic neurons prevents degeneration of grafted raphé neurons in the cerebellum. *Brain Research,* **507**, 301–8.

ZHOU, F. C., LI, Y. & RAISMAN, G. (1989) Embryonic entorhinal transplants project selectively to the deafferented entorhinal zone of adult mouse hippocampi, as demonstrated by the use of thy-1 allelic immunohisto-chemistry. Effect of timing of transplantation in relation to deafferentation. *Neuroscience*, **32**, 349–62.

ZUDDAS, A., CORSINI, G. U., BARKER, J. L., KOPIN, I. J. & diPORZIO, U. (1991) Specific reinnervation of lesioned mouse striatum by grafted mesencephalic dopaminergic neurons. *European Journal of Neuroscience*, **3**, 72–85.

CHAPTER 8

Clinical results of transplanting fetal

pancreas

B. E. TUCH

CONTENTS

THE IDEA OF TRANSPLANTING HUMAN FETAL PANCREAS into diabetic humans in order to normalize blood glucose levels was first seriously entertained in 1977, when the initial use of the vascularized pancreas (Sutherland, 1981) and the islet (Najarian *et al.*, 1975) proved to be unsuccessful. What prompted the move in this direction were the elegant studies of Brown and his group in California, demonstrating that the rat fetal pancreas, when isografted at 17 days gestation into an adult diabetic recipient, was capable of normalizing the blood glucose levels within 4–6 weeks of transplantation (Brown *et al.*, 1974). Subsequent studies by Mandel in Melbourne, Australia, showed that the fetal mouse pancreas behaved in a similar manner when isografted (Mandel, 1984). Several years later, in 1985, the human fetal pancreas was shown to be capable of reversing diabetes when xenografted in the immunoincompetent athymic, or nude, mouse (Tuch *et al.*, 1985*b*). This and other studies demonstrated that human fetal pancreatic explants, when grafted into these animals, reversed diabetes within one to three months (Hullett *et al.*, 1987; Tuch *et al.*, 1988*b*) (Figure 8.1). The apparent universal potential of grafted fetal pancreas to reverse diabetes gained further support with the demonstration, in 1988, of the successful normalization of blood glucose levels in the athymic mouse by explants of pig fetal pancreas (Walthall *et al.*, 1988) and, in 1990, proislets, or islet-like cell clusters, of this tissue (Simeonovic *et al.*, 1990; Korsgren *et al.*, 1991).

215

Figure 8.1. Reversal of diabetes in athymic mice by human fetal pancreatic explants grafted beneath the renal capsule. The diabetes was induced by injection of 275 mg/kg streptozotocin (STZ) three weeks after the tissue was implanted – STZ is not toxic to the human fetal beta cell (Tuch *et al.*, 1989). Note the length of time required before normalization of blood glucose levels varied between 50 and 100 days.

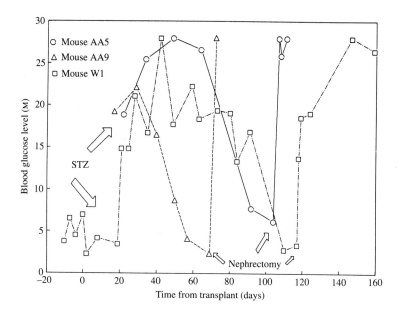

Source of human fetal tissue

In the Western world, human fetal pancreas is obtained from termination of pregnancies performed up to the twenty fourth week of gestation (Jovanovic-Peterson *et al.*, 1988). In some countries, such as Australia, the guidelines are stricter, prohibiting the termination of pregnancies after 20 weeks (National Health & Medical Research Council of Australia Medical Research Ethics Committee, 1983). In the People's Republic of China, where there is a policy of one child per family, termination, which is an accepted form of contraception, may be performed at a relatively late stage of pregnancy, thus making it possible to utilize pancreas obtained in the third trimester (Hu *et al.*, 1985).

For the purpose of transplantation, the human fetal pancreas is generally not used before 11 weeks of gestation, although pancreatic buds appear on the dorsal and ventral surfaces of the primitive gut at the fourth week of gestation (Davies & Davies, 1962); fuse during the seventh week; and contain endocrine tissue from the eighth week (Stefan *et al.*, 1983). The major reason for this is the small size of the fetal pancreas, the length of a 12-week pancreas being 2 mm and an 18-week organ being 14 mm (Figure 8.2), as compared to 120–180 mm for an adult pancreas (Davies & Davies, 1962). The practical implications involve not only handling a tiny fetal pancreas, but also in identifying the organ if the termination is carried out by suction curettage.

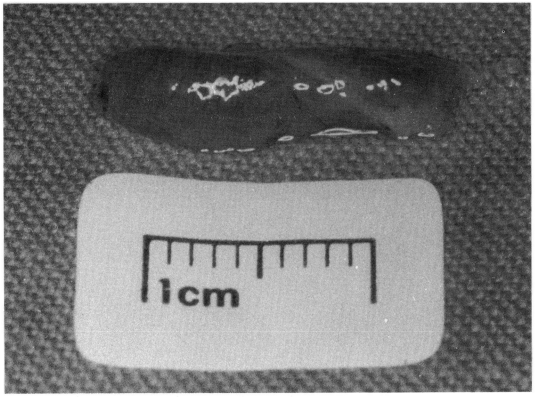

Figure 8.2. Human fetal pancreas of 18 weeks gestation. The length of the pancreas was 14 mm.

The major advantage in using human fetal pancreas up to 18-weeks of gestation is the comparative absence of acini, containing digestive enzymes (Falin, 1967). Before this age the pancreas consists of fibrous tissue, ducts, which are the precursors of both acini and islets (Pictet & Rutter, 1972), as well as endocrine cells, which are present as single cells, groups of cells, and islets (Jaffe *et al.*, 1982) (Figure 8.3). Mesenchyme represents 64% of the organ, with epithelial cells constituting the rest (B. E. Tuch, unpublished data). A small component of the gland consists of blood vessels and lymphocytes, the latter located at the periphery. Endocrine cells constitute 35% of all epithelial cells present (B. E. Tuch, unpublished data), the majority being beta cells containing insulin (Stefan *et al.*, 1983). A morphometric study carried out at the University of Sydney showed that the percentage of beta, delta and alpha cells was 53%, 24%, and 21% respectively. Pancreatic polypeptide (PP) cells were sparse, constituting 2% of all endocrine cells, although the number was more numerous in the selective PP-region of the organ. Pancreases in fetuses older than 18 weeks of gestation contain acini in addition to the other components (Falin, 1967).

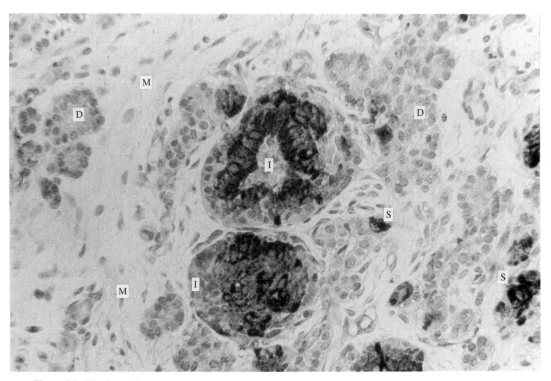

Figure 8.3. Histology of a human fetal pancreas of 17 weeks gestation. Note the presence of ducts (D), mesenchyme (M), and beta cells (dark stain) both in islets (I) and as single cells and small clumps (S). Immunoperoxidase stain for insulin, × 200.

Viable fetal pancreas can be obtained from any of four methods of termination used throughout the world: hysterotomy, suction curettage, mechanical induction (by saline or a water bag), and prostaglandin administration. The last method has resulted in tissue that is poorly viable in some (Otonkoski *et al.*, 1988) but not all, centres (Tuch & Turtle, 1987). To reduce anoxic damage to the tissue, it is advisable to remove the pancreas as soon after termination as possible, preferably in less than four hours and divide it into explants sized 1 mm^3 (Figure 8.4) within a further four hours (Tuch & Turtle, 1987).

In vitro handling of tissue

Most of the tissue grafted into diabetic humans has been in the form of these explants, for it is possible to maintain the viability of most of the tissue in organ culture for several weeks (Tuch & Turtle, 1987) with diffusion of oxygen (Andersson *et al.*, 1984) and nutrients across this distance (Figure 8.4). This tissue continues to secrete insulin, both acutely in response to 10 mmol theophylline (Hoffman *et al.*, 1982), and chronically (Tuch & Turtle, 1987). The amount of insulin secreted increases proportionately to the gestational age of the pancreas, probably because of the greater number of beta cells present in the

218

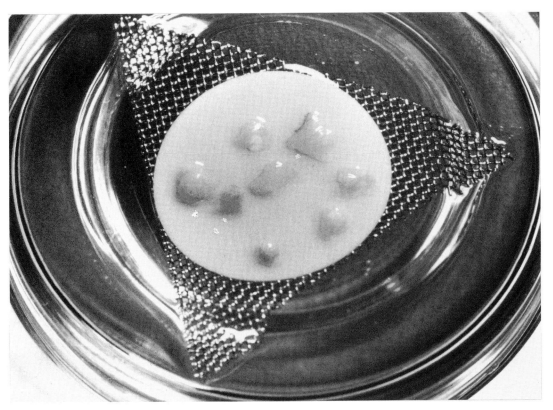

Figure 8.4. 1 mm³ explants of human fetal pancreas in organ culture. The tissue has been placed on filter paper, which rests on a stainless steel grid. Nutrients diffuse into the tissue, which is at an air–liquid interface.

older pancreases. For example, average insulin secretion from a 14-week pancreas is 3.2×10^{-3} units/day, whereas from an 18-week pancreas it is 15.2×10^{-3} units/day. Morphologically, the percentage of epithelial to stromal tissue remains unchanged during this time, being 55% before culture, 57% at two weeks and 59% at four weeks. Beta cells remain the predominant endocrine cell throughout this period of culture, constituting 23% of epithelial cells initially and 19% after four weeks in culture. The percentage of alpha and delta cells is not significantly different, both being 11% initially and 13% and 16% respectively after four weeks. Culturing of this tissue for periods longer than three weeks usually results in extensive loss of viable tissue because of ischaemic necrosis (Table 8.1). Tissue that has been cultured for such long periods survives less well than that cultured for shorter periods when it is implanted into athymic mice (B. E. Tuch, unpublished data).

The ability to culture a human fetal pancreas for up to three weeks before transplanting it makes it possible to ascertain that the explants are continuing to secrete insulin, and that there are no aerobic and anaerobic bacteria, mycoplasma, fungi or viruses contaminating the

Table 8.1. *Effect of duration of culture on the viability of human fetal pancreatic explants in organ culture*

These data were collected from six pancreases of gestational age 17–19 weeks, that were cultured for seven weeks. Whilst all organs were viable up to at least three weeks of culture, only two of them were still alive at seven weeks.

Duration of culture (weeks)	Diameter of explants mm (mean ± standard error of the mean)	Viable tissue (%)	Necrotic tissue (%)
0	0.96 ± 0.08	100	0
1	0.83 ± 0.09	95	5
2	0.78 ± 0.08	84	16
3	0.71 ± 0.09	79	21
4	0.76 ± 0.08	37	63
5	0.71 ± 0.11	25	75
6	0.93 ± 0.09	21	79
7	0.82 ± 0.08	22	78

culture medium, which might be transmitted at the time of grafting. A number of pathogenic viruses, such as hepatitis B, and other microorganisms, such as *Treponema pallidum*, which will be difficult to discern in such examinations, are more likely to be detected by examining maternal serum for antibodies to these agents (Voss *et al.*, 1989). In a study conducted at the University of Sydney between 1981 and 1986, the presence of antibodies to hepatitis B surface antigen in 129 samples of sera was nil. Antibodies to *Treponema pallidum* and the human immunodeficiency virus also were absent, whereas recent exposure to cytomegalovirus and toxoplasmosis occurred in 10% and 20% of samples respectively. One further examination that may be conducted during the period of organ culture is histocompatibility typing of the fetal tissue (Mandel *et al.*, 1982; Danilovs *et al.*, 1983; Tuch *et al.*, 1985*a*). The need for matching donor tissue and recipient is likely to be meaningful, however, only when a single fetal pancreas is grafted, unless an organ bank of fetal pancreases is available.

Several groups have used an alternative approach to the grafting of 1 mm³ slices of human fetal pancreas (Shumakov *et al.*, 1983; Farkas & Karácsonyi, 1985; Walthall *et al.*, 1988). All these groups have used collagenase or a similar enzyme to digest the tissue into single cells. The Hungarian group then maintains their cells freely floating in culture for up to ten weeks before grafting (Farkas & Karácsonyi, 1985). Shumakov in the Soviet Union cultures his cells for a much shorter period (Shumakov *et al.*, 1983), whilst the group in San Francisco

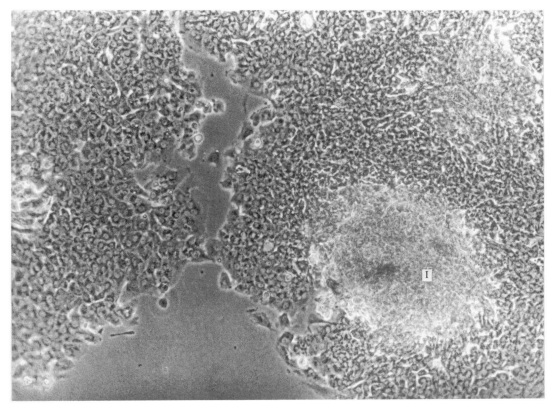

Figure 8.5. Islet-like cell cluster (I) obtained by partial digestion of human fetal pancreas of 19 weeks gestation. This tissue has attached to the culture well, and is spreading out to form monolayers which are rich in beta cells. Photograph kindly supplied by A. M. Simpson. Magnification × 40.

culture their cells in a three-dimensional matrix in order to increase the number of cells available for transplantation (Walthall *et al.*, 1988). A third method, soon to be utilized in humans, is the use of islet-like cell clusters, or proislets (Figure 8.5), which are obtained by partial digestion of the original pancreas (Sandler *et al.*, 1985). From a single pancreas, it is possible to obtain 200 islet-like cell clusters, only a small percentage of which are beta cells (Otonkoski *et al.*, 1988; Sandler *et al.*, 1989). It is possible to increase the component of beta cells in these clumps, up to 51%, by forming a monolayer of these clusters (Simpson *et al.*, 1991).

Irrespective of whether the fetal beta cell is present in explants, islet-like cell clusters, or monolayers, they behave in a similar physiological manner. They release little insulin in response to the usual physiological stimuli, such as glucose and amino acids (Ågren *et al.*, 1980; Hoffman *et al.*, 1982; Sandler *et al.*, 1985; Tuch *et al.*, 1990*b*; Simpson *et al.*, 1991), but avidly secrete this hormone in response to: agents that increase levels of cyclic AMP, such as theophylline (Milner *et al.*, 1971; Hoffman *et al.*, 1982; Tuch *et al.*, 1990*b*; Simpson *et al.*, 1991); agents

221

that increase intracellular levels of calcium (Tuch *et al.*, 1990*b*; Simpson *et al.*, 1991); and substances, such as phorbol acetate, that activate protein kinase C (Tuch *et al.*, 1990*b*; Simpson *et al.*, 1991). Synergy is observed when theophylline and calcium are used together as stimuli (Tuch *et al.*, 1990*b*). In contrast to their poor ability to secrete insulin in response to glucose, the human fetal beta cell is capable of synthesizing insulin in the presence of glucose (Maitland *et al.*, 1980; Sandler *et al.*, 1985).

Requirements for successful normalization of diabetes in humans

Before hyperglycaemia can be normalized in diabetic humans, there are a number of requirements. These include: the grafting of sufficient tissue; maturation of the insulinogenic response to glucose by the beta cell; the successful vascularization of grafted tissue; and the means of preventing rejection.

Grafting of sufficient amount of tissue

One of the advantages of using human fetal tissue is its remarkable capacity to grow *in vivo* (Figure 8.6). The growth rate of the fetal pancreas is greater the younger the fetal tissue, especially 15 weeks of gestation or less (Tuch *et al.*, 1986). On average, human fetal pancreas of gestational age 14–19 weeks increase in size fifteen-fold in one year when grafted into the athymic mouse, the insulin content increasing fifty-one-fold in this period (Tuch *et al.*, 1986). The increase in the number of beta cells in the graft is likely to be due to increased differentiation of the immature precursor duct cells, rather than from previously committed beta cells, since this is the usual method of beta cell formation in the fetus (Pictet & Rutter, 1972). Interestingly acini do not appear, even though they are also thought to stem from the duct cell. Despite this growth advantage of fetal over adult tissue, the amount of pancreas grafted into a diabetic athymic mouse is an important determinant of the time for normalization of blood glucose levels to occur, this period ranging from one to three months (Tuch, 1991). As little as one-eighth of a fetal pancreas can normalize blood glucose levels in these mice, but an entire pancreas will achieve this goal faster. Reversal of diabetes in athymic mice is usually achieved with 1 mm^3 explants of human fetal pancreas that have been cultured for periods of up to several days (Tuch *et al.*, 1988*b*), although it is possible for normoglycaemia to be achieved in these animals if the tissue is cultured for three weeks (Tuch & Osgerby, 1990). As was mentioned

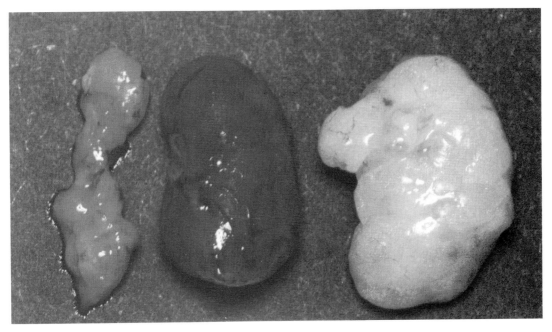

1 cm

Figure 8.6. Human fetal pancreatic graft (right) removed from beneath the capsule of the kidney (centre) of an athymic mouse 97 weeks after it was implanted. The mouse pancreas (left) is shown for comparison. In this experiment the mouse was not rendered diabetic. The human pancreas graft was of 13 weeks gestation and weighed 16 mg; its weight when removed from the mouse was 356 mg. Despite the large size of the graft the mouse remained normoglycaemic at all times.

previously, culturing the explants for longer periods is deleterious to its ability to survive in the athymic mouse. Treatment of tissue with nicotinamide before transplantation also may reduce the time required to achieve normoglycaemia, as has been the case with fetal pig islet-like cell clusters (Korsgren *et al.*, 1990). How many fetal pancreases will be needed to reverse diabetes in humans is not known, but the use of multiple organs would seem to be more advantageous. The same conclusion was reached regarding the successful grafting of cadaveric adult islets into diabetic humans (Scharp *et al.*, 1990).

Maturation of response to glucose

The human fetal beta cell must be able to release insulin in response to glucose, if it is to be successful in normalizing blood glucose levels in diabetic patients. As previously mentioned, the human fetal beta cell releases insulin poorly, if at all, in response to glucose. For this cell to respond to glucose it has to mature, something that normally occurs over a period of many months. Some response to glucose is observed in preterm infants of 34 weeks of gestation (Grasso *et al.*, 1975) and in

223

full-term infants with an increase after the first day of life (Grasso *et al.*, 1983). An adult-type response is observed between 1 and 6 months of life (von Euler *et al.*, 1964). In the case of the grafted human fetal beta cell, there is reason to believe that maturation will occur after the tissue is transplanted into a diabetic human, since some maturation does occur in such tissue grafted into the immunoincompetent athymic mouse, rendered diabetic with streptozotocin (Tuch *et al.*, 1985*b*, 1988*b*). Normalization of blood glucose levels in these animals is achieved more rapidly the older, and presumably the more mature, the grafted tissue is (Tuch, 1991). These data, together with the positive effect of the amount of tissue grafted, suggest that reversal of diabetes in humans is likely to be achieved most rapidly if many fetal pancreases, that are as 'old' as possible, are transplanted. Interestingly, a physiological biphasic response to glucose is not required for normalization of blood glucose levels in grafted athymic mice, the presence of only the second phase being compatible with normoglycaemia (Tuch *et al.*, 1988*b*).

Successful vascularization of grafted tissue

The site at which the human fetal pancreas is likely to function best is not known. Studies contrasting the grafting of this tissue into a peripheral site versus a central one have shown that tissue placed beneath the renal capsule grows faster and contains more insulin than that placed subcutaneously (Tuch *et al.*, 1986). Subsequent studies contrasting a portal with a systemic site showed no advantage of the liver or spleen over the renal capsule (Tuch *et al.*, 1987*a*), although more elegant studies with fetal rodent pancreas showed portal drainage to be more beneficial (Brown *et al.*, 1979). Whatever the site chosen, a prominent vascular supply should have developed a few days after transplantation (Brown *et al.*, 1974) and be complete by ten days (Menger *et al.*, 1990).

Prevention of rejection

It needs to be understood that human fetal pancreatic tissue is immunogenic, a single cell suspension of the collagenase-digested pancreas stimulating proliferation of allogeneic lymphocytes in a mixed lymphocyte culture (Tuch *et al.*, 1988*a*; Simpson *et al.*, 1991). Further, if such tissue is xenografted into an immunocompetent mouse, lymphocytic infiltration occurs and the graft is destroyed. This immunogenicity of human fetal pancreatic tissue should not be confused with the immature immunological system of the fetus

(Bernales & Bellanti, 1982), which results in the unborn child being unable to mount an adult-type response to foreign antigens.

The reason for the immunogenicity of the tissue is a result of the presence of histocompatibility antigens, the presentation of these antigens, especially class II, in conjunction with antigen presenting cells being what initiates a cellular immune response (Lafferty *et al.*, 1983). Most fetal pancreatic cells express class I antigens, but few normally express class II antigens (Campbell *et al.*, 1986), this occurring in dendritic cells distributed throughout the parenchyma and interstitial connective tissue, and foci of lymphocytes, usually in the periphery of the organ (Danilovs *et al.*, 1982). Expression of these class II antigens is, however, induced during rejection of allografted tissue in humans (Tuch *et al.*, 1988c) and by exposure to the cytokine, interferon-γ (Campbell *et al.*, 1986).

Expression of these antigens, as well as the presence of other tissue antigens, can be reduced by culturing the tissue or cells *in vitro* (Thomson *et al.*, 1983; Simpson *et al.*, 1991). Despite the reduction in tissue antigens by culturing, it seems a trifle unrealistic to expect cultured human fetal pancreas to be grafted successfully into diabetic humans without the recipients also being immunosuppressed, just as is the case with allografts of cultured mouse fetal pancreas (Burkhardt *et al.*, 1989).

Clinical transplants of human fetal pancreas

History records that the first attempt at normalizing blood glucose levels in a diabetic human was in 1928, when pancreatic tissue from three fetuses was placed beneath the tunica vaginalis of the testis, as well as intramuscularly and preperitoneally in an 18-year-old diabetic male. This experiment was a failure; the patient dying of ketoacidosis three days after being transplanted (Downing, 1984). More systematic attempts at grafting human fetal pancreas into diabetic humans began in 1977, with thirty transplants being performed in six centres between then and 1981 (Sutherland *et al.*, 1981). Initial reports were encouraging with claims that two recipients were able to cease their exogenous insulin 2–5 months after transplantation (Chastan *et al.*, 1980; Valente *et al.*, 1980). In a number of other cases, C-peptide rises were reported in blood (Valente *et al.*, 1980) and urine (Groth *et al.*, 1980), with a concomitant reduction in insulin requirements in some. These results enthused many groups throughout the world, so that as of June 1990, 1582 cases of engraftment of human fetal tissue from a total of sixty centres were reported to the International Islet Transplant Registry in Giessen, West Germany (Hering *et al.*, 1988). The majority of these cases were carried out in: the Soviet Union (1000 cases); People's Republic of China (436 cases) (Hu *et al.*, 1989); and the Hana multicentre series in the United States (36 cases) (Voss *et al.*, 1989). Unfortunately, the results from all these clinical trials have not matched the enthusiasm of the people conducting these experiments.

It is extremely difficult to be absolute about what conclusions can be drawn from all these data, despite the excellent attempt at recording relevant information by Dr Bernhard Hering, who manages the International Islet Transplant Registry. There are numerous claims of graft function, as determined by measurement of human C-peptide in blood, and a further nineteen claims for being able to cease all exogenous insulin requirements. A factor that compounds the assessment of many of these claims is the failure to carry out appropriate endocrinological studies on the recipients before transplantation. The minimum tests necessary include measurement of C-peptide, by a reproducible assay, with a defined lower limit of detection, in the fasting state and after a pharmacological challenge, for example, 1 mg glucagon or sustacal; and a 24-hour urinary C-peptide level. The histology of the grafted tissue, for example at biopsy, would be ideal, but is difficult to obtain if the graft was functioning. The need for tissue analysis is illustrated by the single report of four patients grafted with human fetal pancreas, in whom insulin requirements were said to be reduced by 71% to 100% and C-peptide levels rose. But biopsy of the graft site showed only non-specific inflammation and no evidence of beta cells (Jovanovic-Petersen *et al.*, 1988). One further safeguard that is necessary is to ascertain prior to transplantation that the patient was not overinsulinized, and hence was suppressing secretion of C-peptide from naturally occurring beta cells.

There are two centres who have been successful in demonstrating the survival of human fetal pancreas at the engrafted site. These are the University of Sydney in Australia (Tuch *et al.*, 1988c) and the Barbara Davis Centre in Denver, Colorado (Lafferty *et al.*, 1989). In the former centre, explants of human fetal pancreas, cultured for up to twenty one days, were implanted in the forearm muscle, as well as a number of other sites, including portal vein, omentum, and beneath the renal capsule (Figure 8.7). In three of the four cases where immunosuppression was used, some of the original tissue was recovered in the forearm one year after transplantation had occurred. This consisted of ducts interspersed with endocrine cells, either as single cells or clumps, or an islet, surrounded by fibrous tissue (Figure 8.8). Small numbers of alpha, beta and delta cells, in that order of magnitude, were identified by immunoperoxidase stains. Lymphocytes of recipient origin were seen to be infiltrating the graft in two patients, the majority of these

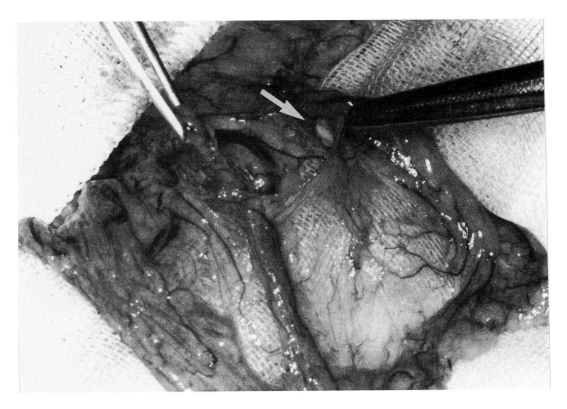

Figure 8.7. Pooled explants from one human fetal pancreas of 15 weeks gestation (arrowed) being implanted into an omental loop of an insulin-dependent diabetic person. Whilst the fate of this tissue is unknown, a portion of the explants of a second pancreas, grafted at the same time into the forearm muscle of this person, was located and removed one year later.

cells being T cells; in one case most of these were CD4$^+$, and in the other CD8$^+$. In one of these patients, B lymphocytes in germinal centres were also identified, as were HLA class II antigens on duct cells and on activated T lymphocytes, indicating that either rejection or the autoimmune destruction of the tissue was slowly occurring. Antibodies to both islet cells and the 64K antigen were unmeasurable in this patient. Further, in three of the recipients who had renal transplants, rejection of the grafted kidney did not occur. In Denver, diced human fetal pancreas, cultured for 5–10 days, was grafted beneath the renal capsule of a donor kidney immediately after the transplantation of this organ. One month later, a biopsy of the kidney showed the presence of beta cells in an islet (Lafferty *et al.*, 1989). Less precise confirmation of the presence of human fetal pancreas at the site of grafting has been obtained by magnetic resonance imaging of tissue placed in the forearm (Tuch *et al.*, 1988*c*) and beneath the renal capsule (Voss *et al.*, 1989).

Despite the obvious presence of beta cells in these four cases, there was no detectable plasma or urinary C-peptide to suggest that these cells were functioning. Perhaps the most convincing evidence supporting

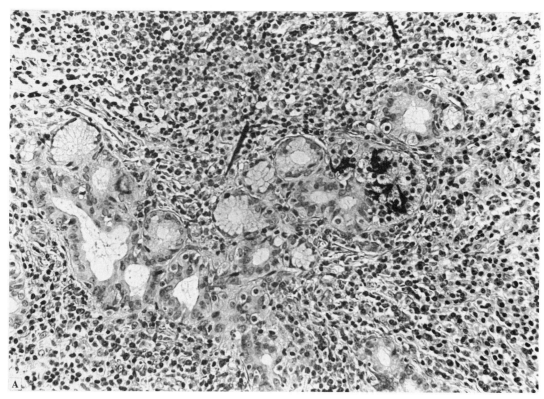

Figure 8.8. Human fetal pancreatic tissue removed from an insulin-dependent diabetic person one year after engraftment of six fetal pancreases in the forearm muscle. Note the presence of numerous ducts and endocrine cells, including both beta cells staining for insulin (A) and alpha cells staining for glucagon (B). Examination of these two consecutive sections indicates that most of the endocrine cells are in an islet. A. Immunoperoxidase stain for insulin, × 100. B. Immunoperoxidase stain for glucagon, × 100. (From B. E. Tuch, A. R. G. Sheil, A. B. P. Ng, J. R. Trent & J. R. Turtle, Recovery of human fetal pancreas after one year of implantation in the diabetic patient. *Transplantation, 46,* 865–70, © by Williams & Wilkins, 1988.)

the idea that functioning will occur in time, comes from the Swedish data in 1980 (Groth *et al.*, 1980). This group was able to detect urinary C-peptide in a patient, who was previously C-peptide negative, one month after the intraportal injection of the cultured microfragments of six human fetal pancreases. The levels rose progressively until at four months, at the same time as islet cell surface antibodies were detected, the levels fell abruptly and became unmeasurable (Groth *et al.*, 1980). Strangely, despite the presence of as much as 1200 pmol C-peptide during a twenty four hour period, plasma C-peptide remained undetectable. In the Sydney experience, plasma but not urinary C-peptide was measurable in one recipient 3 months after transplantation, during a glucagon challenge (Tuch *et al.*, 1988c); this hormone was undetectable either before or after this time. The Hungarian experience from Szeged looks promising, with C-peptide being detected for at least one year after the intraportal injection of collagenase-digested beta cells, cultured for ten weeks (Farkas & Karácsonyi, 1985). All these patient were C-peptide negative before being grafted; the possibility of their being overinsulinized has yet to be excluded. The data from thirty hospitals in the People's Republic of

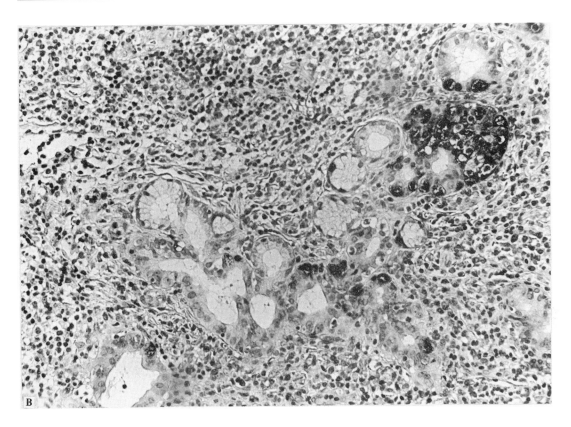

China indicate that there was an overall rise in plasma C-peptide after surgery, suggesting that the graft was functioning, in some cases in the absence of any form of immunosuppression (Hu *et al.*, 1989). It would be advantageous in assessing these data if results for individual patients were made available, and if a control group of patients could be monitored for plasma C-peptide function. Unfortunately, it is not possible to assess adequately the claims from the largest group of recipients in the Soviet Union, since sufficient data are not available (Shumakov *et al.*, 1983; Suskova *et al.*, 1989).

It would be incorrect to take away the impression that grafting human fetal pancreas into diabetic humans will be a waste of time. After all, history has revealed that, after fifteen years of trials with islets taken from an adult cadaver (Scharp *et al.*, 1990), it is now possible, only as of 1990, to reverse diabetes in humans. The success enjoyed by surgeons who transplant vascularized pancreas took almost two decades to realize, since the first unsuccessful transplant in 1966 (Kelly *et al.*, 1967). Progress has occurred in the past decade in our understanding of the human fetal beta cell. It will reverse diabetes in an animal if rejection is not a problem. There is improved knowledge of

229

methods to optimize the amount of tissue required for this purpose: demonstrating that maturation of the beta cell will occur after transplantation; showing the lack of toxicity of immunosuppressive agents including cyclosporine A (Tuch *et al.*, 1987*b*; Leonard *et al.*, 1989); and making the tissue available in purer preparations, either as islet-like cell clusters (Sandler *et al.*, 1985) or monolayers (Simpson *et al.*, 1991). Human studies have demonstrated that: the tissue will survive for up to one year in an immunosuppressed recipient; some function may occur several months after grafting; and a grafted kidney is not more likely to be rejected irrespective of whether tissue is implanted beneath the capsule of this kidney or elsewhere.

Ethics

It would be remiss not to conclude this chapter with a brief comment on the ethics of using human fetal tissue. Ethical guidelines have been established by a number of Ethical Groups, e.g. the National Health & Medical Research Council of Australia Medical Research Ethics Committee (1983) and other groups (Vawter *et al.*, 1990), some of their main points are:

(i) the research group shall not be involved in the clinical decision to terminate pregnancy
(ii) the research shall not be carried out in proximity to the clinical ward
(iii) maternal consent shall be obtained for the use of the tissue for medical research, particularly for purposes such as culturing and transplantation of the tissue
(iv) the clinician involved shall gain no pecuniary benefit from providing the tissue for research purposes
(v) researchers with ethical objections to working with the tissue shall not be compelled to do so

It is understandable that some people have difficulty in distinguishing between the termination of pregnancy and utilizing tissue so obtained for the purposes of medical research (Murphy, 1989). If the decision is taken to use such tissue then, at least in the Western world, guidelines such as those detailed above seem reasonable and appropriate. In one centre where these guidelines are applied, an analysis of the ethics and morals of researchers handling the tissue showed no difference from those of a matched group of similar people who did not (Tuch *et al.*, 1990*a*).

The future

For the next clinical trial of grafting human fetal pancreas into diabetic people, it seems certain that tissue will need to be cryopreserved in order that multiple organs are available for transplantation. The technique for doing this has been perfected and implemented in a number of centres (Sandler *et al.*, 1982; Brown *et al.*, 1980; see Chapter 12, this volume). Much the same storage of tissue is now occurring with adult islets in some centres, so that there are sufficient numbers available for clinical needs. The human fetal pancreatic tissue to be used will be either sliced fragments, or more purified preparations of islet-like cell clusters or monolayers. Even if these transplants are successful, it seems unlikely that there will ever be sufficient supply in the Western world to meet the demand. For this reason the xenografting of pig fetal beta cells, either as microfragments or islet-like cell clusters, is envisaged. One such graft has already occurred in Sweden in 1990 (A. Andersson, personal communication). Increasing evidence suggests that xenotransplantation may be successful, the most convincing evidence so far coming from the acceptance of pig fetal proislets by mice transiently immunosuppressed with anti-CD4 antibodies (Simeonovic *et al.*, 1990). The possibility of autoimmune rejection of grafted fetal beta cells cannot be ignored, since such a phenomenon has occurred in grafted vascularized pancreases (Sibley & Sutherland, 1987). It might be theorized, however, that this will not occur, since the human fetal beta cell is resistant to such beta cell toxins as streptozotocin (Tuch *et al.*, 1989), and, unlike the adult beta cell, is not destroyed by the cytokines tumour necrosis factor α and interferon-γ (Tuch *et al.*, 1991).

Of course, the goal with fetal pancreas transplantation, as in all forms of pancreatic grafting, is to be able to normalize blood glucose levels early in the course of diabetes whilst utilizing only a brief period of immunosuppression of the recipient. This remains an elusive goal for the present not only for the more established vascularized pancreatic transplants but also for the islets obtained from adult cadavers. The success rate with the vascularized grafts transplanted into diabetic people with chronic renal failure has been increasing over the last decade (Sutherland & Moudry-Munns, 1990) with most recipients being able to cease injections of insulin. In August 1990, at the International Transplantation Meeting held in San Francisco, the one-year graft survival was reported to be 75%, a figure similar to that for renal transplants (D. E. R. Sutherland, personal communication). In general, the success rate for patients grafted earlier in the course of diabetes, when complications were minimal or absent, is poor, even though immunosuppressive agents are used. It may be that the immunosuppressive effect of renal failure itself is a necessary supplement to the drugs used. In support of this concept, reversal of diabetes has recently been reported for the first time using adult cadaveric islets grafted into diabetic patients with chronic renal failure (Scharp *et al.*, 1990). It remains to be seen whether such islet grafts can be of benefit to patients earlier in the course of diabetes. Until the complete clinical role of this form of transplantation, as well as the vascularized graft, is determined, it is paramount that the potential of the human fetal beta cell to reverse diabetes should be explored. It may well be that there are separate clinical situations in which the three types of pancreatic transplants will be used.

Acknowledgments

I am indebted to Dr Bernhard Hering from Giessen in West Germany for the data stored in the International Islet Transplant Registry. The research conducted in my laboratory at the University of Sydney over the past decade was made possible by the support of the following bodies: National Health and Medical Research Council of Australia; Juvenile Diabetes Foundation International; Kellion Diabetes Foundation; Diabetes Youth Foundation; Rebecca L. Cooper Medical Research Foundation; Foundation Diabetes; Lions Save Sight Foundation; Juvenile Diabetes Foundation Australia; Hoechst Diabetes Foundation; Ramaciotti Research Foundation; Apex/Diabetes Australia Research Foundation; Sir Zelman Cowen Universities Fund. The assistance of the following technicians in carrying out this work is gratefully acknowledged: Rebecca Gauci, Annette Jones, Jenny Nicks, Samantha Grigoriou, Zambela Palavidis, Judy Lissing, Yvonne Osborne, Kate Osgerby, Karen Darby, Kate Lenord, Sandy Beynon, Roger Monk, Halina Motyka, and Julia Beretov.

References

ÅGREN, A., ANDERSSON, A., BJÖRKEN, C., GROTH, C-G., GUN-NARSSON, R., HELLERSTRÖM, C., LINDMARK, G., LUNDQVIST, G., PETERSSON, B., SWENNE, I. (1980) Human fetal pancreas: culture and function *in vitro*. *Diabetes*, **29**, Supplement 1, 64–9.

ANDERSSON, A., CHRISTENSEN, N., GROTH, C-G., HELLER-STRÖM, C., PETERSSON, B. & SANDLER, S. (1984) Survival of human fetal pancreatic explants in organ culture as reflected in insulin secretion and oxygen consumption. *Transplantation*, **37**, 499–503.

BERNALES, R. & BELLANTI, J. A. (1982) Fetal and neonatal immunology. In: *Fetal and Maternal Medicine*, pp. 267–314. Eds. E. J. Quilligan & N. Kretchmer. J. Wiley & Sons, New York.

BROWN, J., KEMP, J. A., HURT, S. & CLARK, W. R. (1980) Cryopreservation of human fetal pancreas. *Diabetes*, **29**, Supplement 1, 70–3.

BROWN, J., MOLNAR, I. G., CLARK, W. & MULLEN, Y. (1974) Control of experimental diabetes mellitus in rats by transplantation of fetal pancreases. *Science*, **184**, 1377–9.

BROWN, J., MULLEN, Y., CLARK, W. R., MOLNAR, I. G. & HEIN-INGER, D. (1979) Importance of hepatic portal circulation in streptozoto-cin-diabetic rats transplanted with fetal pancreases. *Journal of Clinical Investigation*, **64**, 1688–94.

BURKHARDT, K., CHARLTON, B. & MANDEL, T. E. (1989) The synergistic effect of anti-CD4 monoclonal antibodies and cyclosporin A on murine fetal islet allograft survival. *Transplantation Proceedings*, **21**, 2663–4.

CAMPBELL, I. L., BIZILJ, K., COLMAN, P. G., TUCH, B. E. & HARRI-SON, L. C. (1986) Interferon-γ induces the expression of HLA-A,B,C but not HLA-DR on human pancreatic beta cells. *Journal of Clinical Endocrinology & Metabolism*, **62**, 1101–9.

CHASTAN, Ph., BERJON, J. J., GOMEZ, H. & MEUNIER, J. M. (1980) Treatment of an insulin-dependent diabetic by homograft of fetal pancreas removed before the tenth week of pregnancy: one-year follow up. *Transplantation Proceedings*, **12**, Supplement 2, 218–22.

DANILOVS, J. A., BROWN, J., TERASAKI, P. I. & CLARK, W. R. (1983) HLA-DR and HLA-A, B, C typing of human fetal tissue. *Tissue Antigens*, **21**, 296–308.

DANILOVS, J. A., HOFMAN, F. M., TAYLOR, C. R. & BROWN, J. (1982) Expression of HLA-DR antigens in human fetal pancreas tissue. *Diabetes*, **31**, Supplement 4, 23–8.

DAVIES, D. V. & DAVIES, F. (Eds) (1962) *Gray's Anatomy: Descriptive and Applied*, 33rd edition. Longmans, Green & Co Ltd, London.

DOWNING, R. (1984) Historical review of pancreatic islet transplantation. *World Journal of Surgery*, **8**, 137–42.

FALIN, L. I. (1967) The development and cytodifferentiation of the islets of

Langerhans in human embryos and foetuses. *Acta Anatomica*, (*Basel*), **68**, 147–68.

FARKAS, Gy. & KARÁCSONYI, S. (1985) Clinical transplantation of fetal human pancreatic islets. *Biomedica Biochimica Acta*, **1**, 155–9.

GRASSO, S., DISTEFANO, G., MESSINA, A., VIGO, R. & REITANO, G. (1975) Effect of glucose priming on insulin response in the premature infant. *Diabetes*, **24**, 291–4.

GRASSO, S., FALLUCCA, F., MAZZONE, D., GIANGRANDE, L., ROMEO, M. G. & REITANO, G. (1983) Inhibition of glucagon secretion in the human newborn by glucose infusion. *Diabetes*, **32**, 489–92.

GROTH, C. G., ANDERSSON, A., BJÖRKEN, C., GUNNARSSON, R., HELLERSTRÖM, C., LUNDGREN, G., PETERSSON, B., SWENNE, I. & OSTMAN, J. (1980) Attempts at transplantation of fetal pancreas to diabetic patients. *Transplantation Proceedings*, **12**, Supplement 2, 208–12.

HERING, B. J., BRETZEL, R. G. & FEDERLIN, K. (1988) Current status of clinical islet transplantation. *Hormone and Metabolic Research*, **20**, 537–45.

HOFFMAN, L., MANDEL, T. E., CARTER, W. M., KOULMANDA, M. & MARTIN, F. I. R. (1982) Insulin secretion by human fetal pancreas in organ culture. *Diabetologia*, **23**, 426–30.

HU, Y., HONG, Z., ZANG, H., ZANG, H., SHAO, A., LI, L. ZHOU, H. ZHAO, B. & ZHOU, Y. (1985) Culture of human fetal pancreas and islet transplantation in 24 patients with type I diabetes mellitus. *Chinese Medical Journal*, **98**, 236–43.

HU, Y-f., GU, Z-f., ZHANG, H-d. & YE, R-s. (1989) Fetal islet transplantation in China. *Transplantation Proceedings*, **21**, 2605–7.

HULLETT, D. A., FALANY, J. L., LOVE, R. B., BURLINGHAM, W. J., PAN, M. & SOLLINGER, H. W. (1987) Human fetal pancreas – a potential source for transplantation. *Transplantation*, **43**, 18–22.

JAFFE, R., HASHIDA, Y. & YUNIS, E. J. (1982) The endocrine pancreas of the neonate and infant. *Perspectives in Pediatrics & Pathology*, **7**, 137–65.

JOVANOVIC-PETERSON, L., WILLIAMS, K., BRENNAN, M. FUHR-MANN, K., RASHBAUM, W., WALKER, L. & PETERSON, C. M. (1988) Studies of transplantation of human fetal tissue in man. In: *Fetal Islet Transplantation: Implications for Diabetes*, pp. 184–95. Eds. C. M. Peterson, L. Jovanovic-Peterson, & B. Formby. Springer Verlag, New York.

KELLY, W. D., LILLEHEI, R. C., MERKEL, F. K., IDEZUKI, Y. & GOETZ, F. C. (1967) Allotransplantation of the pancreas and duodenum along with the kidney in diabetic nephropathy. *Surgery*, **61**, 827–37.

KORSGREN, O., JANSSON, L., EIZIRIK, D. & ANDERSSON, A. (1991) Functional and morphological differentiation of fetal porcine islet-like cell clusters after transplantation into nude mice. *Diabetologia*, **34**, 379–86.

KORSGREN, O., SANDLER, S. & ANDERSSON, A. (1990) Nicotinamide-stimulated porcine fetal pancreatic B-cells as a source for transplantation in diabetes mellitus. *International Congress of the Transplantation Society*, **13**, 710.

LAFFERTY, K. J., HAO, L., BABCOCK, S. K. & SPEES, E. (1989) Is there a future for fetal pancreas transplantation? *Transplantation Proceedings*, **21**, 2611–13.

LAFFERTY, K. J., PROWSE, S. J. & SIMEONOVIC, C. J. (1983) Immunobiology of tissue transplantation: A return to the passenger leucocyte concept. *Annual Reviews in Immunology*, **1**, 143–73.

LEONARD, D. K., LANDRY, A. S., SOLLINGER, H. W. & HULLETT, D. A. (1989) Prednisone, azathioprine, and cyclosporine A toxicity on human fetal pancreas. *Journal of Surgical Research*, **46**, 625–32.

MAITLAND, J. E., PARRY, D. G. & TURTLE, J. R. (1980) Perifusion and culture of human fetal pancreas. *Diabetes*, **29**, Supplement 1, 57–63.

MANDEL, T. E. (1984) Growth of organ-cultured fetal mouse pancreas isografts in diabetic and non-diabetic recipients. *Australian Journal of Experimental Biological & Medical Science*, **61**, 497–508.

MANDEL, T. E., JACK I. & TAIT, B. D. (1982) HLA-DR typing of fetal human spleen and liver lymphoblastoid cells transformed by Epstein–Barr virus. *Transplantation*, **34**, 50–3.

MENGER, M. D., JÄGER, S., WALTER, P., HAMMERSEN, F. & MESSMER, K. (1990) The microvasculature of xenogeneic transplanted islets of Langerhans. *Transplantation Proceedings*, **22**, 802–3.

MILNER, R. D. G., BARSON, A. J. & ASHWORTH, M. A. (1971) Human fetal pancreatic secretion in response to ionic and other stimuli. *Journal of Endocrinology*, **51**, 323–32.

MURPHY, J. B. (1989) The ethics of research using human fetal tissue. *New England Journal of Medicine*, **321**, 1608.

NAJARIAN, J. S., SUTHERLAND, D. E. R., STEFFES, M. W., SIMMONS, R. L. & GOETZ, F. C. (1975) Human islet transplantation: A preliminary report. *Transplantation Proceedings*, **7**, Supplement 1, 611–13.

NATIONAL HEALTH & MEDICAL RESEARCH COUNCIL OF AUSTRALIA MEDICAL RESEARCH ETHICS COMMITTEE (1983) *Ethics in Medical Research Involving the Human Fetus and Human Fetal Tissue*. Australian Government Publishing Service, Canberra.

OTONKOSKI, T., KNIP, M., PANULA, P., ANDERSSON, S., WONG, I., GOLDMAN, H. & SIMELL, O. (1988) Morphology, yield and functional integrity of islet-like cell clusters in tissue culture of human fetal pancreata obtained after different means of abortion. *Acta Endocrinologica*, **118**, 68–76.

PICTET, R. & RUTTER, W. J. (1972) Development of the embryonic pancreas. In: *Handbook of Physiology*, Section 7: *Endocrinology*, vol. 1, pp. 25–66. Ed. S. R. Geiger. Williams & Wilkins Co, Baltimore.

SANDLER, S., ANDERSSON, A., HELLERSTRÖM, C., PETERSSON, B., SWENNE, I., BJÖRKÉN, C. & GROTH, C.-G. (1982) Preservation of morphology, insulin biosynthesis, and insulin release of cryopreserved human fetal pancreas. *Diabetes*, **31**, 238–41.

SANDLER, S., ANDERSSON, A., KORSGREN, O., TOLLEMAR, J., PETERSSON, B., GROTH, C-G. & HELLERSTRÖM, C. (1989) Tissue culture of human fetal pancreas: effects of nicotinamide on insulin production and formation of isletlike cell clusters. *Diabetes*, **38**, Supplement 1, 168–71.

SANDLER, S., ANDERSSON, A., SCHNELL, A., MELLGREN, A., TOLLEMAR, J., BORG, H., PETERSSON, B., GROTH, C-G. & HELLERSTRÖM, C. (1985) Tissue culture of human fetal pancreas: development and function of β-cells *in vitro* and transplantation of explants to nude mice. *Diabetes*, **34**, 1113–19.

SCHARP, D. W., LACY, P. E., SANTIAGO, J. V., McCULLOUGH, C. S.,

WEIDE, L. G., FALQUI, L., MARCHETTI, P., GINGERICH, R. L., JAFFE, A. S., CRYER, P. E., ANDERSON, C. B. & FLYE, M. W. (1990) Insulin independence after islet transplantation into type I diabetic patient. *Diabetes*, **39**, 515–18.

SHUMAKOV, V. I., BLUMKIN, V. N., IGNATENKO, S. N., SKALETSKY, N. N., KAURICHEVA, N. I., SEID-GUSEINOV, A. Y. & SLOVESNOVA, T. A. (1983) Transplantation of islet cell cultures of the pancreas of human fetuses to diabetes mellitus patients. *Klin Med (Mosk)*, **61**, 46–51.

SIBLEY, R. K. & SUTHERLAND, D. E. R. (1987) Pancreas transplantation: An immunohistologic and histopathologic examination of 100 grafts. *American Journal of Pathology*, **128**, 151–70.

SIMEONOVIC, C. J., CEREDIG, R. & WILSON, J. D. (1990) Effect of GK1.5 monoclonal antibody dosage on survival of pig proislet xenografts in CD4$^+$ T cell-depleted mice. *Transplantation*, **49**, 849–56.

SIMPSON, A. M., TUCH, B. E. & VINCENT, P. C. (1991) Characterization of endocrine-rich monolayers of human fetal pancreas that display reduced immunogenicity. *Diabetes*, **40**; 800–9.

STEFAN, Y., GRASSO, S., PERRELET, A. & ORCI, L. (1983) A quantitative immunofluorescent study of the endocrine cell populations in the developing human pancreas. *Diabetes*, **32**, 292–301.

SUSKOVA, V. S., MATSULENKO, E. N., SLOVESNOVA, T. A., SHALNEV, B. I., BLYUMKIN, V. N. & IGNATENKO, S. N. (1989) Levels of blood C-peptide in type I diabetes mellitus patients after pancreatic islet cell transplantation. *Diabetes*, **38**, Supplement 1, 313.

SUTHERLAND, D. E. R. (1981) Pancreas and islet transplantation: II. Clinical trials. *Diabetologia*, **20**, 435–50.

SUTHERLAND, D. E. R., GOETZ, F. C. & NAJARIAN, J. S. (1981) Review of world's experience with pancreas and islet transplantation and results of intraperitoneal segmental pancreas transplantation from related and cadaver donors at Minnesota. *Transplantation Proceedings*, **13**, 291–7.

SUTHERLAND, D. E. R. & MOUDRY-MUNNS, K. C. (1990) International pancreas transplantation registry analysis. *Transplantation Proceedings*, **22**, 571–4.

THOMSON, N. M., HANCOCK, W. M., LAFFERTY, K. J., KRAFT, N. & ATKINS, R. C. (1983) Organ culture reduces Ia-positive cells present within the human fetal pancreas. *Transplantation Proceedings*, **15**, 1373–6.

TUCH, B. E. (1991) Reversal of diabetes by human fetal pancreas: Optimization of requirements in the hyperglycaemic nude mouse. *Transplantation*, **51**, 557–62.

TUCH, B. E., DORAN, T. J., MESSEL, N. & TURTLE, J. R. (1985a) Typing of human fetal organs for the histocompatibility antigens – A, B and DR. *Pathology*, **17**, 57–61.

TUCH, B. E., DUNN, S. M. & de VAHL DAVIS, V. (1990a) The effect on researchers of handling human fetal tissue. *Transplantation Proceedings*, **22**, 2109–10.

TUCH, B. E., GRIGORIOU, S. & TURTLE, J. R. (1986) Growth and hormonal content of human fetal pancreas passaged in athymic mice. *Diabetes*, **35**, 464–9.

TUCH, B. E., GRIGORIOU, S. & TURTLE, J. R. (1987a) Comparison of liver, spleen and kidney as sites for xenografting human fetal pancreas in the nude mouse. *Transplantation Proceedings*, **19**, 2902–9.

TUCH, B. E., JONES, A. & TURTLE, J. R. (1985*b*) Maturation of the response of human fetal pancreatic explants to glucose. *Diabetologia*, **28**, 28–31.

TUCH, B. E., LISSING, J. R. & SURANYI, M. G. (1988*a*) Immunomodulation of human fetal cells by the fungal metabolite gliotoxin. *Immunology & Cell Biology*, **66**, 307–12.

TUCH, B. E. & OSGERBY, K. J. (1990) Maturation of insulinogenic response to glucose in human fetal pancreas with retinoic acid. *Hormone & Metabolic Research*, Supplement 25, 233–8.

TUCH, B. E., OSGERBY, K. J. & TURTLE, J. R. (1988*b*) Human fetal pancreas grafted into non-diabetic nude mice normalizes blood glucose levels once diabetes is induced. *Transplantation*, **46**, 608–11.

TUCH, B. E., OSGERBY, K. J. & TURTLE, J. R. (1990*b*) The role of calcium in insulin release from the human fetal pancreas. *Cell Calcium*, **11**, 1–9.

TUCH, B. E., SHEIL, A. R. G., NG, A. B. P., TRENT, R. J. & TURTLE, J. R. (1988*c*) Recovery of human fetal pancreas after one year of implantation in the diabetic patient. *Transplantation*, **46**, 865–70.

TUCH, B. E., SIMPSON, A. M. & CAMPBELL, I. L. (1991) Role of tumour necrosis factor-α and interferon-γ as growth factors to the human fetal beta cell. *Journal of Clinical Endocrinology & Metabolism*, **73**, 1044–50.

TUCH, B. E. & TURTLE, J. R. (1987) Long-term organ culture of large numbers of human fetal pancreases: Analysis of their insulin secretion. *Diabetic Medicine*, **4**, 116–21.

TUCH, B. E., TURTLE, J. R. & SIMEONOVIC, C. J. (1989) Streptozotocin is not toxic to the human fetal beta cell. *Diabetologia*, **32**, 678–84.

TUCH, B. E., VIKETOS, S., GRIGORIOU, S. & TURTLE, J. R. (1987*b*) Lack of toxicity of Cyclosporin A on human fetal pancreas. *Transplantation Proceedings*, **19**, 1257–8.

VALENTE, U., FERRO, M., BAROCCI, S., CAMPISI, C., PARODI, F., CATALDI, L., ARCURI, V. & TOSATTI, E. (1980) Report of clinical cases of human fetal pancreas transplantation. *Transplantation Proceedings*, **12**, Supplement 2, 213–17.

VAWTER, D. E., KEARNEY, W., GERVAIS, K. G., CAPLAN, A. L., GARRY, D. & TAUER, C. (1990) *The use of human fetal tissue: scientific, ethical, and policy concerns*. Centre for Biomedical Ethics, University of Minnesota.

von EULER, U., LARSSON, Y. & PERSSON, B. (1964) Glucose tolerance in the neonatal period and during the first six months of life. *Archives of the Diseases of Childhood*, **39**, 393–6.

VOSS, F., BREWIN, A., DAWIDSON, I., LAFFERTY, K., SPEES, E., COLLINS, G. & BRY, W. (1989) Transplantation of proliferated human pre-islets into diabetic patients with renal transplants. *Transplantation Proceedings*, **21**, 2751–6.

WALTHALL, B. J., ELIAS, K., GODFRY, W. L., McHUGH, Y. E., MOSS, P. S., NOONAN, R. A., ZAYAS, J. R. & VOSS, H. F. (1988) Rodent xenografts of human and porcine fetal tissue. In: *Fetal Islet Transplantation: Implications for Diabetes*, pp. 93–110. Eds. C. M. Peterson, L. Jovanovic-Peterson & B. Formby. Springer Verlag, New York.

CHAPTER 9

The suitability of fetal and infantile donors for corneal transplantation

H. J. VÖLKER-DIEBEN

CONTENTS

THE NORMAL CORNEA is clear and avascular. An opaque cornea interferes with good visual acuity and such patients are candidates for a corneal transplant. Corneal transplantation is the replacement of the central 7 to 8 mm of the diseased organ. The clarity of the graft is used as the parameter for defining graft survival. However, a crystal-clear cornea with an uncorrectable refractive error does not constitute a successful transplant, since visual acuity is not restored. It is the challenge for the ophthalmic surgeon to achieve a clear cornea with curvature that is as close as possible to normal.

Factors affecting the success of corneal transplantation

Endothelial cell density

Numerous factors affect the success of corneal transplantation: i.e. selection and storage of donor corneas, surgical techniques and postoperative therapy. The importance of good donor tissue has been appreciated from the very beginning of corneal surgery. As early as 1906, Zirm stated in his rules for grafting: 'use a human donor cornea, which should be young and healthy' (Zirm, 1906). Corneal surgeons have traditionally preferred young donor corneas because of their high endothelial cell density.

Figures 9.1 to 9.4 show the endothelial cell densities in four donor corneas of different ages: 5400, 3500, 2800 and 1200 cells/mm² at the age of 2 months, 2 years, 20 years and 79 years respectively. There is no regeneration of endothelial cells and the importance of the number and viability of the endothelial cells in maintaining corneal clarity is generally accepted. The high endothelial cell density in corneas of

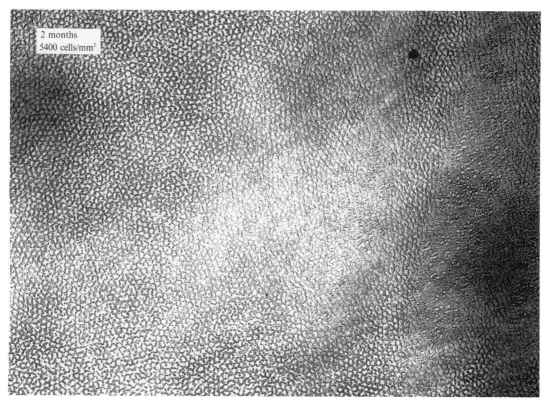

Figure 9.1. Endothelial cell density of 5400 cells/mm² in a 2-month-old corneal donor. (By courtesy of Dr E. Pels.)

young donors provides a greater buffer against perioperative cell loss and consequently leads to better graft survival. However, the Medical Standards of the Eye Bank Association of America state that the lower age limit for donor corneal tissue is fullterm birth. A majority of the American Eye Banks and corneal surgeons accepts tissue from donors as young as 6 months old. For many European corneal surgeons the lower limit for acceptance is one year. Beveridge even maintained in 1972 that 'eyes of young children (under five years of age) are unsuitable, because of steep corneal curvature and lack of rigidity (Beveridge, 1972).

In our records of 1643 corneal transplants the endothelial cell density of 839 donor corneas which were accepted for transplantation was noted. The highly significant correlation between cell density and age is clear ($p < 0.001$) (Figure 9.5), the data being obtained from counts on corneal sceral buttons stained with trypan blue (Pels & Schuchard, 1983). These results confirm and extend the report of Schimmelpfennig (1986) who observed a weak correlation between donor age and endothelial cell density. In 20 of the 30 donors who were under the age of 16 years, cell densities of more than 3000 cells/mm² were counted.

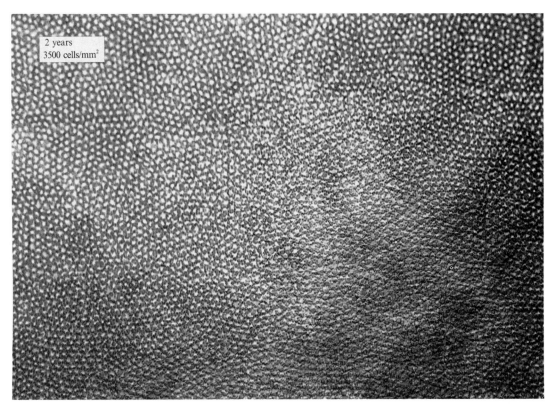

2 years
3500 cells/mm²

Figure 9.2. Endothelial cell density of 3500 cells/mm² in a 2-year-old corneal donor. (By courtesy of Dr E. Pels.)

Four of the eyes from donors who were under the age of 2 years (one at 7 weeks, two at 6 months and one at 15 months) revealed cell counts of 4100 to 3600 cells/mm², with an average of 3825 cells/mm². The four donors of 2 or 3 years old varied from 3700 to 2900 cells with an average of 3555 cells/mm². The assumption that a greater endothelial cell density is correlated with an improved graft survival becomes clear in Figure 9.6. The correlation between these two factors was analysed in 839 corneal transplants with a follow-up of 5 years. Although the correlation was not statistically significant, the best graft survival was seen when donor corneas with more than 3000 cells/mm² were used.

In 706 corneal grafts of which the preoperative endothelial cell density was unknown, the relation between donor age and graft survival was analysed (Figure 9.7). The linear correlation between these two factors is statistically significant. The younger the donor cornea, the better is the chance of graft survival.

On the basis of these observations it is evident that younger donor corneas should be preferred for corneal transplantation. However, the very young donors, i.e. below the age of one year, are associated with technical problems. As early as 1943, Ehlers reported the difficulty in

241

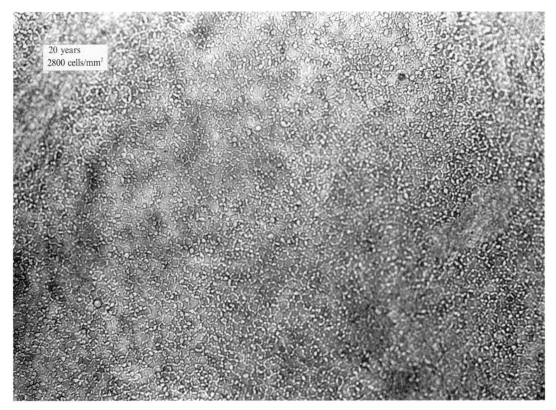

20 years
2800 cells/mm²

Figure 9.3. Endothelial cell density of 2800 cells/mm² in a 20-year-old corneal donor. (By courtesy of Dr E. Pels.)

avoiding scleral fibres and remnants of conjunctiva while trephining a small diameter cornea of a stillborn baby donor (Ehlers, 1943).

The myopic shift

The postoperative myopic shift was reported by Ehlers (1943) to be an advantage for the poor-sighted patient. Vannas (1950) recognized severe postoperative myopia as a complication of penetrating kerato-plasty when donor tissue was obtained from stillborn babies. Belyaev & Veretnikova (1972) reported on the correction of aphakia by using fetal donor corneas for transplants in patients with aphakic bullous keratopathy. Pfister & Breaud (1983) analysed the refractive error of 18 eyes transplanted with corneas from premature, neonatal and infant donors respectively. They also found that aphakic correction was possible with corneas from newborn donors. Koenig *et al.*, (1982) performed transplants in five patients using corneas from donors aged between 5 days and 3 months. They observed a large myopic shift postoperatively and consequently a severe anisometropia up to 19 diopters in their patients. Wood & Nissenkorn (1981) summarized the

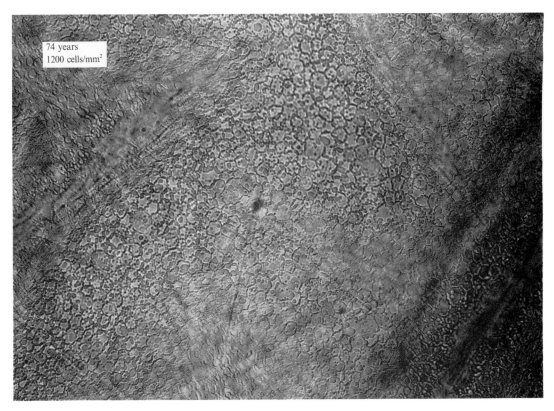

Figure 9.4. Endothelial cell density of 1200 cells/mm² in a 74-year-old corneal donor (By courtesy of Dr E. Pels.)

refractive errors of patients who received corneal grafts from donors who were less than 2 years of age. They concluded that the steepness of the infant cornea is the cause of the unpredictable refractive error postoperatively.

It is not certain when the corneal curvature attains adult levels, and this probably occurs in the second six months of life (Sorsby & Sheridan, 1953). Whether the curvature of very young donor corneas stays normal after transplanting into the grown adult patient depends on the rigidity of this donor material which is certainly not comparable to the rigidity of the mostly adult recipient cornea. Consequently, it is to be expected that the curvature of the young donor cornea above the age of 1 year will become steeper under the influence of the normal eye pressure.

In our experience with four corneas from donors under 2 years of age and four corneas from donors between 32 and 42 months of age, a myopic shift was observed in seven of the eight recipients. The myopic shift was the result of an increase in the dioptric power of the cornea caused by the steepness of the corneal curvature. In Table 9.1 the refractive error and keratometer readings of these eight patients are

243

Figure 9.5. The relation between endothelial cell density and age in 839 donor corneas ($p < 0.000\,001$). The horizontal bar shows the mean endothelial cell count for each group; above the mean is high and below the mean is low.

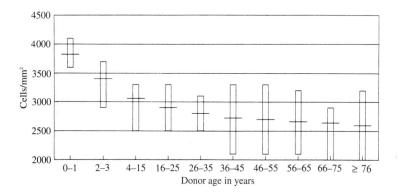

Figure 9.6. The relation between endothelial cell density and corneal graft survival ($p = $ ns.).

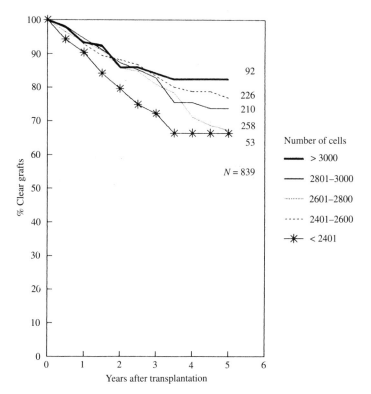

listed. The youngest donor cornea of a 7-week-old donor developed a curvature of $58.0 \times > 60.5$ diopters. The two donor corneas from the six-month-old donor were transplanted to a 74-year-old and a 71-year-old female recipient. The 74-year-old recipient developed a glaucoma in the first six months postoperation. The myopic shift in this eye was as much as 21 diopters, possibly under the influence of the elevated ocular pressure, since, after glaucoma surgery the myopic shift was reduced to 14 diopters, the corneal curvature was 57.5×60.5. The reduction of the myopia from 21 to 14 may be due to the capability of stretching in

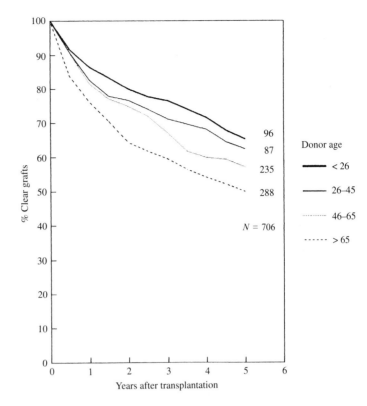

Figure 9.7. The relation between donor age and corneal graft survival ($p = 0.008$).

response to mechanical stresses within the physiologic range (Nyquist, 1968). The 71-year-old recipient gradually reached 11 diopters myopia in three postoperative years; the dioptric power of her cornea was 52.5×55.0. The 33-year-old recipient became 10 diopters myopic with a corneal curvature of 52.0×60.0. However, this patient suffered from recurrent epithelial defects which healed with superficial stromal scarring and an irregular corneal surface. None of these patients was myopic before transplantation.

On theoretical grounds, the myopic shift observed in eyes that were transplanted with corneas from infant donors (25 to 48 months of age) should be less compared with those described above (see also Table 9.1). A 23-year-old recipient developed a myopia of 7 diopters eight years postoperatively, while the preoperative refraction had been -1.0. A 75-year-old recipient made a shift from -0.75 to -5.0 in six years postoperatively. An 86-year-old aphakic recipient needed only $+7.0$ (spherical equivalent) diopters correction, i.e. 5 diopters below the expected refractive error. Only the 81-year-old recipient demonstrated the expected aphakic correction of $+11.0$ (spherical equivalent) diopters. We conclude that even corneas from donors aged from 2 to 4 years old show, in the majority of cases, a myopic shift in

Table 9.1. *Myopic shift and keratometer readings in patients who received very young donor corneas*

Donor age	Recipient's age (years)	Myopic shift (diopters)	K readings (diopters)
7 weeks	80	?	58.0×60.5
6 months	74	21——→14	57.5×60.5
6 months	71	11	52.5×55.0
19 months	33	10	52.0×60.5
34 months	23	7	43.5×51.5
35 months	75	5	47.5×53.0
42 months	86	5	48.0×52.0
32 months	81	0	41.5×45.0

Note:
The first recipient had a severe macular degeneration so the refractive error was not measurable.

postoperative years. This conclusion is in concordance with the statement of Beveridge (1972) that was quoted previously.

The incomplete development of corneal rigidity may explain the tendency towards steep corneal curvatures in these donor corneas. The consistency of these observations by several authors leads to the conclusion that young donors (below the age of 4 years) should be used only in aphakic eyes and/or in monocular patients (Ehlers, 1943; Vannas, 1950; Belyaev & Veretnikova, 1972; Wood & Nissenkorn, 1981; Koenig *et al.*, 1982; Pfister & Breaud, 1983).

Technical problems

The elasticity, thinness and small diameter of the infant cornea may cause surgical problems, as described by Ehlers (1943) and confirmed by others. The elasticity results in the steep curvature of the cornea when transplanted. The thinness and pliability of the infant cornea complicates the transfer of the donor button to the host corneal bed, since the cornea may fold upon itself. Graft–host thickness disparity will cause overriding of the recipient cornea at the wound margin and may result in poor apposition between the Descemet's membranes of the donor and host corneas. Accurate placement of the sutures is more difficult because of the thinness and flexibility of the infant cornea. Deep sutures cause microperforations with potential complications of wound leak, flat anterior chamber and endophthalmitis. Shallow sutures may cut through the tissue, ultimately loosen and produce high astigmatism. Disparity between the steep curvature of the infant cornea and the flat radius of the standard teflon punch block, which is used for punching the donor button from the endothelial side, may result in an oversized button with bevelled edges. To avoid this, Pfister & Breaud (1983) advised using the whole globe and trephining the donor button from the epithelial side. This interferes with short-term or medium-term storage methods and with the organ culture method for donor cornea preservation in which corneal scleral buttons are used. Storage or preservation methods are essential when the advantages of tissue typed and matched donor corneas are indicated for the patient (Ehlers & Kissmeyer-Nielsen, 1973; Gibbs *et al.*, 1974; Vannas *et al.*, 1976; Völker-Dieben *et al.*, 1978; Foulks & Sanfilippo, 1982; Boisjoly *et al.*, 1986; Völker-Dieben & D'Amaro, 1989). The use of the globes of newborn infants that are stored in a moist chamber carries the risk of transfer to the recipient of infectious processes acquired in utero or during vaginal delivery.

Endothelial cell transplantation

A logical solution for the two conflicting factors, namely the advantage of the high endothelial cell density and the disadvantage of the insufficient corneal rigidity in very young donor corneas would be to use the rigid mature donor corneas which are denuded of their senior endothelial cells and seeded with very young endothelial cells. The senior donor corneas are more readily available and cultured corneal endothelial cells may be kept in stock under laboratory conditions. The ability of human corneal endothelium to undergo mitosis and to regenerate a new layer in organ culture indicates that it may be possible to replace or graft endothelium to injured or diseased corneas by using endothelial cells grown in tissue culture. Pure endothelial cell cultures have been described by Stocker *et al.* (1958). Gospodarowicz *et al.* (1979) reported that successful penetrating keratoplasty had been carried out on cats and monkeys by applying corneal discs from the host, from which the Descemet's membrane was scraped off and coated with cultured endothelium. Although rabbit and bovine corneal endothelial cultures have been developed by many laboratories, the growth of human corneal endothelium in culture has proved to be more difficult, with about half the cultures becoming contaminated with fibroblasts (Nayak & Binder, 1984). Skelnik *et al.* (1985) reported clear grafts in cats when cat donor corneas that were seeded with cultured human endothelial cells were used. Similar observations were made by Insler & Lopez (1986) who transplanted donor corneas, which were denuded of their native endothelium and seeded with cultured human neonatal endothelial cells, into rhesus monkeys. However, retrocorneal opacities developed two weeks postoperatively and stromal opacities three to four weeks postoperatively because of host immune response directed against bovine endothelium (Bahn *et al.*, 1982).

The immune competence of endothelial cells has been known for years. The rejection, or 'Khodadoust', line on corneal endothelium in cases of immunological rejection of the graft has been described as one of the major signs of an immunological event in the cornea (Khodadoust & Silverstein, 1969). In that respect, numerous publications described the benefits of HLA-matched donor corneas (Ehlers & Kissmeyer-Nielsen, 1973; Gibbs *et al.*, 1974; Vannas *et al.*, 1976; Völker-Dieben *et al.*, 1978; Foulks & Sanfilippo, 1982; Boisjoly *et al.*, 1986; Völker-Dieben & D'Amaro, 1989). Clinical application of this approach requires stocks of neonatal and fetal endothelial cell lines with different HLA types or the development of methods to eliminate or minimize the immunogenicity of the endothelial cells.

Conclusions

In view of the large numbers of corneal transplants performed each year (40 000 per year in Europe and the USA) (Völker-Dieben, 1989) and the very few publications about the small numbers of corneal transplants performed with very young donors, we may conclude that fetal, premature, neonatal and infant donor corneas have been used very rarely since 1943 (Ehlers, 1943). The unpredictable and severe myopia resulting from the very steep corneal curvature postoperatively are the main disadvantages of the use of this donor material. These disadvantages overrule the advantage of the very high endothelial cell density and consequently the greater chance of a clear graft. Attempts have been made to seed cultured endothelial cells from very young donors on denuded mature corneas in order to combine the desired high endothelial cell density with mature corneal rigidity. Additional studies in this area of transplantation are needed before this technique can be used for patients.

The problem described above reflects the unique double goal in corneal transplantation. A perfectly-functioning (clear) graft is not sufficient, for optical function is restored only when the refractive power of the transplanted cornea approaches that of the normal cornea.

Acknowledgments

I wish to express my thanks to Dr E. Pels from the Netherlands Ophthalmic Research Institute, Amsterdam, The Netherlands, for generously providing the photographs for Figures 9.1 to 9.4. My gratitude is also due to Dr J. D'Amaro from the Department of Immunohaematology and Blood Bank, Leiden University Hospital, Leiden, The Netherlands, for his many helpful comments during the preparation of this chapter. This work was partly supported by the Dutch Cornea Foundation and the Dutch Foundation for Medical Research and Health Research.

References

BAHN, C. F., MacCALLUM, D. K., LILLIE, J. H., MAYER, R. F. & MARTONYI, C. L. (1982) Complications associated with bovine corneal endothelial cell-lined homografts in the cat. *Investigative Ophthalmology and Visual Science*, **22** (1), 73–90.

BELYAEV, V. S. & VERETNIKOVA, V. V. (1972) Refractive keratoplasty using fetal donor corneas. *Vestnik Ophthalmologii*, **6**, 47–50.

BEVERIDGE, B. F. (1972) Eye banking. In: *Corneal Grafting*, pp. 11–37. Ed. T. A. Casey. Butterworths, London.

BOISJOLY, H. M., ROY, R., DUBE, I., *et al.* (1986) HLA-A,B and DR matching in corneal transplantation. *Ophthalmology*, **93**, 1290–5.

EHLERS, H. (1943) 5 Tilfaelde af hornhindetranplantation. *Soertryk af Ugesktift for Loeger*, **30**, 762, 1–7.

EHLERS, N. & KISSMEYER-NIELSEN, F. (1973) *Corneal graft failure.* Ciba Foundation Symposium. Associated Scientific Publishers, Amsterdam; London; New York. pp. 307–22.

FOULKS, G. N. & SANFILIPPO F. (1982) Beneficial effects of histocompatibility in high risk corneal transplantation. *American Journal of Ophthalmology*, **94**, 622–9.

GIBBS, D. C., BATCHELOR, J. R., WERB, A., *et al.* (1974) The influence of tissue type compatibility on the fate of full-thickness corneal grafts. *Transactions Ophthalmological Society United Kingdom*, **94**, 101–26.

GOSPODAROWICZ, D., GREENBERG, G. & ALVAREDO, J. (1979) Transplantation of cultured bovine corneal endothelial cells in species with non regenerative endothelium. *Archives of Ophthalmology*, **97**, 2163–9.

INSLER, M. S. & LOPEZ, J. G. (1986) Transplantation of human neonatal-endothelium. *Current Eye Research*, **5**, 12, 967–72.

KHODADOUST, A. A. & SILVERSTEIN, A. M. (1969) Transplantation and rejection of individual cell layers of the cornea. *Investigative Ophthalmology*, **8**, 180–95.

KOENIG, S., GRAUL, E. & KAUFMAN, H. (1982) Ocular refraction after penetrating keratoplasty with infant donor corneas. *American Journal of Ophthalmology*, **94**, 534–9.

NAYAK, S. & BINDER, P. S. (1984) The growth of endothelium from human corneal rims in tissue culture. *Investigative Ophthalmology and Visual Science*, **25**, 1213–16.

NYQUIST, G. W. (1968) Rheology of the cornea. Experimental techniques and results. *Experimental Eye Research*, **7**, 183–8.

PELS, E. & SCHUCHARD, Y. (1983) Organ culture of human corneas. *Documenta Ophthalmologica*, **56**, 147–53.

PFISTER, R. & BREAUD, S. (1983) Aphakic refractive penetrating keratoplasty using newborn donor corneas. *Ophthalmology*, **90**, 1207–13.

SCHIMMELPFENNIG, B. H. (1986) Tissue storage. In: *Corneal Surgery*, pp. 60–75. Ed. E. S. Brightbill. The C. V. Mosby Company, St Louis; Washington DC; Toronto.

SKELNIK, D. L., LINDSTROM, R. L., MINDRUP, E. A. & TORIS, C. B. (1985) Culturing and application of HCE cells in human corneal endothelial enhancement Arvo supplement. *Investigative Ophthalmology and Visual Science*, **26**, 147.

SORSBY, S. & SHERIDAN, M. (1953) Changes in refractive power of the cornea during growth. *British Journal of Ophthalmology*, **37**, 555–7.

STOCKER, F. W., EIRING, A., GEORGIADE, R. & GEORGIADE, N. (1958) A tissue culture technique for growing corneal epithelial, stromal, and endothelial tissues separately. *American Journal of Ophthalmology*, **46**, 294–8.

VANNAS, M. (1950) Remarks on the technique of corneal transplantation. *American Journal of Ophthalmology*, **33** (supplement), 70–6.

VANNAS, S., KARJALAINEN, P., RUUSUVAARA, A., *et al.* (1976) HLA compatable donor for the prevention of allograft reaction. *Albrecht von Graefes Archive Klinische Ophthalmologi*, **198**, 217–22.

VÖLKER-DIEBEN, H. J., KOK-VAN ALPHEN, C. C. & KRUIT, P. J. (1978) Advances and disappointments, indications and restrictions regarding HLA matched corneal grafts in high risk cases. *Documenta Ophthalmologica*, **46**, 219–26.

VÖLKER-DIEBEN, H. J. & D'AMARO, J. (1989) Corneal transplantation: a single center experience in 1976 to 1988. In: *Clinical Transplants 1988*, pp. 249–61. Ed. P. Terasaki. UCLA Tissue Typing Laboratory, Los Angeles.

VÖLKER-DIEBEN, H. J. (1989) Corneal transplantation: state of the art. *Transplantation Proceedings*, **21**, 1, 3116–19.

WOOD, T. O. & NISSENKORN, I. (1981) Infant donor corneas for penetrating keratoplasty. *Ophthalmic Surgery*, **12**, 7, 500–2.

ZIRM, E. (1906) Eine erfolgreiche totale Keratoplastiek. *Albrecht von Graefes Archive Ophthalmologi*, **64**, 580–5.

CHAPTER 10

Transplantation of ovaries and testes

R. G. GOSDEN

CONTENTS

FEW SUBJECTS IN EXPERIMENTAL SURGERY have attracted as much public interest or professional controversy as the transplantation of testes and ovaries. At one time hailed as a cure-all for old age, clinical transplantation of gonads was eventually overtaken by advances in chemical endocrinology and transplantation biology and is now regarded mainly as one of the blind alleys of science. The legacies of the so-called rejuvenators have effectively smothered further consideration of transplantation as a potential treatment for hypogonadism.

The first authenticated record of gonadal transplantation is attributed to an eighteenth century Scottish anatomist and surgeon, John Hunter, who grafted chicken testes and ovaries to the body cavity of hosts of either the same or opposite sex. Full details of this work have not survived and it is difficult to evaluate his claims but, since he used allografts, it seems doubtful that he could have been successful. Persistent scar tissue or hypertrophy of host gonads that were incompletely extirpated may explain his claims to success. Such dangers of misinterpretation can account for many false positive findings in a later era and for much of the confusion that followed.

It is the Gottingen biologist, Berthold (1849), who should be credited with the first successful testicular transplants, since, by using autografts, he luckily avoided the risk of rejection. When he replaced the testes of capons in their own body cavity he found that the growth of comb, plumage and courting behaviour, all of which are androgen dependent, were maintained. The transplantation of ovaries was pioneered in France by Bert (1865), but several decades passed until interest in either technique became widespread.

The turn of the century signalled an explosion of interest in gonadal transplantation. One causal factor was the dawning of the new science of endocrinology and the opportunities that transplantation offered for experimentally testing hormone secretion and action. Knauer

(1896) autotransplanted rabbit ovaries to the broad ligament and peritoneal cavity and obtained evidence of normal function, including ovulation and prevention of uterine atrophy. Like most of his contemporaries, he regarded allografting as potentially successful, but failed to provide any convincing evidence to support this assumption. The first investigator to transplant fetal ovarian tissue was Foà in 1900. He made the important discovery that immature organs undergo accelerated maturation in an adult environment. Interest in transplanting fetal tissue has been revived from time to time by the erroneous belief that it resembles cancer tissue in evading surveillance by the host's immune system (Dameron, 1950).

A second factor promoting interest in gonadal transplantation was the widespread misapprehension that somatic ageing is due to withdrawal of sex hormones. This old idea received impetus from a paper given in 1889 at the Société de Biologie in Paris by an eminent neurologist and endocrinologist, Brown-Séquard (Borell, 1976). At the age of seventy-two, and after a decade of deteriorating vigour, he injected himself with aqueous extracts of dog and guinea-pig testes. His genuine belief that he had rejuvenated himself caused a public sensation and gave impetus to a search for the sex steroids, though this would take forty years to succeed. In the meantime, however, many attempts were made to confirm his claims by testing organ extracts and, when those failed, by transplanting whole or partial gonads. These neatly coincided with improved surgical techniques and a general upsurge of interest in organ transplantation. Carrel was developing methods for anastomosing blood vessels which he used with brilliant effect in a series of organ transplants, including ovaries (Carrel & Guthrie, 1906), and for which he was rewarded with a Nobel Prize in 1912. He was convinced, unlike some others, that only autografts had any chance of success.

About 1913 a Chicago surgeon, after experimenting on himself, began a small but well-publicized series of testicular transplantations in his patients (Lydston, 1916). Like their predecessor, Brown-Séquard, Lydston and others who followed him believed that transplanted sex glands produce a hormone that was a 'cell stimulant, nutrient and regenerator' (Lydston, 1916, p. 1541) which could prolong life, restore waning sexual functions, combat senile dementia, atherosclerosis and other infirmities of mid and late life. Organs were obtained from young men who had died accidentally or by judicial execution; sometimes they were available from patients who had maldescended testes when a short vas deferens prevented orchiopexy. There was no serious debate about the use of fetal organs, which were unavailable. Because of the unpredictable supply, testes were sometimes stored in refrigerators for up to two or three days before grafting (Thorek, 1924). Organs were grafted whole (after scarifying the tunica albuginea to aid penetration of blood vessels), as slices or by injecting minced tissue into rectus muscle (Stanley, 1922). Despite the charlatans who were attracted into this field, a number of respectable doctors of the day were convinced of the value of these developments.

The excess demand for testis grafts over the supply of donor organs led Voronoff (1923) to use chimpanzee and baboon organs for treating patients presenting signs of early senility. This fad was taken up by other surgeons and became known as the 'monkey gland campaign' because the American press could not publish the word 'testicle' in their newspapers. Despite the doubts of Carrel and other authorities, there was widespread optimism that allografts, and even xenografts between closely related species, could be successful. None of the rejuvenators used microsurgery to join blood vessels of the graft to the host's circulation, and as a result ischaemic necrosis preceded rejection. Nevertheless, they reassured themselves that the lump that could be palpated in the scrotum of patients was a surviving graft rather than a scar, and many patients did profess to feeling better. Voronoff had gained experience of transplantation techniques from his earlier work on rams and bulls which began in 1917. He reported dramatic improvements in wool growth and virility of prize livestock and even suggested that these traits were heritable. Such large claims invited critical attention and in 1927 an international delegation of European scientists and veterinary surgeons visited him in Algiers (Figure 10.1). With the exception of the British group (Marshall *et al.*, 1928), who expressed reservations about the experimental protocols, the national representatives returned home with glowing reports of Voronoff's work and its commercial significance for animal breeding (Hamilton, 1986).

By the time transplantation of testes was attracting public attention, that of ovary grafting was already established as a method for treating a number of gynaecological problems and even senility (Pettinari, 1928). In 1895 Morris autotransplanted a fragment of ovary in a woman suffering from a pelvic inflammatory disease to the stump of one fallopian tube. The patient was reported to have become pregnant shortly afterwards, though spontaneous abortion occurred at the end of her first trimester. Morris also reported a transient phase of menstrual cyclicity after transplanting an ovarian allograft to a woman aged 30 years who had amenorrhoea and an infantile uterus; and in another case a child was delivered four years after an operation.

255

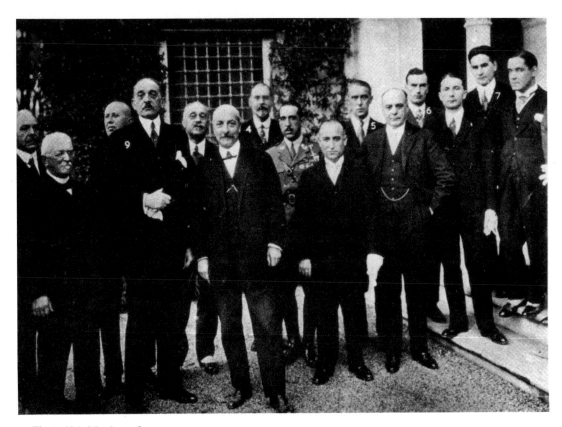

Figure 10.1. Members of an
international delegation of
scientists and veterinary
surgeons investigating
Voronoff's claims, Algiers
1927 (Parkes (1966).
Reproduced with the kind
permission of *Journal of
Endocrinology*.)

Comparable transplants with varying outcomes were described in the
following years by a number of clinicians (e.g. Martin, 1908; Davidson,
1912; reviewed by Woodruff, 1960).

But the 1930s brought nemesis for the so-called rejuvenators.
Carefully conducted grafting trials failed to confirm former claims (see
Hamilton, 1986); the new synthetic sex steroids were shown not to
affect the lifespan of experimental animals (Parkes, 1966); and, finally,
skepticism about the survival of allografts and xenografts was
confirmed (Neaves & Billingham, 1979).

Even when immunologically compatible, whole testes are unfavour-
able candidates for transplantation. They can tolerate only about two
to four hours of cold ischaemia before irreversible changes occur;
ovaries may do slightly better. Remarkably successful testicular
transplantation can be achieved when ischaemia time is reduced to less
than one hour by vascular anastomosis using dogs (Attaran *et al.*,
1966) and inbred rats (Lee *et al.*, 1971; Gittes *et al.*, 1972). The first
convincing demonstration of human testis transplantation was published comparatively recently (Silber, 1978). An anorchic man was

256

grafted with a testis from his genetically identical twin brother and, after microsurgically joining blood vessels and vasovasostomy, serum testosterone levels were rapidly raised and the ejaculate presented good sperm motility and a sperm count of 15 million per ml. The stringent requirements for success have, however, precluded a surge in demand for this operation.

Woodruff (1960, pp. 494–5) concluded about the early clinical and experimental studies that 'much of it . . . is of little value because many papers fail to state clearly the conditions of the experiment and many others report observations which cannot be reproduced or conclusions which appear to be based on a misinterpretation of the findings presented'. The lack of histocompatibility of donor and host was perhaps the most serious general limitation of those studies, although some investigators used autografts and others chose immunologically privileged sites, such as the anterior chamber of the eye (Dameron, 1950, 1951). Woodruff (1960, pp. 497–8) concludes, however, 'It is almost impossible . . . after reading critically the early literature on the subject, to escape the conclusion that ovarian homotransplants (allografts) may survive for weeks or even months in various different species'. Careful studies indicated that the ovary may carry a minor degree of privilege compared with skin grafts of comparable immunological diversity (Billingham & Parkes, 1955). Whether the explanation is a paucity of lymphocytes in the ovary, poor lymphatic drainage or weak antigenicity of follicular cells is not clear, but limited confidence should be placed in assumptions about immunological privilege because other, well-documented studies show that survival of ovarian allografts is brief unless rats are immunosuppressed (Cornier *et al.*, 1985). A number of attempts have been made to evade graft recognition and infiltration by isolating ovarian tissues in porous capsules to exclude T lymphocytes. Unfortunately, cell viability was compromised under these conditions (Sturgis & Castellanos, 1958; Shaffer & Hulka, 1969). In most experimental studies, the use of inbred animal strains or immunodeficient hosts should be mandatory.

Scope for gonadal transplantation

Setting aside the errors of the rejuvenators, gonadal transplantation can still be regarded as having clinical potential. The main beneficiaries would be the significant numbers of women with gonadal dysgenesis or premature menopause. The simplicity of a single, minor operation involving cell transfer leading to long-term recovery of menstrual cycles with fertile potential is likely to be attractive to women who are dissatisfied with existing hormone replacement therapy and the

Table 10.1. *Potential applications for gonadal cell transplantation*

Restoration of sex steroid secretion:
Transfer of ovarian follicles or their stem cells to overcome gonadal
dysgenesis and premature menopause
Transfer of testicular interstitial cells to hypogonadal men

Restoration of fertility to sterile patients

Transsexual grafting

Replacement of germ cells in patients transmitting genetic disease

---

obtrusion into private sex life of some reproductive technologies.
Whether it would be possible or even desirable to postpone the normal
age of menopause to the sixth decade of life or later has, as yet, received
very little consideration. The undiminished ability of postmenopausal
women to produce ovulatory surges of gonadotrophins indicates that
restitution of cycles is, in principle, feasible (Karande *et al.*, 1990).
Transplantation would be less likely to succeed in patients with
histories of autoimmune oophoritis.

Gonadal tissue transplants could find a number of other applications (Table 10.1). For example, carriers of genetic diseases could
receive normal germ cells from donors. Animal studies have shown
that there is no theoretical obstacle to transferring cells between sexes,
althouth H-Y histoincompatibility poses a potential problem for male
female combinations. Ovaries transplanted to adult male rodents
produce oestrogens continuously from anovulatory follicles because
neuroendocrine mechanisms are masculinized shortly after birth. But
there is apparently no such problem in primates. Ovaries transplanted
to male macaque monkeys who were treated with cyclosporin A to
suppress organ rejection showed normal follicular development,
ovulatory luteinizing hormone surges and luteinization (Norman &
Spies, 1986), demonstrating the possibility of establishing ovarian
cycles by grafting ovaries in transsexual men.

Certain types of gonadal transplantation already have a long record
of clinical practice. Before the advent of in vitro fertilization and
embryo transfer, ovaries were transplanted to the resected stump of the
fallopian tube to restore fertility (Estes' operation), although the
probability of pregnancy was only comparable to the failure rates of
some contraceptives (7 per 100 woman-years) (Adams, 1979). In the
male, orchiopexy can restore fertile potential by adjusting maldescended testes (Hargreave *et al.*, 1984; Kumar *et al.*, 1989). Success is
partly attributable to the absence of transplantation immunity.
Sterility caused by the absence of germ cells is, however, a more

intractable problem and, until immature germ cells can be used to repopulate sterile gonads, donor insemination and oocyte donation techniques will remain therapeutic mainstays (Cornet *et al.*, 1990; Rotszteyn *et al.*, 1990).

Endocrine glands are, in a number of respects, ideal subjects for transplantation because their functions are, with the notable exception of the pituitary gland and a few special circumstances (see below), not topographically specific. Isolation and synthesis of hormones have provided highly dependable means of treating endocrine hypofunction and have consequently reduced the need for transplantation. Nevertheless, cellular replacement remains attractive because hormone levels would be under normal physiological control and any pathological effects of endogenous hormones should be minimal. In theory, androgen deficiency should be treatable by transplanting one cell type only, namely the Leydig cell, whereas the endocrinology of the menstrual cycle requires an intact follicle, which comprises three cell types. When only granulosa cells are transferred to rat hosts, progestins are the only significant steroidal products (Farookhi *et al.*, 1982). The technical problems of gonadal tissue transplantation are, therefore, different in the two sexes.

Methods that have proved to be effective in inbred laboratory animals do not necessarily indicate clinical opportunities. Grafted gonadal cells, unlike ejaculated spermatozoa and mature oocytes, may be rejected by the host before they are effective, except in rare instances where identical twins are involved. Unless graft immunogenicity is reduced or the host is tolerant, immunosuppression is likely to be required. Some existing immunosuppressive drugs are neither teratogenic nor compromise gonadal hormone secretion (Handelsman *et al.*, 1984), but, in view of possible side effects (notably cancer), it is arguable whether such treatment should be offered to patients who are, apart from their infertility, young and healthy.

The possibility of using fetal tissue increases the prospects for a clinical method because of the ready availability of material under existing abortion legislation in many countries. Other authors in this volume have drawn attention to the advantages and problems of using fetal organs. In the case of fetal ovaries, a major advantage is the abundance of germ cells (Baker, 1963); organs from one abortus would be sufficient to repopulate the ovaries of a number of children and young women. However, the developmental potential of these cells after transfer to postnatal ovaries is still uncertain. There is little prospect of joining fine blood vessels of fetal gonads to those of the host, but the delicacy of the organs favours rapid revascularization of grafted slices or disaggregation for storage and transfer of isolated cells.

Before fetal tissues can be used in orthodox medicine there are, in

addition to technical hurdles, important ethical and legal considerations (see Chapter 13, this volume). The possibility of transplanting
fetal germ cells to sterile human ovaries has been raised only recently
(Edwards, 1989) and, although some patients profess interest, public
reactions are difficult to predict. For fetal tissue grafting, germ cells
present the unique problem of being involved potentially in reproduction and therefore transmitting genes to children.

In the following sections, I have selected, from a vast body of
literature, experimental evidence with the most relevant bearing on the
possibilities for transplantation of human fetal gonadal tissues. To
date, there have been comparatively few studies of this technique in any
species and I have, therefore, had to draw on many studies of postnatal
organs. This is not a serious drawback because birth is not a
particularly important milestone for gonadal development, as far as we
are aware. Moreover, the developmental schedules in the major
experimental models, mice and rats, are such that in infant animals the
gonads are comparable to those in human fetuses at midgestation.
Thus, much of the experimental animal evidence is pertinent to the
theme of this chapter.

Transplantation of ovarian tissues

The experimental extirpation of endocrine glands and their replacement has been one of the cornerstones of classical endocrine
investigation for decades (see Krohn, 1977). Ovarian grafts in inbred
mice have been very successful; as many as 17 litters and 79 offspring
have been delivered from a single animal (Krohn, 1965). Mice and rats
have been favoured subjects because inbred strains are available, but
virtually all common laboratory mammals have been used.

Small ovaries have tended to be grafted whole, trusting to rapid
revascularization before necrosis becomes extensive. With larger
ovaries from dogs (Dempster, 1954; Wingate et al., 1970) and farm
animals (Goding et al., 1967) it is necessary to use vascular anastomosis
to minimize ischaemic damage. Cotransplantation by vascular microsurgery of fallopian tube with its neighbouring ovary has led to
successful rabbit pregnancies (Winston & McClure Browne, 1974).

Ovaries generally resume cycles of normal length in heterotopic
locations provided that a good blood supply is available, but there are a
few exceptions. For guinea pig ovaries, for instance, the proximity of
the uterus permits the action of a local luteolytic agent, prostaglandin
$F_{2\alpha}$, and separation leads to extended oestrous cycles (Bland &
Donovan, 1968). The behaviour of ovarian transplants is likely to be
disturbed in the spleen, omentum and other sites with portal venous

Figure 10.2. A bisected mouse ovary that had been grafted under the kidney capsule of an ovariectomized host. Normal follicular development with ovulations (arrow) and corpus luteum formation is occurring (haematoxylin and eosin, × 35).

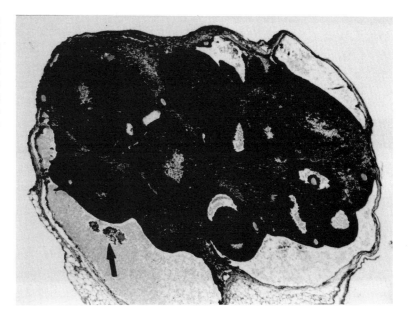

drainage. In ovariectomized rats with splenic implants, hepatic clearance of steroid hormones reduces negative feedback on pituitary gonadotrophin secretion and causes implants to become hyperstimulated and polyfollicular. Ovarian tumours appear after the disppearance of follicular parenchyma (Biskind *et al.*, 1950).

Even under optimal conditions, it is rare for more than 50% of the total follicle population to survive transplantation, unless vascular anastomosis is carried out (Green *et al.*, 1956; Jones & Krohn, 1960; Felicio *et al.*, 1983). Primordial follicles are virtually the sole survivors of the ischaemic phase of grafting (Bland & Donovan, 1968) and atresia of large follicles delays the reappearance of signs of oestrogenization for at least two weeks. The differential survival of small follicles is probably attributable to their peripheral location in the ovarian cortex and lower metabolic requirements. Since oocytes are postmitotic and cannot be replaced, their loss is of far greater significance than that of any other cell type, some of which dedifferentiate as a consequence of oocyte death (granulosa and thecal cells). Cell survival is poor in both subcutaneous and adipose tissue compared with better vascularized sites such as the renal capsule, which also provides a convenient pocket for anchorage (Figure 10.2).

Experimental ovarian transplantation has been used to investigate whether the maximum reproductive lifespan of rodents is limited by ovarian ageing, as is plainly the case in humans (Gosden, 1985). Whereas human menopause coincides approximately with the exhaustion of follicular stores (Richardson *et al.*, 1987), most animal ovaries contain substantial numbers of follicles at all developmental stages after the final ovulation has occurred (Jones, 1970). Ovaries transplanted from old anovulatory rats to young hosts were capable of cyclic activity whereas the reciprocal combination failed (Aschheim, 1965; Peng & Huang, 1972). These results imply that the neuroendocrine mechanism controlling ovulation is impaired before fecundity is lost, although a more recent study indicates ovarian ageing contributes to anovulation in this species too (Sopelak & Butcher, 1982). In the CBA strain, Krohn (1962) used young ovaries to restore cycles. The reduced ability of a reciprocal combination to produce cycles was because this strain loses follicles precociously, a situation reminiscent of human ovaries (Jones & Krohn, 1961). Using a more fecund strain (C57Bl/6J), Felicio *et al.* (1983) found that both ovarian and hypothalamo-pituitary factors were responsible for acyclicity at midlife, the latter being related to oestrogen exposure during life (Finch *et al.*, 1984). Comparable studies have not been appropriate in subhuman primates because menopause occurs late in life, if at all.

Studies of laboratory rodents have shown that grafts become progressively less effective with age because primordial follicles become scarcer and the organ accumulates dense fibrous tissue. In addition to the advantage of abundant germ cells, fetal and neonatal organs provide opportunities for transferring isolated germ cells and/or small follicles. This strategy permits a greater degree of control and better prospects for banking gonadal cells (see below).

Naked germ cells and primordial follicles can be recovered readily from fetal and infant rodent ovaries, respectively, by disaggregation in medium containing collagenase (type I) (Roy & Greenwald, 1985; Torrance *et al.*, 1989). Human fetal ovaries at 12–18 weeks of gestation are readily isolated in this way. At later ages, enzyme digestion times are protracted and the quality and yield of oocytes are reduced. Larger follicles that are recovered during the process tend to be damaged, have little capacity for self-repair and are unsuitable for transfer.

Optimal methods for transferring cell or follicle suspensions to host animals vary with species. Since cells injected into small rodent ovaries are poorly retained, we reaggregated them in a fibrin clot or collagen gel before grafting (Gosden, 1990; Telfer *et al.*, 1990). In larger species, problems of retention may be less serious or the larger antra of non-ovulating follicles may provide suitable receptacles for injected cells from which colonization could begin. Vehicles for cell transfer can be loaded with thousands of small follicles harvested from neonatal mice (Figure 10.3). After one to two days in culture, fibrin clots contract to produce compact masses which can be pipetted readily or held with fine forceps (Figure 10.4). These grafts have been transferred to the ovaries

Figure 10.3. Thousands of primordial follicles from infant mouse ovaries have been reaggregated in this plasma clot for grafting into a sterilized host (Phase contrast, × 66). (Reproduced from Gosden (1990) with the permission of *Human Reproduction*.)

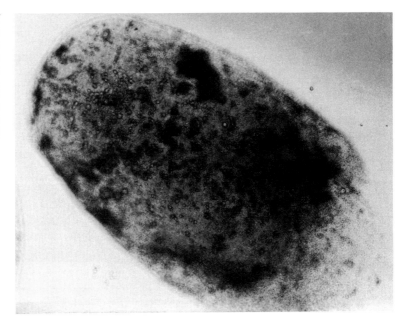

Figure 10.4. After 24 hours in culture, clots containing follicles and other ovarian cells contract to dense masses. Prolonged culture leads to cellular necrosis at the centre and enlargement of oocytes at the periphery of the grafts (haematoxylin and eosin, × 50).

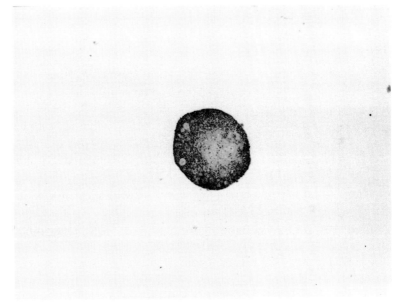

of young adult mice which had been given a low dose of X-irradiation to sterilize them (0.5 Gy). The primordial follicles rapidly grew to dominate the host organ, producing Graafian stages and even ovulations within three weeks (Figure 10.5). The scrambled follicles and other cells, presumably including thecal precursors, restore the appropriate cellular associations that were lost by digesting connective

Figure 10.5. Primordial follicles grafted into a X-ray sterilized mouse ovary grow to Graafian dimensions within three weeks; some may subsequently ovulate and restore fertility (haematoxylin and eosin, × 50). (Reproduced from Gosden (1990) with the permission of *Human Reproduction*.)

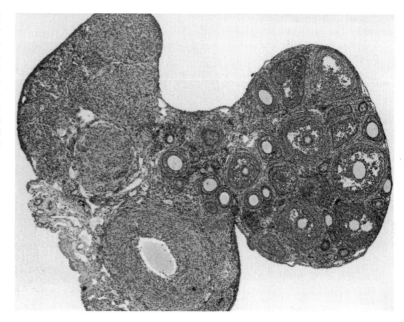

Figure 10.6. Clotted follicles placed in the evacuated ovarian capsule of ovariectomized hosts grow and develop to Graafian size (haematoxylin and eosin, × 50). (Reproduced from Gosden (1990) with the permission of *Human Reproduction*.)

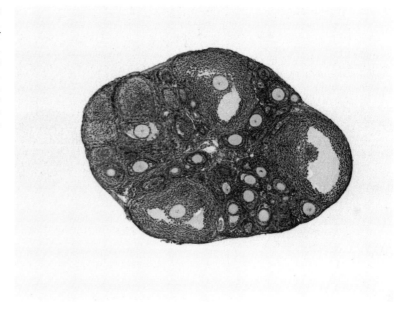

tissues. The host ovary is not required for successful grafting, since morphologically normal ovaries can form from grafts inserted in the evacuated capsules of ovariectomized animals (Figure 10.6). The numbers of follicles surviving for more than a month is very variable (Table 10.2); low viability and premature recruitment of follicles is a

Figure 10.7. Variation in vaginal cornification (oestrogen index) in X-ray sterilized mice receiving either sterile grafts or grafts containing primordial follicles (R. G. Gosden, unpublished).

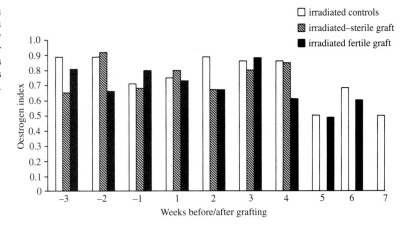

□ irradiated controls
▨ irradiated–sterile graft
■ irradiated fertile graft

Oestrogen index

Weeks before/after grafting

Figure 10.8. Primordial follicles grow to Graafian dimensions when grafted to the sterile ovaries of old mice (haematoxylin and eosin, × 66). This host animal, which was 14 months old and CBA strain, was past the normal age range for fecundity (Jones & Krohn, 1961).

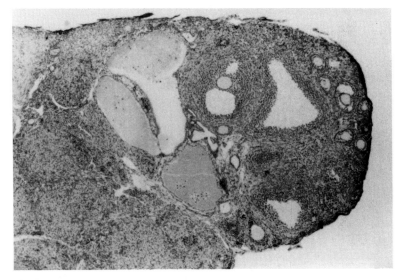

major limitation on the long-term performance of grafts (Gosden, 1990). Unfortunately, it is not possible to monitor successfully the restoration of cycles in X-irradiated mice by the standard method of vaginal smearing because the afollicular host ovary continues to produce oestrogens (Figure 10.7). There can be no doubt, however, that grafts are functional since pregnancies and offspring have been obtained from sterilized animals (Table 10.2). And there is no reason to assume that only young hosts may be grafted successfully. In a study of CBA strain mice which had passed the age of sterility (about 1 year of age), grafts were able to restore Graafian follicles, though without ovulation, in a majority of animals (Figure 10.8).

265

Table 10.2. *Restoration of fertility to X-irradiated mice by transferring primordial ovarian follicles*

Group	No. animals	Total no. of follicles[a]	No. mated	Litter size
Control (no graft)	5	0–1	1	0
Control (sterile graft)	7	0	2	0
Fertile graft	10	8–537	6	1,3,4,6,8

Note: [a]Range.
Source: Adapted from Gosden (1990).

Table 10.3. *Gestational age at onset of stages of meiotic prophase and folliculogenesis in human fetal oocytes*

Stage	Weeks of gestation
Leptotene	9–11
Pachytene	13–19
Diplotene (and folliculogenesis)	12–28

Note: zygotene is brief and rarely observed.
Sources: Baker (1963); Manotaya & Potter (1963); Kurilo (1981); Speed (1985).

Transplantation of primordial follicles is particularly attractive because these units consist simply of an oocyte and pregranulosa cells. If pretheca cells were absent from the graft, they might be available for recruitment from stroma of sterile host ovaries, reducing the likelihood of immunological rejection. But it is unlikely that this strategy can be applied clinically because primordial follicles are rare or absent in abortuses at the gestational ages at which most terminations take place, and current attitudes and technology are encouraging earlier abortion. Germ cells around the end of the first trimester and the beginning of the next are either in various stages of the protracted process of meiotic prophase or at earlier mitotic stages (oogonia) (Table 10.3). An understanding of the developmental potency of human prefollicular germ cells with their accompanying somatic cells, is a *sine qua non* if clinical grafting is to become an option.

Fetal rodent ovaries can be successfully grafted to adult animals (Arrau *et al.*, 1983; Taketo-Hosotani & Sinclair-Thompson, 1987). Germ cells continue to develop normally to diplotene of meiosis, when they become arrested and form follicles. The endocrine environment of adults promotes early, and sometimes, explosive growth of follicles when grafted to X-irradiated ovaries (compare Figures 10.9 and 10.10).

Figure 10.9. Typical X-irradiated host ovaries are small, atrophic and sterile when receiving grafts of isolated primordial follicles (cf. Figure 10.5) or fetal ovary fragments (cf. Figure 10.10) (haematoxylin and eosin, × 66).

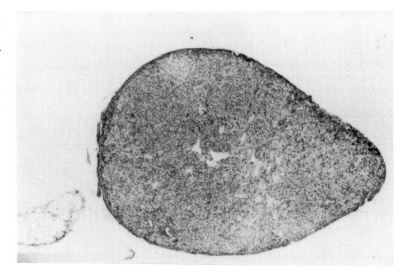

Figure 10.10. This mouse ovary, which was excised from a fetus at 19 days of gestational age (about 1 day before birth) and grafted into a sterilized host ovary, has developed large, secretory follicles in three weeks (haematoxylin and eosin, × 66).

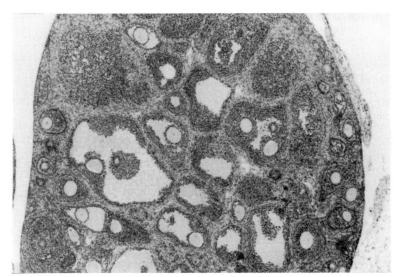

Preclinical trials have demonstrated the viability of human fetal germ cells after transplantation. The SCID mouse, which lacks both T and B lymphocytes (see Chapter 3, this volume), tolerates xenografts and provides a new model for ovarian studies. For instance, when fragments of feline ovarian cortex containing small follicles were grafted under the renal capsule of ovariectomized mice, vaginal cornification and endometrial hyperplasia occurred within a month (Figure 10.11). The sources of oestrogens were Graafian follicles, which had attained mature sizes (2–3 mm diameter) under the influence of host gonadotrophic hormones (Figure 10.12).

The same host and site have been used for transplanting ovarian

Figure 10.11. Longitudinal section of the uterus of an ovariectomized mouse carrying a fragment of cat ovary. The greater oestrogen production by the xenograft than by a set of normal mouse follicles has resulted in cystic glandular hyperplasia (haematoxylin and eosin, × 40).

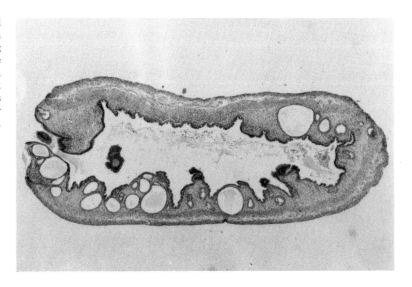

Figure 10.12. Graafian follicle development occurs in xenografted ovaries under the kidney capsule of ovariectomized SCID mice. In this example, cat follicles have taken one month to grow to the mature size which is typical for this species (haematoxylin and eosin, × 40).

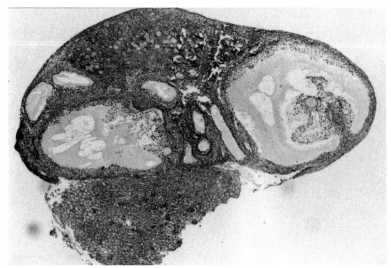

fragments and isolated germ cells from human fetuses approximately 16 weeks old. The grafts vascularized rapidly and can persist as healthy, growing tissue for six months (R. G. Gosden, unpublished). Germ cells in mitosis and at all stages of meiotic prophase were abundant, whereas diplotene cells were less common and few, if any, follicles had formed even after many months (Figure 10.13). Despite the lack of progression to more advanced stages, these results indicate that tissue obtained under routine conditions in a general hospital remains sufficiently viable for grafting purposes.

Conflicting claims have been made about the expression of

Figure 10.13. Human fetal oogonia continue to multiply and enter meiosis under the kidney capsule of the SCID mouse. Tissue from a 16-week-old fetus two weeks after grafting (haematoxylin and eosin, × 260).

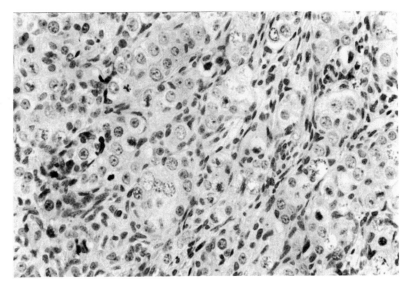

histocompatibility antigens by fetal cells. Since the genes are not silent (Seigler & Metzgar, 1970), fetal cells are liable to undergo allograft rejection. Endocrine cells have often been regarded as relatively weakly antigenic (Krohn, 1965) and immunohistochemical studies have shown that mouse granulosa cells and oocytes do not express H-2 antigens of either class I or II, or only weakly (Ponder *et al.*, 1983; Goldbard *et al.*, 1985; R. G. Gosden & A. Murray, unpublished). According to Dohr *et al.* (1987), human oocytes do not express HLA antigens. In the same study, granulosa cells were found to express class II strongly as well as class I antigens, which is surprising and contrary to our findings. The antigenicity or otherwise of these cells is, perhaps, only marginally relevant, since whole or disaggregated organs will contain endothelial cells which do express class I antigens. Moreover, the release of γ-interferon caused by infiltrating leucocytes may lead to the expression of genes for histocompatibility antigens. As the search continues for methods of safely encouraging host tolerance it is likely that the problems of rejection will eventually be overcome. Recent experiments show that a state of unresponsiveness to cardiac allografts is induced by pretreating recipients with blood cells expressing donor-specific histocompatibility antigens or by DNA-mediated transfer of relevant genes (Madsen *et al.*, 1988). A less elaborate method involving simple culture before organ grafting, which eliminates passenger leucocytes (Lafferty & Gill, 1989), may even be effective in prolonging survival of ovarian allografts.

Transplantation of testicular tissues

The problems arising from the size of the testis and its fibrous capsule led some pioneer gland transplanters to use sliced or minced organs. The most plausible case was produced by Kearns (1941) who reimplanted testicular tissue subcutaneously in a victim of accidental castration. Subsequent examination of the mass and secretions of the prostate gland indicated that testosterone was being produced by the autograft. It is very difficult, however, to envisage how germ cell transfer could restore spermatogenesis. The highly complex architecture of the seminiferous epithelium and the need to maintain patency of excurrent ducts preclude simple grafting, and the prospect of injecting spermatogonial stem cells from donor testes into atrophic tubules is daunting. In women, only one mature oocyte is required per month whereas testes must produce tens of millions of spermatozoa per day to be fertile; besides, other pathological changes in the testis often coexist with oligospermia and azoospermia.

For these reasons, efforts to develop tissue grafting for the purpose of improving testosterone levels in hypogonadal men are more likely to be rewarding than attempts to restore fertility. This goal would appear to be deceptively simple, since it requires merely the transfer of interstitial cells, which are readily isolated from donor testes using collagenase. Moreover, the number of cells can be expanded either *in vitro* before grafting or *in vivo* afterwards. Growth occurs from mesenchymal stem cells or by Leydig cell mitosis, depending on age (Kerr *et al.*, 1987; Hardy *et al.*, 1989). There are two distinct generations of Leydig cells in the testis: fetal and adult; and, although the former have greater steroidogenic potential (Tapanainen *et al.*, 1984), both are potentially suitable for transplantation.

Interstitial cells grafted to heterotopic sites in castrated rodents have resulted in mild androgenization: partial restoration of the weight of the body, seminal vesicles and penis (Fox *et al.*, 1973; Boyle *et al.*, 1976) and serum testosterone levels elevated above controls (Tai *et al.*, 1989). On the other hand, seminiferous tubules failed to maintain complete spermatogenesis and underwent atrophy shortly after transplantation.

A number of vehicles and several implantation sites for interstitial cells have been tried, but none fully replaced testicular androgen production. We isolated interstitial cells from neonatal mice and grafted them in a fibrin clot to the spermatic cord of orchidectomized hosts. This site offers the advantage of a single minor incision; the scrotal environment is not obligatory for Leydig cell function. Grafted tissue grew, much of which was cytologically normal Leydig cells (Figure 10.14), but circulating testosterone levels remained low and

Table 10.4. *The response of castrated adult C57Bl/6 mice five weeks after grafting interstitial cells from immature syngeneic donors*

Group	Number	Seminal vesicle weight (mg)	Serum testosterone (ng/ml)
Intact controls	6	414 ± 56	8.2 ± 2.9
Castrates	6	28 ± 8	< 0.3
Castrated and grafted	6	48 ± 4	< 0.3

Note: Means ± standard error of means are given.
Source: R. G. Gosden, A. Murray & H. M. Fraser, unpublished data.

Figure 10.14. Interstitial cells isolated from infant mouse testes form a solid, vascularized structure within two weeks of grafting in a castrated mouse host (haematoxylin and eosin, × 66).

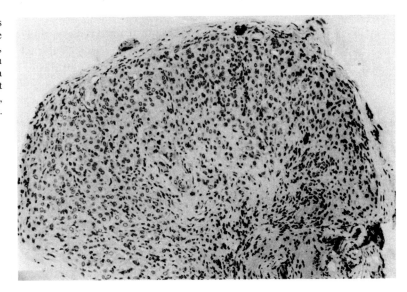

seminal vesicle mass was maintained poorly (though significantly better than controls); nor did it restore libido (Table 10.4).

Such modest results are not surprising when the architecture of the testis and its high blood flow per unit mass is taken into account. In contrast to the clump of cells in these grafts, normal Leydig cells are distributed widely throughout the testicular interstitium, in close proximity to capillaries and have a notable lymphatic drainage (Setchell, 1978). It is unlikely that these conditions can be mimicked by grafting compact masses of cells in subcutaneous and intraperitoneal sites, but proximity to highly vascular areas (e.g. kidney capsules) may be more successful (Tai *et al.*, 1989) and the use of gelatin sponges loaded with cells should encourage rapid ingrowth of vessels (van Dam *et al.*, 1989). The outcomes of attempts to replace Leydig cells have been limited in success, but sufficiently interesting to encourage further research.

Low temperature storage of gonadal cells

The discovery in the late 1940s of the cryoprotective properties of glycerol for storing spermatozoa encouraged attempts to store whole or fragmented testes and ovaries at subzero temperatures. Tubules and interstitial tissue teased from rat testes were frozen in medium containing glycerol to reduce damage from ice crystal formation. Some Leydig cells had evidently survived because thawed tissue was able to stimulate seminal vesicle growth in castrated recipient animals (Parkes & Smith, 1954). More surprisingly, another study presented cytological evidence that spermatogenesis continued after freeze–thawing (Deanesly, 1954b). Comparable results following freezing have been obtained with ovarian tissues. Although many more oocytes disappeared than could be accounted for by ischaemia during revascularization, it was found that slow cooling reduced the damage (Parkes & Smith, 1953; Deanesly, 1954a; Green et al., 1956). After orthotopically transplanting frozen–thawed mouse ovaries, Parrot (1960) obtained pregnancies and live offspring. These modest successes were probably due to the location of small oocytes in the cortex, which is soon reached by slowly penetrating cryopreservation medium.

Successful frozen storage of spermatozoa, oocytes and preimplantation embryos of a number of species demonstrates the advantages of using cells in isolation or small clusters. While considerable effort has been devoted to frozen storage of freshly ovulated oocytes because of the needs of clinical embryology (Whittingham, 1977; Friedler et al., 1988), comparatively little attention has been paid to preovulatory oocytes and germ cells. On the one hand, the absence of a metaphase spindle should reduce the risks of cooling damage to their cytoskeleton: on the other, these early stages require follicle cells for optimal development after thawing. Recently, murine preovulatory oocytes enclosed in cumulus cells and at the germinal vesicle stage have been frozen successfully in medium containing dimethylsulfoxide (Schroeder et al., 1990).

Ovaries possess few preovulatory oocytes at any given time whereas thousands of primordial ones remain in reserve. Bulk storage of small follicles and germ cells is highly desirable, and would assist the development of transplant programmes. Little attention has been given to fetal ovaries, but the feasibility of storing primary follicles isolated from infant mouse ovaries was demonstrated recently (Carroll et al., 1990). The viability of frozen–thawed follicles was tested by transferring them to the kidney capsule, where Graafian follicles formed. Oocytes that were recovered from the follicles were able to resume meiosis, undergo fertilization and cleave *in vitro*. When the resultant 2-cell embryos were transferred to pseudopregnant hosts, normal pups were born. In view of these results, it seems likely that methods can be devised for storing simpler stages: primordial follicles and prefollicular germ cells, and even testicular interstitial cells should the need arise.

Conclusions

The transplantation of gonadal tissue has had a long history and, despite being side-tracked in the futile pursuit of rejuvenation, continues to be of potential clinical value for hypogonadism and related disorders. The transplantation of whole organs, with or without vascular anastomosis, and of organ fragments is now being joined by grafting of isolated germ and somatic cells. This should: reduce problems of transplant ischaemia; allow more control of what is transferred; and open the possibility of tissue banking.

Laboratory studies have shown that when primordial follicles and fetal ovarian germ cells are transferred, follicle maturation, oestrogen secretion and even fertility can be restored to sterilized hosts. Full restitution of serum androgen levels by grafting testicular interstitial cells in castrated males has not yet been achieved, though this aim is much more realistic than restoring fertility by transferring spermatogonial stem cells. These studies have been carried out mainly with postnatal tissue from inbred animals and need refinement. Nevertheless, they indicate potential opportunities for using fetal tissue for disorders of human reproductive endocrinology and fertility.

Acknowledgments
The author thanks the Wellcome Trust and the Galton Institute (London) for funding his research and Alison Murray and Kay Grant for excellent technical assistance.

References

ADAMS, C. E. (1979) Consequences of accelerated ovum transport, including a re-evaluation of Estes' operation. *Journal of Reproduction & Fertility*, **55**, 239–46.

ARRAU, J., ROBLERO, L., CURY, M. & GONZALEZ, R. (1983) Effect of exogenous sex steroids upon the number of germ cells and the growth of foetal ovaries grafted under the kidney capsule of adult ovariectomized hamsters. *Journal of Embryology and Experimental Morphology*, **78**, 33–42.

ASCHHEIM, P. (1965) Résultats fournis par la greffe héterochrone des ovaires dans l'étude de la regulation hypothalamo-hypophyso-ovarienne de la ratte sénile. *Gerontologia*, **10**, 65–75.

ATTARAN, S. E., HODGES, C. V., CRARY, L. S., Jr, VANGALDER, G. C., LAWSON, R. K. & ELLIS, L. R. (1966) Homotransplants of the testis. *Journal of Urology*, **95**, 387–9.

BAKER, T. G. (1963) A quantitative and cytological study of germ cells in human ovaries. *Proceedings of the Royal Society, B*, **158**, 417–33.

BERT, P. (1865) Sur la greffe animale. *Comptes Rendus des Séances et Memoires de la Société de Biologie*, **61**, 587.

BERTHOLD, A. A. (1849) Transplantation der Hoden. *Archiv für Anatomie, Physiologie und wissenschaftliche Medicine*, **16**, 42–6.

BILLINGHAM, R. E. & PARKES, A. S. (1955) Studies on the survival of homografts of skin and ovarian tissue in rats. *Proceedings of the Royal Society, B*, **143**, 550–60.

BISKIND, G. R., KORDAN, B. & BISKIND, M. S. (1950) Ovary transplanted to spleen in rats: the effect of unilateral castration, pregnancy, and subsequently castration. *Cancer Research*, **10**, 309–18.

BLAND, K. P. & DONOVAN, B. T. (1968) The effect of autotransplantation of the ovaries to the kidneys or uterus on the oestrous cycle of the guinea pig. *Journal of Endocrinology*, **41**, 95–103.

BORELL, M. (1976) Brown-Séquard's organotherapy and its appearance in America at the end of the Nineteenth Century. *Bulletin of the History of Medicine*, **50**, 309–20.

BOYLE, P. F., FOX, M. & SLATER, D. (1976) Transplantation of interstitial cells of the testis: effect of implant site, graft mass and ischaemia. *British Journal of Urology*, **47**, 891–8.

BROWN-SÉQUARD, C. E. (1989) Des éffets produits chez l'homme par des injections souscutanées d'un liquide retire des testicules frais de cobaye et de chien. *Comptes Rendus Hebdomaidaires de Séances et Mémoires de la Société de Biologie*, **1**, (9th ser.), 415–19.

CARREL, A. & GUTHRIE, C.-C. (1906) Technique de la transplantation homoplastique de l'ovaire. *Comptes Rendus des Séances de la Société de Biologie*, **6**, 466–8.

CARROLL, J., WHITTINGHAM, D. G., WOOD, M. J., TELFER, E. &

GOSDEN, R. G. (1990) Extraovarian production of mature viable mouse oocytes from frozen primary follicles. *Journal of Reproduction & Fertility*, **90**, 321–7.

CORNET, D., ALVAREZ, S., ANTOINE, J. M., TIBI, Ch., MANDEL-BAUM, J., PLACHOT, M. & SALAT-BAROUX, J. (1990) Pregnancies following ovum donation in gonadal dysgenesis. *Human Reproduction*, **5**, 291–3.

CORNIER, E., SIBELLA, P. & CHATELET, F. (1985) Études histologiques et devenir fonctionnel des greffes de trompe et d'ovaire chez la ratte (isogreffes et allogreffes traitteés par cyclosporine A). *Journal de Gynecologie, Obstetrique et Biologie de la Reproduction*, (Paris), **14**, 567–73.

DAMERON, J. T. (1950) Homologous transplantation of fetal endocrine tissue to adult non-related host. *Proceedings of the Society of Experimental Biology & Medicine*, **73**, 343–5.

DAMERON, J. T. (1951) The anterior chamber of the eye for investigative purposes. A site for transplantation of fetal endocrine tissues and cancer, and for the study of tissue reaction. *Surgery*, **30**, 787–99.

DAVIDSON, H. S. (1912) Transplantation of the ovary in the human being: record of three cases. *Edinburgh Medical Journal*, **3**, 441–9.

DEANESLY, R. (1954a) Immature rat ovaries grafted after freezing and thawing. *Journal of Endocrinology*, **11**, 197–200.

DEANESLY, R. (1954b) Spermatogenesis and endocrine activity in grafts of frozen and thawed rat testis. *Journal of Endocrinology*, **11**, 201–6.

DEMPSTER, W. J. (1954) A technique for the study of the behaviour of the autotransplanted kidney, adrenals and ovary of the dog. *Journal of Physiology*, **124**, xv–xvi.

DOHR, G. A., MOTTER, W., LEITINGER, S., DESOYE, G., URDL, W., WINTER, R., WILDERS-TRUSCHNIG, M. M., UCHANSKA-ZIEGLER, B. & ZIEGLER, A. (1987) Lack of expression of histocompatibility leukocyte antigen class I and class II molecules on the human oocyte. *Journal of Immunology*, **138**, 3766–70.

EDWARDS, R. G. (1989) *Life Before Birth*, p. 81. Hutchinson, London.

FAROOKHI, R., KEYES, P. L. & KAHN, L. E. (1982) A method for transplantation of luteinizing granulosa cells: evidence for progesterone secretion. *Biology of Reproduction*, **27**, 1261–6.

FELICIO, L. S., NELSON, J. F., GOSDEN, R. G. & FINCH, C. E. (1983) Restoration of ovulatory cycles by young ovarian grafts in aging mice: potentiation by long-term ovariectomy decreases with age. *Proceedings of the National Academy of Sciences, USA*, **80**, 6076–80.

FINCH, C. E., FELICIO, L. S., MOBBS, C. V. & NELSON, J. F. (1984) Ovarian and steroidal influences on neuroendocrine aging processes in female rodents. *Endocrine Reviews*, **5**, 467–97.

FOÀ, C. (1900) La greffe des ovaires en relation avec quelques questions de biologie generale. *Archives Italiennes de Biologie*, **34**, 43–73.

FOX, M., BOYLE, P. F. & HAMMONDS, J. C. (1973) Transplantation of interstitial cells of the testis. *British Journal of Urology*, **45**, 696–701.

FRIEDLER, S., GIUDICE, L. C. & LAMB, E. J. (1988) Cryopreservation of embryos and ova. *Fertility & Sterility*, **49**, 743–64.

GITTES, R. F., ALTWEIN, J. E., YEN, S. S. C. & LEE, S. (1972) Testicular transplantation in the rat: long-term gonadotropin and testosterone radioimmunoassays. *Surgery*, **72**, 187–92.

275

GODING, J. R., McCRACKEN, J. A. & BAIRD, D. T. (1967) The study of ovarian function in the ewe by means of a vascular autotransplantation technique. *Journal of Endocrinology*, **39**, 37–52.

GOLDBARD, S. B., GOLLNICK, S. O. & WARNER, C. M. (1985) Synthesis of H-2 antigens by preimplantation mouse embryos. *Biology of Reproduction*, **33**, 30–6.

GOSDEN, R. G. (1985) *Biology of Menopause: the Causes and Consequences of Ovarian Ageing*. Academic Press, London.

GOSDEN, R. G. (1990) Restitution of fertility in sterilized mice by transferring primordial ovarian follicles. *Human Reproduction*, **5**, 499–504.

GREEN, S. H., SMITH, A. U. & ZUCKERMAN, S. (1956) The numbers of oocytes in ovarian autografts after freezing and thawing. *Journal of Endocrinology*, **13**, 330–4.

HAMILTON, D. (1986) *The Monkey Gland Affair*. Chatto & Windus, London.

HANDELSMAN, D. J., McDOWELL, I. F. W., CATERSON, I. D., TILLER, D. J., HALL, B. M. & TURTLE, J. R. (1984) Testicular function after renal transplantation: comparison of Cyclosporin A with azathioprine and prednisone combination regimes. *Clinical Nephrology*, **22**, 144–8.

HARDY, M. P., ZIRKIN, B. R. & EWING, L. L. (1989) Kinetic studies on the development of the adult population of Leydig cells in testes of the pubertal rat. *Endocrinology*, **124**, 762–70.

HARGREAVE, T. B., ELTON, R. A., WEBB, J. A., BUSITTIL, A. & CHISHOLM, G. D. (1984) Maldescended testes and fertility: a review of 68 cases. *British Journal of Urology*, **56**, 734–9.

JONES, E. C. (1970) The ageing ovary and its influence on reproductive capacity. *Journal of Reproduction & Fertility*, Supplement, **12**, 17–30.

JONES, E. C. & KROHN, P. L. (1960) Orthotopic ovarian transplantation in mice. *Journal of Endocrinology*, **20**, 135–46.

JONES, E. C. & KROHN, P. L. (1961) The relationships between age, numbers of oocytes and fertility in virgin and multiparous mice. *Journal of Endocrinology*, **21**, 469–95.

KARANDE, V. C., SCOTT, R. T., Jr & ARCHER, D. F. (1990) The relationship between serum estradiol-17β concentrations and induced pituitary luteinizing hormone surges in postmenopausal women. *Fertility & Sterility*, **54**, 217–21.

KEARNS, W. (1941) Testicular transplantation. Successful autoplastic graft following accidental castration. *Annals of Surgery*, **114**, 886–90.

KERR, J. B., BARTLETT, J. M. S., DONACHIE, K. & SHARPE, R. M. (1987) Origin of regenerating Leydig cells in the testes of the adult rat. An ultrastructural, morphometric and hormonal assay study. *Cell and Tissue Research*, **249**, 367–77.

KNAUER, E. (1896) Einige Versuche über Ovarientransplantation bei Kaninchen. *Zentralblatt Gynäkolfür*, **20**, 524–8.

KROHN, P. L. (1962) Review Lectures on Senescence. II. Heterochronic transplantation in the study of ageing. *Proceedings of the Royal Society, B*, **157**, 128–47.

KROHN, P. L. (1965) Transplantation of endocrine organs. With special reference to the ovary. *British Medical Bulletin*, **21**, 157–62.

KROHN, P. L. (1977) Transplantation of the ovary. In: *The Ovary*, Vol. II.

Physiology, pp. 101–28. 2nd edition. Eds. Lord Zuckerman & B. J. Weir. Academic Press, New York; London.

KUMAR, D., BREMNER, D. N. & BROWN, P. W. (1989) Fertility after orchiopexy for cryptorchidism: a new approach to assessment. *British Journal of Urology*, **64**, 516–20.

KURILO, L. F. (1981) Oogenesis in antenatal development in man. *Human Genetics*, **57**, 86–92.

LAFFERTY, K. J. & GILL, R. G. (1989) Is there a clinical future for the modulation of donor organ immunogenicity? In: *Organ Transplantation: Current Clinical and Immunological Concepts*, pp. 167–76. Eds. L. Brent & R. A. Sells. Balliere Tindall, London.

LEE, S., TUNG, K. S. & ORLOFF, M. J. (1971) Testicular transplantation in the rat. *Transplantation Proceedings*, **3**, 586–90.

LYDSTON, G. F. (1916) Sex gland implantation. Additional cases and conclusions to date. *Journal of the American Medical Association*, **66**, 1540–3.

MADSEN, J. C., SUPERINA, R. A., WOOD, K. J. & MORRIS, P. J. (1988) Immunological unresponsiveness induced by recipient cells transfected with donor MHC genes. *Nature*, **332**, 161–4.

MANOTAYA, T. & POTTER, E. L. (1963) Oocytes in prophase of meiosis from squash preparations of human fetal ovaries. *Fertility & Sterility*, **14**, 378–92.

MARSHALL, F. H. A., CREW, F. A. E., WALTON, A. & MILLER, W. C. (1928) Report on Dr. Serge Voronoff's experiments on the *Improvement of Livestock*. Ministry of Agriculture & Fisheries and Board of Agriculture for Scotland. 24/108. HMSO, London.

MARTIN, F. H. (1908) Transplantation of ovaries. *Surgery, Gynecology & Obstetrics*, **7**, 7–21.

MORRIS, R. T. (1895) The ovarian graft. *New York Medical Journal*, **62**, 436.

NEAVES, W. B. & BILLINGHAM, R. E. (1979) Transplantation of the testis. *Transplantation*, **28**, 163–5.

NORMAN, R. L. & SPIES, H. G. (1986) Cyclic ovarian function in a male macaque: additional evidence for a lack of sexual differentiation in the physiological mechanisms that regulate the cyclic release of gonadotropins in primates. *Endocrinology*, **118**, 2608–10.

PARKES, A. S. (1966) The rise of reproductive endocrinology, 1926–1940. *Journal of Endocrinology*, **34**, xx–xxxii.

PARKES, A. S. & SMITH, A. U. (1953) Regeneration of rat ovarian tissue grafted after exposure to low temperatures. *Proceedings of the Royal Society, B*, **140**, 455–70.

PARKES, A. S. & SMITH, A. U. (1954) Storage of testicular tissue at very low temperatures. *British Medical Journal*, **1**, 315–16.

PARROT, D. M. V. (1960) The fertility of mice with orthotopic ovarian grafts derived from frozen tissue. *Journal of Reproduction & Fertility*, **1**, 230–41.

PENG, M. & HUANG, H. (1972) Aging of the hypothalamic-pituitary-ovarian function in the rat. *Fertility & Sterility*, **23**, 535–42.

PETTINARI, V. (1928) *Greffe ovarienne et action endocrine de l'ovaire*. Doin, Paris.

PONDER, B. A. J., WILKINSON, M. M., WOOD, M. & WESTWOOD, J. H. (1983) Immunohistochemical demonstration of H2 antigens in mouse tissue sections. *Journal of Histochemistry & Cytochemistry*, **31**, 911–19.

RICHARDSON, S. J., SENIKAS, V. & NELSON, J. F. (1987) Follicular depletion during the menopausal transition: evidence for accelerated loss and ultimate exhaustion. *Journal of Clinical Endocrinology & Metabolism*, **65**, 1231–7.

ROTSZTEYN, D. A., REMOHI, J., WECKSTEIN, L. N., ORD, T., MOYER, D. L., BALMACEDA, J. P. & ASCH, R. H. (1990) Results of tubal embryo transfer in premature ovarian failure. *Fertility & Sterility*, **54**, 348–50.

ROY, S. K. & GREENWALD, G. S. (1985) An enzymatic method for dissociation of intact follicles from the hamster ovary: histological and quantitative aspects. *Biology of Reproduction*, **32**, 203–15.

SCHROEDER, A. C., CHAMPLIN, A. K., MOBRAATEN, L. E. & EPPIG, J. J. (1990) Developmental capacity of mouse oocytes cryopreserved before and after maturation *in vitro*. *Journal of Reproduction & Fertility*, **89**, 43–50.

SEIGLER, H. F. & METZGAR, R. S. (1970) Embryonic development of human transplantation antigens. *Transplantation*, **9**, 478–86.

SETCHELL, B. P. (1978) *The Mammalian Testis*, pp. 10–12. Paul Elek, London.

SHAFFER, C. F. & HULKA, J. F. (1969) Ovarian transplantation. Graft–host interactions in corneal encapsulated homografts. *American Journal of Obstetrics & Gynecology*, **103**, 78–85.

SILBER, S. J. (1978) Transplantation of a human testis for anorchia. *Fertility & Sterility*, **30**, 181–7.

SOPELAK, V. M. & BUTCHER, R. L. (1982) Contribution of the ovary versus hypothalamus–pituitary to termination of estrous cycles in aging rats using ovarian transplants. *Biology of Reproduction*, **27**, 29–37.

SPEED, R. M. (1985) The prophase stages in human foetal oocytes studied by light and electron microscopy. *Human Genetics*, **69**, 69–75.

STANLEY, L. L. (1922) An analysis of one thousand testicular substance implantations. *Endocrinology*, **6**, 787–94.

STURGIS, S. H. & CASTELLANOS, H. (1958) Ovarian homografts in the primate: experience with Millipore filter chambers. *American Journal of Obstetrics & Gynecology*, **76**, 1132–47.

TAI, J., JOHNSON, H. W. & TZE, W. J. (1989) Successful transplantation of Leydig cells in castrated inbred rats. *Transplantation*, **47**, 1087–9.

TAKETO-HOSOTANI, T. & SINCLAIR-THOMPSON, E. (1987) Influence of the mesonephros on the development of fetal mouse ovaries following transplantation in adult male and female mice. *Developmental Biology*, **124**, 423–30.

TAPANAINEN, J., KUOPIO, T., PELLINIEMI, L. J. & HUHTANIEMI, I. (1984) Rat testicular endogenous steroids and number of Leydig cells between the fetal period and sexual maturity. *Biology of Reproduction*, **31**, 1027–35.

TELFER, E., TORRANCE, C. & GOSDEN, R. G. (1990) Morphological study of cultured preantral ovarian follicles of mice after transplantation under the kidney capsule. *Journal of Reproduction & Fertility*, **89**, 565–71.

THOREK, M. (1924) Experimental investigations of the role of the Leydig, seminiferous and Sertoli cells and effects of testicular transplantation. *Endocrinology*, **8**, 61–90.

TORRANCE, C., TELFER, E. & GOSDEN, R. G. (1989) Quantitative study of the development of isolated mouse pre-antral follicles in collagen gel culture. *Journal of Reproduction & Fertility*, **87**, 367–74.

van DAM, J. H., TEERDS, K. J. & ROMMERTS, F. F. (1989) Transplantation and subsequent recovery of small amounts of isolated Leydig cells. *Archives of Andrology*, **22**, 123–9.

VORONOFF, S. (1923) *Greffes Testicularies*. Doin, Paris.

WHITTINGHAM, D. G. (1977) Fertilization *in vitro* and development to term of unfertilized mouse oocytes previously stored at − 196 °C. *Journal of Reproduction & Fertility*, **49**, 89–94.

WINGATE, M. B., KARASEWICH, E., WINGATE, L., LAUCHIAN, S. & RAY, M. (1970) Experimental uterotubovarian homotransplantation in the dog. *American Journal of Obstetrics & Gynecology*, **106**, 1171–6.

WINSTON, R. M. L. & McCLURE BROWNE, J. C. (1974) Pregnancy following autograft transplantation of fallopian tube ovary in the rabbit. *Lancet*, **ii**, 494–5.

WOODRUFF, M. F. A. (1960) *The Transplantation of Tissues and Organs*. C. C. Thomas, Springfield, Illinois.

CHAPTER 11

Cell grafting and gene therapy in metabolic diseases

M. ADINOLFI

CONTENTS

THE LONG-TERM PROSPECTS FOR A SUCCESSFUL CORRECTION of inherited lysosomal enzymatic deficiencies by the transplantation of enzymatically normal cells depend on a series of interconnected factors (Nadler, 1980; Desnick & Grabowski, 1981). The most important condition is the availability of donor cells capable of producing and secreting specific enzymes, whilst not expressing histocompatibility antigens which may induce an immunological rejection. The donor cells should also be immunologically incompetent and, consequently, unable to trigger graft-versus-host (GVH) reactions. Another essential factor is that the lysosomal enzyme released by the donor cells should be taken up by the enzymatically deficient cells of the host via specific receptors.

In this chapter, I will analyze these and other requirements for achieving a successful transplant and summarize the results of studies performed to correct selected enzymatic deficiencies, particularly in patients with mucopolysaccharidoses (MPS), by transplanting normal fetal fibroblasts or amniotic epithelial cells. Alternative strategies, such as the use of somatic gene therapy, will be outlined briefly in view of their possible future applications.

Grafting fibroblasts or amniotic epithelial cells

The rationale for choosing fibroblasts or amniotic epithelial cells

'The willingness to risk failure is an essential component of most successful initiatives. The unwillingness to face the risk of failure – or an excessive zeal to avoid all risks – is, in the end an acceptance of . . . abdication' (Shapiro, 1990, p. 609).

Perhaps these words best summarize the hesitations and doubts which accompanied some of the early attempts performed in order to correct selected lysosomal enzymatic deficiencies by transplanting normal fibroblasts or amniotic epithelial cells. Both types of cells were known to have intrinsic disadvantages when compared to bone marrow cells, which divide and spread rapidly – ultimately producing larger quantities of a specific enzyme – but may be rejected, if HLA incompatible, or induce GVH reactions (Hirschhorn, 1980; Parkman, 1986). On the other hand, the most important incentive for grafting fibroblasts or amniotic epithelial cells was the knowledge that these cells were not going to be harmful to the transplanted patient, since they lack, or produce only small quantities of, major histocompatibility complex (MHC) antigens and do not transform readily into cancer cells. In fact, previous investigations had shown that the amniotic epithelial membranes could be inserted under the skin of patients or could be used to protect the peritoneal cavity after major surgical interventions, without producing any adverse reaction (Trelford & Trelford-Sander, 1977*a*, *b*; Mathews *et al.*, 1982).

Plans for the transplantation of these cells were also based on circumstantial evidence that patients with selected MPS could benefit from the transfusion of whole blood, leucocytes or plasma (DiFerrante *et al.*, 1971; Dekaban *et al.*, 1972; Dean *et al.*, 1973; Moser *et al.*, 1974; Nadler, 1980; Desnick & Grabowski, 1981; Brady *et al.*, 1982). These results implied that even small quantities of a specific enzyme could alleviate the disease or slow down its progressive deterioration.

Of course, an essential condition for performing the experimental trials was the documentation that the enzymatic deficiency could be corrected *in vitro* by incubating the fibroblasts of each patient in a medium obtained from cultures of normal donor fibroblasts or amniotic epithelial cells (Neufeld & Ashwell, 1980; Neufeld, 1980; Benson & Fensom, 1982). In fact, an indispensible requisite for the successful correction of enzymatic deficiencies is that the affected cells should express on their surface a receptor which would mediate endocytosis of the missing enzyme.

Mammalian cells produce two mannose 6-phosphate receptors (MPRs), responsible for the transport of newly synthesized soluble lysosomal proteins to lysosomes. They bind their ligands within the secretory route and transfer them to the endocytic route, where the ligands are released and delivered to the lysosomes, whilst the receptors recycle to the secretory route (von Figura & Hasilik, 1986; Kornfeld & Hellman, 1989; Chao *et al.*, 1990). The two MPRs, with respective molecular weights of 46 000 and 300 000 (MPR46 and MPR300), appear to bind the same ligands, albeit with different affinities and pH optima. However, two major functional differences have been observed. MPR300 mediates endocytosis of mannose 6-phosphate-containing molecules – and thus lysosomal enzymes – besides binding the insulin growth factor II (IGF II) in several, but not all, species (Morgan *et al.*, 1987). MPR46, although present on the cell surface, does not mediate endocytosis (Stein *et al.*, 1987). In vitro studies of the uptake of soluble lysosomal enzymes, which are secreted by normal cells, into deficient cells must be undertaken for each patient before performing any transplant.

Even if the in vitro tests suggest that the deficiency can be corrected, the in vivo clinical effects of the grafted cells may be limited, because the released enzyme does not reach all organs, and particularly the central nervous system (CNS). In fact, lysosomal storage disorders character-ized by neurological impairment may not benefit from the transplan-tation procedures, since plasma proteins do not readily cross the blood–brain–cerebrospinal-fluid barrier in normal adults. Although it has been suggested that monocytes and macrophages – which have the potential to act as donors of lysosomal enzymes to a wide range of receptor cells – may gain access to the brain from peripheral blood, the transplanted fibroblasts and amniotic cells can be beneficial only by releasing specific enzymes in plasma from the site of the transplant.

Some concern has also been expressed about the risk that enzymes produced by the grafted cells may induce an immune response. If the metabolic genetic disorder is due to a point mutation, usually a biologically inactive enzyme is produced. If, instead, the disorder results from a major gene deletion the corresponding protein may not be synthesized. In this case, the grafted cell will release an antigenically 'foreign' enzyme which will sensitize the patient and induce the production of specific antibodies acting as enzymatic 'inhibitors'.

In the course of the various attempts made at correcting enzymatic deficiencies by replacement therapy, much emphasis has been given to the criteria that should be used to assess the biochemical and clinical improvements (Spellacy, 1982). A clinical evaluation of each patient, before and after transplantation, should be carried out by independent observers and fully documented over an extended period of time. Although these principles have often been applied, subjective evalu-ations have inevitably affected the interpretation of some results.

Clinical trials of fibroblast transplantation

Attempts at treating patients with MPS by the administration of whole blood, partially purified enzyme, leucocytes or plasma have given conflicting results (Tager *et al.*, 1980). Clinical improvements or increased glycosaminoglycan (GAG) degradation have been described by some investigators (DiFerrante *et al.*, 1971; Knudson *et al.*, 1971; Dean *et al.*, 1973; Nischioka *et al.*, 1979), whilst others have failed to confirm these findings (Danes *et al.*, 1972; Dekaban *et al.*, 1972; Erickson *et al.*, 1972). In 1975, Dean *et al.* reported that the transplantation of a full-thickness skin graft from a normal individual in a patient with Hunter disease was followed by the excretion in urine of low molecular weight GAGs and oligosaccharide fragments. A 'corrective' factor, which was presumed to be the enzyme, was also detected in urine. It was claimed that the biochemical and clinical improvements persisted even after the graft was rejected. Subsequently, Dean *et al.* (1976, 1979, 1981) reported that the subcutaneous injection of normal fibroblasts, previously cultured *in vitro*, could induce clinical improvements, such as a reduced liver size and the stabilization of mental and physical conditions.

These results were received with a mixture of interest and scepticism. Since the reported biochemical and clinical responses seemed to be in excess of those expected from the relatively low number of the transplanted fibroblasts, the effects could be justified only by assuming that the grafted cells were dividing rapidly, producing large quantities of the specific lysosomal enzymes.

Between 1979 and 1985, Gibbs *et al.*, reported a series of clinical and biochemical trials performed on six patients with Hurler disease (MPS IH), two patients with Hunter syndrome (MPS II) and one patient with Sanfilippo *B* disease (MPS III*B*) who were transplanted with normal fibroblasts (Gibbs, 1982; Gibbs *et al.*, 1979, 1980, 1985).

Before treatment, it was established that the donor cells could correct the metabolic defect in the fibroblasts of each patient *in vitro*. The cultured donor cells (from 5×10^8 to 17×10^8) were injected subcutaneously into 6–8 sites; enzymatic assays were performed on peripheral blood leucocytes and urine samples. Six out of nine patients received immunosuppressive therapy (prednisolone and azathioprine) before the transplant and for about four months afterwards. The results of these studies showed that the grafted fibroblasts did not alter the clinical course of any disorder or induce biochemical improvements in the patients with Hurler disease and Sanfilippo *B* syndromes. Leucocytes from the patients with Hunter disease showed increased activity of α-L-iduronate-sulphate-sulphatase (α-ISS), although these changes were inconsistent over the period of observation. No long-term quantitative or qualitative trends in the excretion of glycosaminoglycans and oligosaccharides were noticed. Extensive immunological tests also demonstrated the absence of specific immune responses against cells or enzymes.

Whilst these studies were in progress, an attempt was made at correcting the specific lysosomal enzymatic deficiencies in seven patients with Hunter or Hurler syndromes by grafting fetal fibroblasts (Adinolfi *et al.*, 1986). These cells, which expressed only small quantities of HLA class I antigens and were HLA class II negative, were cultured in a serum-free medium for forty eight hours before being transplanted. This procedure was followed to remove fetal calf proteins (present in the culture medium used to grow the cells), on the assumption that, once absorbed on the surface of the fibroblasts they could induce an immune response. To avoid rejection by minor histocompatibility antigens, the young patients were transfused with 'stored' red cells, according to a procedure which has been successfully employed to improve survival of incompatible kidney transplants (Persijn *et al.*, 1984; Terasaki, 1984).

The levels of α-L-iduronidase and α-L-iduronate-sulphate-sulphatase were measured in extracts from white cells and in sera collected over a long period of time before and after transplantation.

Despite the fetal origin of the cells and the pretreatment with blood transfusion, the transplanted fibroblasts did not correct the specific enzymatic deficiencies. The absence of suitable markers on the surface of the fetal cells did not allow their fate to be followed, but there was no evidence of a specific immune response in any treated patient.

Transplantation of human amniotic epithelial cells

In the human blastocyst, the amniotic cavity develops within a few days of implantation and almost simultaneously a second cavity appears, known as the primitive yolk sac (Boyd & Hamilton, 1970). The two cavities are separated by a double layer of cells, one of ectodermic and the other of endodermic origin. In a short period of time, the primary yolk sac develops into the extraembryonic coelomic cavity. Later during development, part of the secondary yolk sac becomes enclosed as foregut and hindgut with the remaining part reduced and excluded from the structure of the embryo itself. In humans, the definitive yolk sac becomes slowly atresic, ultimately forming a small vesicle embedded in the inner surface of the chorion.

The amniotic cavity, which is filled with fluid surrounding the embryo, is limited by the amnion, a complex structure formed by several layers of cells (Bourne, 1960). The innermost layer in contact with the amniotic fluid is formed of epithelial cells. They are mostly cuboidal in shape and contain a single nucleus, although multinucleated cellular elements are observed occasionally.

Using monomorphic monoclonal antisera directed against class I

(HLA A, B, C) or class II (HLA DR) major histocompatibility molecules, the absence of these antigens on the surface of the amniotic epithelial cells was documented by immunohistochemical staining of cryostat sections of human amniotic membranes. Similarly, β_2-microglobulin, mostly associated with class I HLA antigens, was shown to be absent from the surface of these cells (Adinolfi et al., 1982).

When the amniotic epithelial cells were cultured in vitro and analyzed after several passages, once again HLA A, B, C and DR antigens could not be detected. However, small quantities of β_2-microglobulin molecules were detected in the supernatants of these cells cultures, suggesting that the amniotic epithelial cells may synthesize an HLA-class-I-like antigen (Adinolfi et al., 1982).

The amniotic epithelial cells were strongly reactive when tested with a rabbit antiserum raised against crude extracts prepared from these cells. The antisera reacted against amniotic epithelial cells cultured in vitro for several weeks but did not react with fibroblasts or cryostat sections prepared from skin obtained from fetuses and adult subjects (Adinolfi et al., 1982).

Further evidence of the absence of MHC antigens on the amniotic epithelial cells was obtained by transplanting a layer of the cells, with the basal membrane, under the skin of seven male volunteers (Akle et al., 1981). Biopsies were taken at intervals varying between twenty and fifty two days after the transplant. The detection of the implanted amniotic cells was facilitated by using rabbit antisera reacting specifically against these epithelial cells. None of the volunteers showed clinical signs of acute rejection. Cryostat and paraffin-embedded sections of the biopsies showed that the implanted cells had survived without signs of necrosis or infiltration of lymphocytes and monocytes. In four volunteers, serological tests confirmed the absence of host reaction toward the transplanted tissue antigens. In fact, antibodies against HLA antigens or amniotic epithelial cells were not present in the sera, even in two subjects who had been deliberately immunized against HLA antigens several years earlier. In vitro tests also provided evidence that lymphocytes from normal adults were not sensitized when incubated with amniotic epithelial cells over a period of three to five days (Akle et al., 1981).

The next step was to demonstrate that lysosomal enzymes were produced and released by freshly collected or in vitro cultured amniotic epithelial cells. Layers of human amniotic cells and underlying basal membrane were collected in sterile conditions from Caesarian deliveries. The epithelial cells were isolated by trypsinization and cultured in RPMI 1640 medium, supplemented with 20% fetal calf serum; the cells were maintained in culture for over twenty weeks and several passages.

Before being tested, the cultured cells were washed several times with RPMI 1640 serum-free medium, and incubated in the same medium for twenty four hours. These supernatants, the extracts from the cultured cells and from freshly collected amniotic epithelial cells were analyzed for the presence of selected lysosomal enzymes (Adinolfi *et al.*, 1982).

Several enzymes, including α-iduronidase, β-galactosidase, α-galactosidase A, α- and β-glucosidase, sphingomyelinase, arylsulphatase A, α-L-iduronate-sulphate-sulphatase and adenosine deaminase (ADA) were detected in extracts from the amniotic epithelial cells and in the supernatants of in vitro cultures. The levels of enzymes were comparable to those detected in fibroblast extracts.

To demonstrate that α-iduronidase and α-ISS produced by the amniotic epithelial cells could correct specific enzymatic deficiencies, fibroblasts from patients with Hurler or Hunter syndromes were cultured in the presence or absence of supernatant from amniotic epithelial cell cultures. The supernatants of the amniotic epithelial cells were shown to correct the abnormal accumulation of specific substrates in the deficient fibroblasts as judged by the uptake of $Na_2^{35}SO_4$.

These findings suggested that the amniotic epithelial cells could be used for transplantation in patients with selected enzymatic deficiencies, provided that substantial quantities of lysosomal enzymes were released *in vivo* by the implanted tissue.

Following transplantation, modest increases of the levels of α-iduronidase or α-ISS were observed in some of the patients. They lasted for a short period of time and seemed to bear no relation to either the methods used to graft the amniotic membranes or to the number of grafted cells (Akle *et al.*, 1985). No evidence of cellular responses was observed in any patient, nor were antibodies against the specific enzymes detected in post-transplantation sera (Adinolfi *et al.*, 1982). Some patients were grafted once again with amniotic membranes; and modest increases of enzymatic activities were detected in the absence of any local immunological reaction. The failure to obtain long-term effects was identified tentatively with the origin of the grafted tissue, which had been collected at the very end of the gestational period when the lifespan of the amniotic cells had reached its physiological end. No attempts have been made at using amniotic cells collected at midgestation due to the unavailability of sterile material.

It was concluded that 'The correction of lysosomal enzyme deficiencies in patients with Hurler's or Hunter's diseases by the transplantation of amniotic epithelial cells is hampered by the transient effects observed in only two of the five patients treated, the impracticality of repeatedly implanting amniotic membranes and the difficulty of producing large numbers of amniotic cells *in vitro* within a short period of time' (Akle *et al.*, 1985, p. 48).

Unsuccessful also was a trial in which two patients with metachromatic leucodystrophy, two with Farber's lipogranulomatosis, one with Hurler–Scheie syndrome and one with GM_1-gangliosidosis were transplanted with amniotic epithelial membranes (Yeager *et al.*, 1985).

In contrast, implantation of amniotic membranes has been claimed to be beneficial in patients with Niemann–Pick disease (Scaggiante *et al.*, 1987; Bembi *et al.*, 1992). In the first patient, who was treated by a series of six implants performed at intervals of up to four months, biochemical and clinical improvements for two to three months after transplantation were observed. Another five patients with Niemann–Pick disease type B were treated by repeated grafting of primary cultures of amniotic epithelial cells and each showed clinical and biochemical improvements. In particular, the treatment 'abolished the recurrent infections . . . and led to a recovery from muscular hypertrophy' (Bembi *et al.*, 1992). In four subjects, who were in the prepubertal stage, there was a pubertal spurt with a concomitant burst of growth. In two cases a sustained normalization of sphingomyelin and total phospholipids in urine was observed. Whether the claimed successes are due to the procedures employed, based on the use of primary cell cultures, or to the particular nature of the disease, is not yet established.

Alternative approaches

The possibility of using other fetal cells, such as bone marrow, thymic and hepatic cells, to correct metabolic diseases is discussed in Chapter 6, this volume. However, the need to search for normal cells – which can be transplanted without being immunologically rejected or inducing unwanted side-effects, such as GVH reactions – may not be necessary if selected inherited biochemical disorders can be corrected by gene therapy. The current efforts to obtain stable correction of genetic deficiencies in somatic cells by gene therapy are based on two main approaches: pharmacological strategies and gene transfer.

Pharmacological attempts have been made, for example, at reactivating enzyme and haemoglobin gene expression in experimental animals and in patients (Dover *et al.*, 1983; Benvenisty *et al.*, 1985; Castellazzi *et al.*, 1986). 5-Azacytidine has been used to 'derepress' the expression of the γ-globin gene (possibly through the demethylation of DNA) in patients with β-thalassaemia or sickle cell anaemia (DeSimone *et al.*, 1982; Ley *et al.*, 1982; Dover *et al.*, 1983; Dover & Charache, 1987). The availability of recombinant erythropoietin has also prompted attempts at treating patients who have sickle cell disease with large doses of this hormone, following evidence that fetal haemoglobin synthesis is induced in baboons when erythropoietin is administered (Al-Khatti *et al.*, 1987). Another, as yet experimental, approach relies on the use of butyrate and its analogues, which inhibit the switch from γ- to β-chain Hb synthesis in sheep; in combination with 5-azacytidine, butyrate has been claimed to reactivate the embryonic Hb gene in the chicken (Perrine *et al.*, 1985, 1987, 1988). However, the switching off and synthesis of the α-fetoprotein gene were not delayed in mice injected with butyrate (Adinolfi *et al.*, 1990). Clinical applications of these procedures in humans await the results of further experimental studies.

Recent advances in molecular genetics may soon offer new and efficient approaches to the therapy of metabolic disorders (Anderson, 1984; Williams & Orkin, 1986; Ledley, 1990; Verma, 1990; Weatherall, 1991). In fact, 'gene transfer' was envisaged as a possible corrective measure in patients with haemoglobinopathies as soon as the globin genes were cloned, but early investigations were hampered by the low efficiency of the in vitro gene transfection.

DNA transfer occurs naturally in the course of viral infections, occasionally producing severe biological alterations of the infected cells which can result in malignant transformation. The basic strategy of gene therapy mimics viral infection, but the vector for the normal gene is a synthetic (or recombinant) virus which cannot be harmful to the host.

The transfected normal gene may either produce the missing protein (e.g. an enzyme) or alter the regulation of the existing dysfunctional gene. Another possibility is that of inducing the repair of the abnormal sequence of the mutant gene. This approach, still at the early stages of investigation, would be particularly useful to modify abnormal dominant genes.

Although gene transfer may be performed using germ cells (germ line therapy) thus preventing transmission of the mutant gene to future generations, for many reasons, particularly ethical ones, this approach is not going to be applied to humans but limited to experimental animals.

Gene transfer into somatic cells (phenotypic gene therapy) affects the treated individual only, and not his/her progeny. The principle of this strategy is to harvest selected cells from patients and infect them *in vitro* with a recombinant virus containing the normal gene; the transfected cells are then transplanted back into the patient. An alternative, as yet experimental, approach would be to inject the patient with the vector containing the normal gene, hoping that it would reach the specific organs.

The selection of the cells to be transfected depends on the nature of the disease: for example, bone marrow stem cells are the ideal targets for the correction of haemoglobinopathies, and lymphocytes for the immunodeficiencies; whilst enzymatic disorders may benefit from the transfection of fibroblasts or hepatocytes (Marx, 1986; Ledley, 1990; Verma, 1990). There are disorders which cannot be cured by somatic gene therapy, such as xeroderma pigmentosum, a disease due to the deficiency of DNA repairing enzymes which are not secreted and transferred to other cells. Disorders associated with mental retardation may require the transfection of glial cells.

Successful gene therapy also relies on the appropriate and efficient design of the vector (Friedman, 1985; Dzierzak *et al.*, 1988; Mansour *et al.*, 1988; Verma, 1990; Weatherall, 1991). In order to achieve expression of the recombinant gene, a vector must contain: an 'open reading frame' comprising the sequence which encodes the gene product; a 'promoter' directing the transcription of DNA into mRNA; a 'polyadenylation' sequence which terminates transcription of the DNA; 'splice sites' which will direct the excision of the introns; a 'start codon' for the translation of mRNA into the beginning of the protein and a 'termination codon' to direct the end of the translation. Retroviruses are particularly useful since they can be manipulated easily to construct defective vectors devoid of sequences coding for viral proteins, and that cannot induce malignancy.

Somatic gene therapy in humans is still in its infancy and many technical problems need to be overcome. For example the prospects of using this approach rely on the possibility of greatly expanding the 'corrected' stem cells in culture whilst avoiding their rapid differentiation.

Research is also in progress to target normal genes to a specific site on the chromosome (Smithies *et al.*, 1985; Capecchi, 1989). If a gene fails to reach the right location it may inactivate an adjacent essential gene. When genes are transfected without attempting to target them, their expression is usually poor because they do not carry all the regulatory sequences needed for normal function.

Genetically engineered cells may fail to continue to synthesize the product of the transfected gene. Palmer *et al.* (1991) have observed that that one month after transplantation mouse fibroblasts containing a transduced human adenosine deaminase (hADA) gene were producing the enzyme at levels 1500 times lower than when initially transplanted. No immune response against the enzyme could be detected in the hosts and suppression was not reversed by reculturing the transplanted fibroblast *in vitro*. However, no suppression was observed when bone marrow cells were used, and production of hADA could be detected five months after the transplant.

Another technical difficulty is how to transfect genes into fully mature, non-dividing cells. In fact until now transfection of normal genes into non-dividing deficient cells has been hampered by the unavailability of an appropriate vector which could deliver the gene inside the postmitotic nuclei. Retrovirus vectors cannot transfect genes into cells which have reached a permanent stage of differentiation and are therefore non-mitotic, like neurons and glial cells. Yet the delivery of normal genes into brain cells has great potential, both as a therapeutic tool and to investigate the particular functions of the nervous system in experimental animals.

Several attempts have been made to isolate vectors which could be used to transfect postmitotic cells. It seems that defective herpes simplex virus (HSV-1) vectors can deliver genes into cells such as neurons or glia in cultures or in adult animals (Geller & Freese, 1990). The prototype HSV-1 vector (pHSV lac) contains a transcriptive unit that places the *lac Z* gene under the control of the HSV-1 promoter that functions in most cells. The expression of the transferred gene can be monitored by the synthesis of a bacterial β-galactosidase, encoded by the *lac Z* gene. When the pHSV lac vector is injected into brain cells of adult rats, β-galactosidase is expressed stably in cells surrounding the site of the injection and by the neurons with axons projecting into the injected site.

Geller *et al.* (1990) have packaged pHSV lac into an HSV-1 deletion mutant (D 30 EBA). This type of temperature-sensitive mutant does not replicate DNA or affect cellular physiology, and, essentially, does not revert to wild-type.

An efficient packaging system for HSV vectors, such as that described by Geller *et al.* (1990), should be a useful tool for investigations of neuronal physiology by, for example, transfecting neurons of experimental animals with genes encoding neurotransmitters. It should also be useful for performing gene therapy. (See note, p. 298.)

Conclusion

> 'But the proper remedy for each disorder cannot be known unless their origins and, as it were, the roots are examined with care and discernment.' (Hugh de la Tour to Hubert of Angers, 1023 (Behrends, 1970).)

Major advances have been made in the elucidation of the molecular pathologies of several metabolic disorders. This has had considerable impact on their treatment, although not all approaches have been successful. Until 1985, enzyme replacement therapy in patients with lysosomal storage disorders, either by the administration of a partially purified enzyme or the transportation of cells from normal donors, appeared to be a promising form of treatment. However, even when, as in the case of the transplantion procedures, the cells which were employed secreted large quantities of enzymes and could induce adverse immunological reactions, the results have been disappointing.

Hopes of treatment in the not too distant future stem mainly from the possibilities of applying the results of new genetic technologies for the production, by recombinant DNA, of large quantitites of specific enzymes *in vitro*, or the transfection of normal genes into a subpopulation of the patient's cells. The delivery of normal genes into hepatic cellular elements or endothelial cells, and the feasibility of directly targeting in vivo complexes of the receptor gene and a protein to the liver, open new avenues for somatic gene therapies (for references see Verma, 1990). However, as outlined in the previous section, many technical difficulties remain to be solved before these procedures can be successfully used in humans. Ironically, perhaps, a special problem in the treatment of some of these fatal inherited disorders arises from the need to develop unique protective measures to safeguard against adverse side-effects. It is also well established that the successful management of some patients with metabolic disorders affecting the central nervous system depends on the prompt implementation of treatment at a very early stage of postnatal life. The results of the first attempts at correcting a few selected cases of genetic disease in humans by somatic gene therapy are awaited eagerly, not only by the scientific and medical communities, but especially by the patients and their relatives.

Acknowledgments
Thanks are due to Adrienne Knight for help in preparation of the manuscript.

References

ADINOLFI, M., AKLE, C., McCOLL, I., FENSOM, A. H., TANSLEY, L., CONNOLLY, P., HSI, B.-L., FAULK, W. P., TRAVERS, P. & BODMER, W. F. (1982) Expression of HLA antigens, β_2-microglobulin and enzymes by human amniotic epithelial cells. *Nature*, **295**, 325–7.

ADINOLFI, M., BECK S. E., SELLER, M. J., FEDOR, T. & McLAREN, A. (1990) Alpha-fetoprotein levels in different strains of mice during development. *Experimental and Clinical Immunogenetics*, **7**, 123–8.

ADINOLFI, M., McCOLL, I., CHASE, D., FENSOM, A. H., WELSH, K., BROWN, S., MARSH, J., THICK, M. & DEAN, M. (1986) Transplantation of fetal fibroblasts and correction of enzymatic deficiences in patients with Hunter's or Hurler's disorders. *Transplantation*, **42**, 271–4.

AKLE, C., ADINOLFI, M., WELSH, K. I., LEIBOWITZ, S. & McCOLL, I. (1981) Immunogeneity of human amniotic epithelial cells after transplantation into volunteers. *Lancet*, **ii**, 1003–5.

AKLE, C., McCOLL, M., DEAN, M., ADINOLFI, M., BROWN, S., FENSOM, A. H., MARSH, J. & WELSH, K. (1985) Transplantation of amniotic epithelial membranes in patients with mucopolysaccharidoses. *Experimental and Clinical Immunogenetics*, **2**, 43–8.

AL-KHATTI, A., VEITH, R. W., PAPAYANNOPOULOU, T., FRITSCH, E. F., GOLDWASSER, E. & STAMATOYANNOPOULOS, G. (1987) Stimulation of fetal hemoglobin synthesis by erythropoietin in baboons. *New England Journal of Medicine*, **317**, 415–20.

ANDERSON, W. F. (1984) Prospects for human gene therapy. *Science*, **226**, 401–9.

BEHRENDS, F. (ed.) (1970) Hugh de la Tour to Hubert of Angers (1023). In: *Letters and Poems of Fulbert of Chartres*. Oxford University Press.

BEMBI, B., COMELLI, M., SCAGGIANTE, B., PINESCHI, A., RAPELLI, S., MONTORFANO, G., BERRA, B., AGOSTI, E. & ROMEO, D. (1991) Treatment of spingomyelinase deficiency by repeated implantations of amniotic epithelial cells. *Journal of Inherited and Metabolic Diseases*, in press.

BENSON, P. F. & FENSOM, A. H. (1982) Prevention and treatment of biochemical genetic disorders. In: *Paediatric Research: A Genetic Approach*, pp. 212–45. Eds. M. Adinolfi, P. F. Benson, F. Giannelli & M. Seller. Heinemann, London.

BENVENISTY, N., SZYF, M., MENCHEV, D., RAZIN, A. & RESHEF, L. (1985) Tissue specific hypomethylation and expression of rat phosphoenolpyruvate carboxykinase gene induced by *in vivo* treatment of fetuses and neonates with 5-azacytidine. *Biochemistry*, **24**, 5015–19.

BOURNE, G. L. (1960) The microscopic anatomy of the human amnion and chorion. *American Journal of Obstetrics & Gynecology*, **79**, 1070–73.

BOYD, J. H. & HAMILTON, W. J. (1970) *The Human Placenta*. W. Heffer and Sons, Cambridge.

BRADY, R. O., BARRANGER, J. A., SCOTT FURBISH, F., MURRAY, G. J., STOWENS, D. W. & GIBBS, E. I. (1982) Therapeutic efficacy of native and storage cell-directed enzymes. In: *Advances in the Treatment of Inborn Errors of Metabolism*, pp. 53–60. Eds. M. d'A Crawfurd, D. A. Gibbs & R. W. E. Watts. John Wiley & Son, Chichester.

CAPECCHI, M. R. (1989) The new mouse genetics: altering the genome by gene targeting. *Trends in Genetics*, **5**, 70–6.

CASTELLAZZI, M., VIELH, P. & LONGACRE, S. (1986) Azacytidine-induced reactivation of adenosine deaminase in a murine cytotoxic T cell line. *European Journal of Immunology*, **16**, 1081–6.

CHAO, H. H.-J., WAHEED, A., POHLMANN, R., HILLE, A. & VON FIGURA, K. (1990) Mannose 6-phosphate receptor dependent secretion of lysosomal enzymes. *EMBO Journal*, **9**, 3507–13.

DANES, B. S., DEGNAN, M., SALK, I. & FLYNN, F. J. (1972) Treatment of Hurler syndrome. *Lancet*, **ii**, 883.

DEAN, M. F., MUIR, H. & BENSON, P. F. (1973) Mobilisation of glycosaminoglycans by plasma infusion in mucopolysaccharidosis type III: two types of response. *Journal of Inherited and Metabolic Diseases*, **1**, 49–53.

DEAN, M. F., MUIR, H., BENSON, P. F. & BUTTON, L. R. (1981) Enzyme replacement therapy by transplantation of HLA-compatible fibroblasts in Sanfilippo A syndrome. *Pediatric Research*, **15**, 959–63.

DEAN, M. F., MUIR, H., BENSON, P. F., BUTTON, L. R., BATCHELOR, J. R. & BEWICK, M. (1975) Increased breakdown of glycosaminoglycans and appearance of corrective enzyme after skin transplants in Hunter Syndrome. *Nature*, **257**, 609–12.

DEAN, M. F., MUIR, H., BENSON, P. F., BUTTON, L. R., BOYLSTON, A. & MOWBRAY, J. (1976) Enzyme replacement therapy by fibroblast transplantation in a case of Hunter Syndrome. *Nature*, **261**, 323–5.

DEAN, M. F., STEVENS, R. L., MUIR, H., BENSON, P. F., BUTTON, L. R., ANDERSON, R. L., BOYLSTON, A. & MOWBRAY, J. (1979) Enzyme replacement therapy by fibroblast transplantations. *Journal of Clinical Investigation*, **6**, 138–46.

DEKABAN, A. S., HOLDEN, K. R. & COSTANTOPOULOS, G. (1972) Effects of fresh plasma or whole blood transfusion on patients with various types of mucopolysaccharidoses. *Pediatrics*, **50**, 688–92.

DeSIMONE, J., HELLER, P., HALL, L. & ZWIERS, D. (1982) 5-Azacytidine stimulates fetal hemoglobin synthesis in anemic baboons. *Proceedings of the National Academy of Science, USA*, **79**, 4428–31.

DESNICK, R. J. & GRABOWSKI, G. A. (1981) Advances in the treatment of inherited metabolic diseases. *Advances in Human Genetics*, **11**, 281–369.

DiFERRANTE, N., NICHOLS, B. L., DONNELLY, P. V., NERI, G., HRGOVCIC, R. & BERGLUND, R. K. (1971) Induced degradation of glycosaminoglycan in Hurler's and Hunter's syndromes by plasma infusion. *Proceedings of the National Academy of Sciences, USA*, **68**, 303–7.

DOVER, G. J. & CHARACHE, S. (1987) Increasing fetal hemoglobin production in sickle cell disease: results of clinical trials. *Progress in Clinical and Biological Research*, **251**, 455–66.

DOVER, G.J., CHARACHE, S., BOYER, S. H., TALBOT, C. C. & SMITH, L. (1983) 5-Azacytidine increases fetal hemoglobin production in a patient with sickle cell disease. *Progress in Clinical and Biological Research*, **134**, 475–80.

DZIERZAK, A., PAPAYANNOPOULOU, T. & MULLIGAN, R. C. (1988) Lineage-specific expression of a human β-globulin gene in murine bone marrow transplant recipients reconstituted with retrovirus-transduced stem cells. *Nature*, **331**, 35–41.

ERICKSON, R. P., SANDMAN, R., ROBERTSON, W. V. B. & EPSTEIN, C. J. (1972) Inefficacy of fresh frozen plasma therapy for mucopolysaccharidosis II. *Pediatrics*, **50**, 693–701.

FRIEDMAN, R. L. (1985) Expression of human adenosine deaminase using a transmissible murine retrovirus vector system. *Proceedings of the National Academy of Sciences, USA*, **82**, 703–7.

GELLER, A. I. & FREESE, A. (1990) Infection of cultured central nervous system neurons with a defective herpes simplex virus 1 vector results in stable expression of *Escherichia coli* β-galactosidase. *Proceedings of the National Academy of Sciences, USA*, **87**, 1149–53.

GELLER, A. I., KEYOMARSI, K., BRYAN, J. & PARDEE, A. B. (1990) An efficient deletion mutant packaging system for defective herpes simplex virus vectors: potential applications to human gene therapy and neuronal physiology. *Proceedings of the National Academy of Science, USA*, **87**, 8950–4.

GIBBS, D. A. (1982) Fibroblast transplantation in lysosomal storage disorders. In: *Advances in the Treatment of Inborn Errors of Metabolism*, pp. 95–103. Eds. M. d'A Crawfurd, D. A. Gibbs & R. W. E. Watts. John Wiley & Son, Chichester.

GIBBS, D. A., ROBERTS, A., SPELLACY, E. & WATTS, R. W. E. (1979) Progress report on the treatment of Hurler's disease by enzyme replacement therapy. *Glycoconjugate Research*, **2**, 885–8.

GIBBS, D. A., SPELLACY, E., ROBERTS, A. & WATTS, R. W. E. (1980) The treatment of lysosomal storage diseases by fibroblast transplantation: some preliminary observations. In: *Birth Defects: Original Article Series*, **16**, *Enzyme Therapy in Genetic Diseases 2*, pp. 457–74. Ed. R. J. Desnick. Alan R. Liss Inc, New York.

GIBBS, D. A., SPELLACY, E., TOMPKINS, R., WATTS, R. W. E. & MOWBRAY, J. F. (1985) A clinical trial of fibroblast transplantation for the treatment of mucopolysaccharidoses. *Journal of Inherited & Metabolic Diseases*, **6**, 62–81.

HIRSCHHORN, R. (1980) Treatment of genetic diseases by allotransplantation. In: *Birth Defects: Original Article Series*, **16**, *Enzyme Therapy in Genetic Diseases 2*, pp. 429–44. Ed. R. J. Desnick. Alan R. Liss Inc, New York.

KNUDSON, A. G., DiFERRANTE, N. & CURTIS, J. E. (1971) Effect of leukocyte transfusion in a child with type II mucopolysaccharidosis. *Proceedings of the National Academy of Sciences, USA*, **68**, 1738–41.

KORNFELD, S. & HELLMAN, I. (1989) The biogenesis of lysosomes. *Annual Review of Cell Biology*, **5**, 483–525.

LEDLEY, F. (1990) Prospects for somatic gene therapy in the management of inborn errors of metabolism. In: *Inborn Metabolic Diseases. Diagnosis and Treatment*, pp. 671–80. Eds. J. Fernandes, J.-M. Sandubray & K. Tade. Springer-Verlag, Berlin.

LEY, T. J., DeSIMONE, J., ANAGNOU, N. P., KELLER, G. H., HUMPHRIES, R. K., TURNER, P. H., YOUNG, N. S., KELLER, P. & NIENHUIS, A. W. (1982) 5-Azacytidine selectively increases gamma-globin synthesis in a patient with β^+ thalassemia. *New England Journal of Medicine*, **307**, 1469–75.

MANSOUR, S. L., THOMAS, K. R. & CAPECCHI, M. R. (1988) Disruption of the proto-oncogene *Int*-2 in mouse embryo-derived stem cells: a general strategy for targeting mutations to non-selectable genes. *Nature*, **336**, 348–52.

MARX, J. L. (1986) Gene therapy. So near and yet so far away. *Science*, **232**, 824–5.

MATHEWS, R. N., FALK, W. P. & BENNETT, J. P. (1982) A review on the role of the amniotic membranes in surgical practice. *Obstetrics & Gynecology Annual*, **11**, 31–58.

MORGAN, D. O., EDWAN, C., STANDRING, D. N., FRIED, V. A., SMITH, M. C., ROTH, R. A. & RUTTER, W. J. (1987) Insulin-like growth factor II receptor as a multifunctional binding protein. *Nature*, **329**, 301–7.

MOSER, H. W., O'BRIEN, J. S., ATKINS, L., FULLER, T. C., KLINMAN, A., JENOWSKA, S, RUSSELL, P. G., BARTSOCAS, C. S., COSINI, B. & DULANEY, J. T. (1974) Infusion of normal HL-A identical leukocytes in Sanfilippo disease type B. *Archives of Neurology*, **31**, 329–37.

NADLER, H. L. (1980) Human trials: direct enzyme replacement – summary and discussion. In: *Birth Defects: Original Article Series*, **16**, *Enzyme Therapy in Genetic Diseases 2*, pp. 425–8. Ed. R. J. Desnick. Alan R. Liss Inc, New York.

NEUFELD, E. F. (1980) The uptake of enzymes into lysosomes: an overview. In: *Birth Defects: Original Article Series*, **16**, *Enzyme Therapy in Genetic Diseases 2*, pp. 74–84. Ed. R. J. Desnick. Alan R. Liss, New York.

NEUFELD, E. F. & ASHWELL, G. (1980) Carbohydrate recognition systems for receptor-mediated pinocytosis. In: *The Biochemistry of Glyco-proteins and Proteoglycans*, pp. 241–66. Ed. W. J. Lennarz. Plenum Press, New York.

NISCHIOKA, I., MUZUSHIMA, T. & ONO, K. (1979) Treatment of mucopolysaccharidosis. Clinical and biochemical aspects of leukocyte transfusion as compared with plasma infusion in patients with Hurler's and Scheie's syndromes. *Clinical Orthopaedic and Related Research*, **140**, 194–203.

PALMER, T. D., ROSMAN, G. J., OSBORNE, W. R. A. & MILLER, A. D. (1991) Genetically modified skin fibroblasts persist long after transplantation but gradually inactivate introduced genes. *Proceedings of the National Academy of Sciences, USA*, **88**, 1330–4.

PARKMAN, R. (1986) The application of bone marrow transplantation to the treatment of genetic diseases. *Science*, **232**, 1373–8.

PERRINE, S. P., GREENE, M. F. & FALLER, D. V. (1985) Delay in the fetal globin switch in infants of diabetic mothers. *New England Journal of Medicine*, **312**, 334–8.

PERRINE, S. P., MILLER, B. A., GREENE, M. F., COHEN, R. A., COOK, K., SHACKLETON, C. & FALLER, D. V. (1987) Butyric acid analogues augment gamma-globin gene expression in neonatal erythroid progenitors. *Biochemical & Biophysical Research Communications*, **148**, 694–700.

PERRINE, S. P., RUDOLPH, A., FALLER, D. V., NORMAN, C., COHEN, R. A., CHEN, S.-Y. & KAN, Y. W. (1988) Butyrate infusions in the ovine fetus delay the biologic clock for globin gene switching. *Proceedings of the National Academy of Sciences, USA*, **85**, 8540–2.

PERSIJN, G. G., D'AURATO, J. & VAN ROOD, J. J. (1984) Pretransplant blood transfusion and long-term renal allograft survival. *Lancet*, **ii**, 1043–5.

SCAGGIANTE, B., PINESCHI, A., SUSTERSICH, M., ANDOLINA, M., AGOSTI, E. & ROMEO, D. (1987) Successful therapy of Niemann-Pick disease by implantation of human amniotic membrane. *Transplantation*, **44**, 59–61.

SHAPIRO, H. T. (1990) The willingness to risk failure. (Editorial) *Science*, **250**, 609.

SMITHIES, O., GREGG, R. G., BOGGS, S. S., KORALEWSKI, M. A. & KUCHERLAPATI, R. S. (1985) Insertion of DNA sequences into the human chromosomal β-globin locus by homologous recombination. *Nature*, **317**, 230–334.

SPELLACY, E. (1982) Assessment of clinical response to therapeutic programmes. In: *Advances in the Treatment of Inborn Errors of Metabolism*, pp. 199–201. Eds. M. d'A. Crawfurd, D. A. Gibbs, & R. W. E. Watts. John Wiley & Son, Chichester.

STEIN, M., ZIJDERHAND-BLEEKEMOLEN, J. E., GEUZE, H., HASILIK, A. & VON FIGURA, K. (1987) Mv 46,000 mannose 6-phosphate specific receptor: its role in targeting lysosomal enzymes. *EMBO Journal*, **6**, 2677–81.

TAGER, J. M., HAMERS, M. N., SCHRAM, A. W., VAN DEN BERGH, F. A. J. T. M., RIETRA, P. J. G. M., LOONENE, C., KOSTER, J. F. & SLEE, R. (1980) An appraisal of human trials in enzyme replacement therapy of genetic diseases. In: *Birth Defects: Original Article Series*, **16**, *Enzyme Therapy in Genetic Diseases*, pp. 343–59. Ed. R. J. Desnick. Alan R. Liss Inc, New York.

TERASAKI, P. I. (1984) The beneficial transfusion effect of kidney graft survival attributed to clonal deletion. *Transplantation*, **37**, 119–24.

TRELFORD, J. D. & TRELFORD-SANDER, M. (1977a) The amnion in surgery, past and present. *American Journal of Obstetrics & Gynecology*, **134**, 833–45.

TRELFORD, J. D. & TRELFORD-SANDER, M. (1977b) Replacement of the peritoneum with amnion following pelvic exenteration. *Surgery in Gynecology & Obstetrics*, **145**, 699–701.

VEGA, M. A. (1991) Prospects for homologous recombination in human gene therapy. *Human Genetics*, **87**, 245–53.

VERMA, I. M. (1990) Gene therapy. *Scientific American*, November, 34–41.

VERMA, I. M. & NAVIAUX, R. K. (1991) Human gene therapy. *Current Opinions in Genetics and Development*, **1**, 54–9.

VON FIGURA, K. & HASILICK A. (1986) Lysosomal enzymes and their receptors. *Annual Review of Biochemistry*, **55**, 167–93.

WEATHERALL, D. J. (1991) Gene therapy in perspective. *Nature*, **349**, 275–6.

WILLIAMS, D. A. & ORKIN, S. H. (1986) Somatic gene therapy. Current status and future prospects. *Journal of Clinical Investigation*, **77**, 1053–6.

YEAGER, A. M., SINGER, H. S., BUCK, J. R., MATALON, R., BRENNAN, S., O'DONNELL O'TOOLE, S. & MOSER, H. W. (1985) A therapeutic trial of amniotic epithelial cell implantation in patients with lysosomal storage diseases. *American Journal of Medical Genetics*, **22**, 347–55.

Note added in proof. Research in the field of gene therapy is progressing so rapidly that, whilst this review was in press, several papers were published and new experimental results presented at scientific meetings documenting the efficiency and versatility of this approach (Culliton, 1991). Several trials to correct ADA deficiency are in progress, and the results are encouraging. In one trial, the enzyme could be detected in at least two patients affected by severe combined immunodeficiency. Following the treatment, humoral and cellular immune responses could be detected in both patients (Matsumoto *et al.*, 1992).

Since the clinical manifestations of cystic fibrosis (CF) are dominated by abnormalities of the airway epithelial cells, a different type of gene therapy has been proposed to help these patients. In vitro studies have shown that transfer of the normal cystic fibrosis gene to epithelial cells derived from individuals with CF can override their abnormalities (Drumm *et al.*, 1990; Rich *et al.*, 1990). In a recent investigation in rats, Rosenfeld *et al.* (1992) have produced evidence that somatic gene therapy – to cure the respiratory manifestations of CF – may be achieved by transferring the normal human gene into non-proliferating lung epithelial cells *in vivo*. Utilizing a recombinant adenovirus containing a human CF cDNA, in vivo transfer and expression of the gene was observed in the epithelial lung cells of the treated animals.

In a previous study a similar approach was used successfully to transfect *in vivo* the human α-1-antitrypsin gene in the respiratory epithelium of experimental animals (Rosenfeld *et al.*, 1991).

These and other studies suggest that '. . . one day in the not too distant future, gene therapy will become a potent new force in medicine, with application to diseases as diverse as heart disease, cancer in its many forms, liver disease and diabetes – among others' (Culliton, 1991), and that it will play an important role in disease prevention, by correcting, for example, deficiencies of enzymes or receptors which predispose to disorders triggered by environmental factors.

CULLITON, B. J. (1991) *Nature*, **354**, 429.
DRUMM, M. L. *et al.* (1990) *Cell*, **62**, 1227–1233.
MATSUMOTO, S. *et al.* (1992) *Immunology Today*, **13**, 4–5.
RICH, D. P. *et al.* (1990) *Nature*, **347**, 358–63.
ROSENFELD, M. A. *et al.* (1991) *Science*, **252**, 431–4.
ROSENFELD, M. A. *et al.* (1992) *Cell*, **68**, 143–55.

CHAPTER 12

The low temperature preservation of fetal cells

M. J. ASHWOOD-SMITH

CONTENTS

A BANK OF CELLS AND TISSUES that are conveniently available for experimentalists and clinicians is clearly desirable. Storage at standard refrigerator temperatures (4 °C) cannot be used for most cells for periods longer than a few hours without serious imbalances in ion concentrations, protein conformation and, in particular, cytoskeletal structure. Microtubules are very temperature sensitive and effects may or may not be reversible, depending on the time and temperature of exposure. Although most of these observations were made with mouse oocytes (Johnson & Pickering, 1987) similar changes in microtubules can be seen with tissue culture cells (M. A. Hammer & M. J. Ashwood-Smith, unpublished observations).

Cryopreservation at temperatures that are lower than -130 °C permits the banking of most individual cells of biological and medical interest (Ashwood-Smith & Farrant, 1980) and has, in recent years, had an important impact on animal breeding and the clinical practice of IVF with the successful preservation of embryos (CIBA Foundation, 1977; Ashwood-Smith, 1986). Before discussing the progress made in fetal tissue cryopreservation a brief overview of cryobiological principles is apposite.

Basic cryobiology

Cells and tissues must be stored at temperatures lower than -130 °C to ensure complete stability, otherwise some reactions and the recrystallization of ice can still occur. Cells may, however, be kept at -70 °C to -80 °C for several months without undue damage. Cryopreserved cells in liquid nitrogen (-196 °C) can be stored for many years.

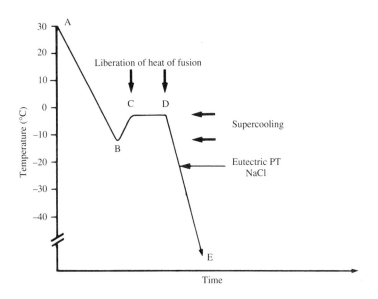

Figure 12.1. Theoretical cooling curve of a balanced salt solution containing 10% DMSO. Axes as labelled: A–B = initial coding plus supercooling; B–C = liberation of heat of fusion (80 cal/g; 1 cal = 4.184 J); C–D = plateau phase as heat of fusion is lost into surrounding fluid; D–E = cooling of frozen sample. In the initial stages this cooling will be faster than that described by line A–B as ice has a higher thermal conductivity than water. However, as the final low temperature is approached the rate will become progressively slower. (Reproduced from Ashwood-Smith (1986) with the permission of *Human Reproduction*.)

However, ten years is the maximum recommended time for human embryos, although this time limit has no scientific basis, since the effects of ionizing radiation (both cosmic and from radioactive isotopes) are so small as to constitute no hazard. A period of 32 000 years of storage at $-196\,°C$ would lead to an accumulated dose of approximately 3.5 Gy (350 rads) which is the LD_{50} for most mammalian cells and over a ten year period in the frozen state an embryo would be exposed to an accumulated and fractionated dose of approximately 0.001 Gy (0.1 rads). These calculations take into account the combined radioprotective effect of temperature and the cryoprotectant (glycerol or dimethyl sulphoxide). Upon cellular resurrection from the frozen state, accumulated damage to the DNA is manifested, since the normal DNA repair enzymes cannot function at cryogenic temperatures (Ashwood-Smith & Grant, 1977).

Freezing and thawing cells is neither mutagenic nor clastogenic and the standard cryoprotectants, when used under the normal conditions necessary for cryopreservation, have no genetic effects (Ashwood-Smith, 1985). Therefore, the possibility that frozen cells might be changed genetically is without foundation. Frozen sperm has been used for artificial insemination in both the cattle breeding industry and medicine for a number of years without reports of birth defects. Frozen animal and human embryos give rise to normal offspring.

The basic cryobiological problem is to cool and warm cells to and from the low temperatures necessary for prolonged storage. The cooling curve of a balanced salt solution is illustrated in Figure 12.1.

When ice is formed, numerous solutes (salts, amino acids, etc.) become increasingly concentrated because there is less water as a solvent. Consequently, the formation and melting of ice has profound effects on cells. Eventually, as the temperature continues to fall during the cooling process, a particular solute will come out of solution at its eutectic temperature; for sodium chloride this is $-21.3\,°C$. Thus, as a cell approaches this temperature, it is exposed to higher and higher concentrations of sodium chloride, and this has osmotic effects and also denaturing effects on the lipoproteins that make up the plasma membrane. Lovelock (1953a, b) suggested that the main cause of freezing damage was in fact high salt concentrations. All cellular solutes will have different eutectic temperatures and, thus, cells must face a barrage of different solute effects as they are cooled. In cells that are in tissue culture media or balanced salt solutions the pH will vary by several pH units, since the different components that make up the buffer will have their individual eutectics. Also, in those systems buffered by carbon dioxide, special problems are presented owing to the increased solubility of gases at low temperature and the high eutectic point of sodium bicarbonate.

Ice rarely forms in a biological system at its freezing point and, therefore, the sample supercools, sometimes by as much as 15 deg.C. Suddenly, ice will be nucleated from the first small ice crystal to form (homogeneous ice nucleation) or from a small particle of debris (heterogeneous ice nucleation). Heat that is associated with the energetics of the phase change is liberated and cells may or may not have intracellular ice. If ice is formed within a cell, and this is more likely when the sample has supercooled, the cell is killed. Thus, severe supercooling is to be avoided and this is best done by adding a small quantity of ice to the specimen at $-6\,°C$ or $-7\,°C$ or by touching the side of the ampoule or straw with a very cold piece of metal. Ice nucleation may also be induced with the use of 'Cryoseeds[R]' which contain a patented non-toxic ice nucleator.

With the relatively slow extracellular formation of ice, the cell will become partly desiccated as the osmotic pressure of the concentrated extracellular solutes draws water from the cell (Figure 12.2). At temperatures in the vicinity of $-30\,°C$ to $-40\,°C$ and with slow cooling rates, cells are very shrunken and can withstand exposure to liquid nitrogen (Figures 12.5 and 12.6). It is possible to keep cells for several minutes at these temperatures to take advantage of the desiccating process; this is known as 'two-step' freezing and results in cell desiccation (Figures 12.5 and 12.6). Cells have different optima for cooling and thawing rates with conventional cryobiological procedures and this is related to cell volume and permeability (Figure 12.3).

Figure 12.2. Shrinkage during cooling. Shrinkage correlates with preservation. Extracellular freezing induces conditions that allow osmotically induced loss of water from cells during slow freezing. This correlates with survival on thawing. Rapidly cooled cells do not have time to shrink, form intracellular ice and are dead on thawing. (Reproduced from Ashwood-Smith & Farrant (1980) with the permission of Churchill Livingstone, UK.)

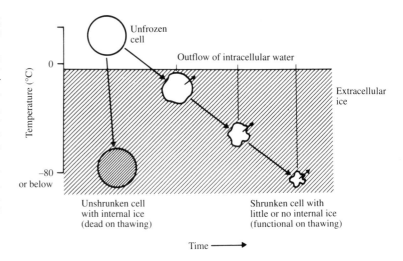

Figure 12.3. Optimum cooling rates for cell survival after freezing. Drawn from data in numerous publications. (Reproduced from Ashwood-Smith (1986) with the permission of *Human Reproduction*.)

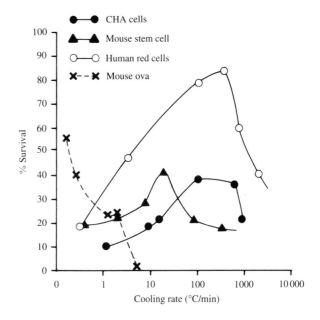

Cryoprotective agents such as methanol, propanediol, dimethyl sulphoxide and glycerol are normally used at concentrations varying from 10–15% (v/v) in the presence of 10% serum. They may be added at room temperature or, in the case of glycerol, at body temperature. Some cells are more sensitive to the toxic effects of these molecules than others. In essence, these molecules act colligatively in that they reduce the amount of solute build up (mostly sodium chloride) that is present in solution at a particular temperature above their eutectic point (Lovelock, 1953*b*). This is illustrated in Figure 12.4.

Figure 12.4. Effect of glycerol on the concentration of salts remaining in the unfrozen water in the presence of ice as a function of temperature. (Reproduced from Ashwood-Smith (1986) with the permission of *Human Reproduction*.) The data have been redrawn from numerous sources, and were based on Farrant (1965).

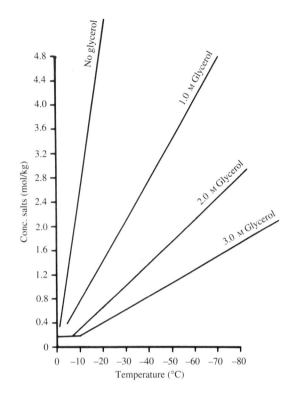

Figure 12.5. Principle of two-step freezing. Cells that are held for a time at a temperature above that at which intracellular ice forms can shrink in response to the conditions produced by the extracellular freezing. The cells can then be cooled rapidly to a very low temperature and survive on thawing. (Reproduced from Ashwood-Smith & Farrant (1980) with the permission of Churchill Livingstone, UK.)

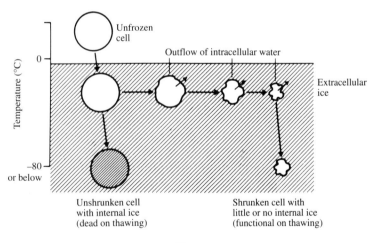

Figure 12.6. Ultrastructural representation of Chinese hamster fibroblasts in dimethyl sulphoxide (5% v/v) after two-step freezing. Rapid cooling induces ice cavities and survival does not occur. In contrast 10 min at -26 °C before cooling to -80 °C allows cellular shrinkage, the absence of obvious intracellular ice and high survival. The cooled cells were examined by freeze-substitution (approximate magnification $\times$ 5400). (Reproduced from Ashwood-Smith & Farrant (1980) with the permission of Churchill Livingstone.)

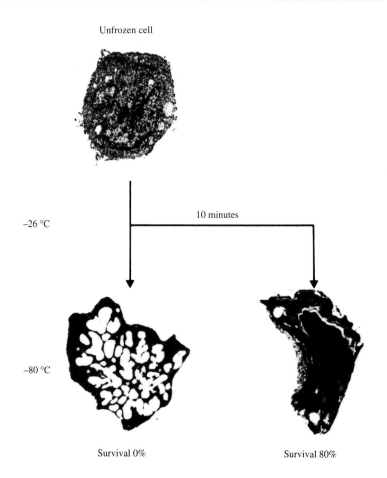

Unfrozen cell

10 minutes

-26 °C

-80 °C

Survival 0%   Survival 80%

Thawing is normally done as rapidly as possible to reduce the probability of intracellular ice formation, and the cryoprotectant is then removed by slow stepwise dilution or by fast dilution in the presence of a sugar solution that acts as an osmotic buffer. Most of the reports on the freezing of fetal tissue and in fact of all cells and tissues have involved protocols of controlled rate slow freezing combined with rapid thawing using either glycerol or dimethyl sulphoxide as the cryoprotectant; dimethyl sulphoxide has been the preferred molecule in most of the studies.

Recently two other methods of cryopreservation have been advocated. The first relies on vitrification, in which water changes directly to a glass without the formation of ice so that problems associated with solute concentration and intracellular ice are avoided. Vitrification requires close attention to freezing and thawing rates, and involves the use of very high concentrations of cryoprotectants such as glycerol, propanediol or dimethyl sulphoxide; complex mixtures of these molecules are often used at final concentrations of 6M. Toxicity is a problem but careful adherence to the published regimens has produced excellent results for animal embryos and other cells (Fahy *et al.*, 1984). MacFarlane & Forsyth (1990) have very recently discussed the role of cryoprotective agents in vitrification.

The second method is based on a short exposure to 3.5M dimethyl sulphoxide to achieve a partial cellular desiccation prior to plunging the cells directly into liquid nitrogen (Trounson *et al.*, 1987). It is too early to tell if this method is as reliable and as universally applicable to cells as the programmed slow freezing method. Should it prove to be so, then expensive controlled rate biological freezers will be things of the past.

Low temperature preservation of fetal cells, tissues and organs

It is apparent from an examination of the literature that fetal cells do not differ from adult cells in how they respond to the damaging effects associated with cooling, freezing and thawing. There is, however, one very important exception, namely the mammalian oocyte. Whether or not it can be considered fetal is open to question. In rodents and in man the second meiotic division is arrested in metaphase until a short time before fertilization and the chromosomes are displayed on the microtubules that make up the spindle. The microtubular cytoskeleton of the oocyte of the spindle consists of polymerized tubulin. Polymerization reactions are easily destabilized by surprisingly small changes in temperature, and a drop of several degrees from body temperature can cause non-reversible changes in mouse and human oocytes (Pickering & Johnson, 1987; Pickering *et al.*, 1988). This has been observed also with Chinese hamster cells in tissue culture but without chromosomal effects. Mouse embryos show increased frequencies of aneuploidy when cryopreserved oocytes are fertilized *in vitro* (Glenister *et al.*, 1986).

The cryopreservation of oocytes is technically possible, since several normal children have been born from cryopreserved oocytes, but is further complicated by the action of the standard cryopreservatives, dimethyl sulphoxide and propanediol. Both compounds have stabilizing and destabilizing effects on oocyte microtubules, *per se*, and propanediol may activate the egg to develop parthenogenetically (Ashorn *et al.*, 1986).

Embryos

Indications that embryos could be cryopreserved came from studies with rabbit embryos in a paper by Smith (1952). Success was very limited and it was nearly twenty years before practical methods for embryo cryopreservation were achieved. Mouse embryos were first cryopreserved in the early part of the seventies when Whittingham (1971), Wilmut (1972) and Whittingham *et al.*, (1972) used slow freezing in the presence of dimethyl sulphoxide. Cooling rates as low as 0.3 °C per minute were used in the most successful protocols and were derived from theoretical considerations associated with cell volume and permeability (Whittingham *et al.* 1972). Fast freezing methods for the preservation of embryos have recently been developed and are based on vitrification (Rall & Fahy, 1985) and desiccation (Trounson *et al.*, 1987). The reliability of these two methods appears to be good but it is, perhaps, a little early to decide whether they should be used for the routine preservation of embryos.

Human embryos that were in the 8-cell stage were cryopreserved with dimethyl sulphoxide and slow cooling (Trounson & Mohr, 1983; Zeilmaker *et al.*, 1984; Downing *et al.*, 1985). The first pregnancy (Trounson & Mohr, 1983) arose from the implantation of a thawed embryo in which only five of the eight blastomeres was intact. Successful cryopreservation of a human blastocyst, using glycerol and slow cooling, was reported in 1985 (Cohen *et al.*, 1985). The human pronucleate embryo (a fertilized oocyte in which both the male and female pronuclei are yet to fuse at syngamy, which is usually 18 hours after fertilization) was first cryopreserved by Lassalle *et al.* (1985) using propanediol as the cryoprotective agent. The majority of the babies born from the implantation of frozen embryos have been frozen by slow cooling with propanediol and thus far there have been no reports of a change in the sex ratio or of increased birth defects arising from the replacement of frozen embryos. In established clinics, about 75% of frozen embryos are recovered intact after thawing and the pregnancy rate per replacement approaches that obtained with fresh embryos.

The success of the cryopreservation methods for embryos has meant that more and more centres are routinely using low temperature preservation as part of their IVF services. On average, with standard stimulation regimen, 6–7 oocytes are recovered per patient. The average fertilization rate is about 60% and this means that one or two embryos are 'spare' after the implantation of three embryos. Most clinics prefer not to implant more than three embryos because of the increased chance of multiple pregnancy and spare embryos can be frozen and replaced in another cycle.

The possibility of separating the recovery cycle from the replacement cycle has considerable scientific merit and was advocated a number of years ago by Robert Edwards who, with Patrick Steptoe, pioneered IVF. Attempts to cryopreserve human embryos were carried out in the seventies by Purdy, Edwards, Steptoe and Whittingham but did not bear fruit. These early trials were reported by Edwards & Steptoe (1980) and Edwards commented (p. 135),

'We could try freezing human embryos. We'd gladly give the fertility drugs as usual to patients, collect the ripening eggs, fertilize them, then when the eggs had divided into sixteen or thirty-two cells we'd freeze them and keep them in store until the effects of the fertility drugs on our patients had long faded away and their menstrual cycles were back to normal. Then we could thaw the embryos out and replace them in their mother'.

Fetal hematopoietic cells

The ability of stem cells to restore a damaged or destroyed hematopoietic system upon grafting has been known for many years and living bone marrow cells and the infant science of cryobiology were used to demonstrate this potential. Mouse bone marrow cells that had been frozen and thawed in the absence of cryoprotection did not prevent the death of lethally X-irradiated mice when administered by intravenous injection after X-irradiation. However, if the donor cells had been frozen with glycerol then the graft was successful, the mice survived and the inference that living cells and not cellular components were involved was proved (Barnes & Loutit, 1955). This was the first reference to the cryopreservation of bone marrow stem cells at low temperature. Dimethyl sulphoxide is the most effective cryoprotective agent for bone marrow cells and was introduced into experimental hematology in 1961 (Ashwood-Smith, 1961).

Stem cells are present not only in bone marrow but in blood and in fetal liver. Their proliferative capacity, *in vitro*, is best measured before and after freezing and thawing by their colony-forming ability in tissue culture in the presence of interleukins and other stimulating factors (see chapters 3 and 6).

The non-frozen preservation of stem cells that are obtained from human bone marrow has been studied by Kohsaki *et al.* (1981). Although stem cells from fetal liver or bone marrow were not investigated, it is likely that the conclusions would be applicable to stem cells from fetal hematopoietic sources. Stem cells were kept in buffered solutions containing 40% fetal calf serum at 4 °C and erythroid stem cells (BFU-e) activity was 84%, 44% and 12% after 2, 4, and 7 days respectively. Cryopreservation is clearly not necessary if cells are to be kept for less than two days.

Although the literature abounds with references to the successful cryopreservation of animal and human bone marrow cells there have been only a few recent studies with stem cells obtained from fetuses. Orlic *et al.* (1982) investigated the morphology of human hepatic erythropoiesis at the level of the electron microscope and was able to demonstrate that it was well established by the tenth week of gestation and that slow cooling and rapid thawing of isolated liver cells in 10% dimethyl sulphoxide (DMSO) left most of the erythroblasts intact. Indeed, the authors commented on the fact that, ten minutes after thawing, erythroblasts looked normal in contrast to the damage to mitochondria and cell membranes suffered by primitive liver cells.

A study by Crowder *et al.* (1980), using mouse fetal liver cells from 14-day embryos, showed that about 40% of the erythroid cell precursers survived slow cooling and rapid thawing in 10% dimethyl sulphoxide; seeding had no effect on the overall survival. In these experiments the incorporation of radioactive ^{59}Fe into hemoglobin was used as a measure of viability.

A comprehensive and well-controlled investigation into the effects of fetal stem cell transplantation and cryopreservation has been conducted by Fleidner and his colleagues (Prummer *et al.*, 1985). Fetal dog liver cells (50 days gestation) were transfused into DLA-compatable sibling dogs that had received three fractionated doses of 3.6 Gy of x-rays. The hematological recovery of irradiated recipients was monitored, a cytological analysis was also performed and the restoration of erythropoiesis, granulopoiesis, and megakarypoiesis was carefully assessed. There were indications that mononuclear cell recovery was poor after cryopreservation but this may have been, in part, due to the handling procedures. Prummer and his colleagues (1985, p. 354) state, 'In conclusion, our results demonstrate that the liver of a single canine fetus at the middle of the third gestational trimester contain enough pluripotent hemopoietic stem cells to restore the radiation-aplastic bone marrow of a histocompatible sibling. They further indicate that this repopulating potential is maintained by cryopreservation, permitting a rapid recovery after transfer without severe GVHD [graft-versus-host-disease] in an outbred species'. The cryopreservation procedures used in these studies were the standard techniques of slow cooling and rapid warming with dimethyl sulphoxide (10%) as the cryopreservative.

The logic of transplanting preimmune fetal stem cells into a preimmune fetal recipient for the treatment of certain congenital hematopoietic diseases is compelling. Harrison *et al.* (1989) have reported the successful in utero transplantation of hematopoietic stem cells (HSCs) obtained from fetal monkey livers.

The donor cells, which were obtained from the livers of fetuses at 59–62 days of gestation, were cryopreserved in 10% dimethyl sulphoxide and then injected, intraperitoneally, into five monkey fetuses (60–62 days of gestation). The donor cells were the opposite sex to the recipients and between 1×10^9 and 1×10^{10} cells were injected per kg (estimated fetal body weight). Four of the five fetal monkeys were engrafted and remained so for two years with no evidence of graft-versus-host-disease. Myeloid, erythroid and lymphoid cells of donor origin coexisted in the blood of the recipient young monkeys, thus establishing chimeric animals.

Harrison et al. (1989, p. 354) concluded their observations with the statements,

> 'Many genetically transmitted diseases that are potentially curable by HSC transplantation (eg. haemoglobinopathies) can now be diagnosed by CVS long before the optimum time for in-utero HSC transplantation (14–18 weeks gestation). The techniques for fetal injection are available; fresh or cryopreserved allogenic HSCs can be used from unmatched donors and fetus-to-fetus transplantation does not require cytoablative procedures or immunosuppression. Thus fetus-to-fetus HSC transplantation may offer the first effective therapy of a genetic disease in-utero'.

The clinical application of techniques of fetal bone marrow transplantation into recipients is discussed in Chapter 1, this volume.

Although not germane to fetal cell cryopreservation, there have been a number of reports demonstrating the successful low temperature storage of adult rat hepatocytes (Gomez-L. et al., 1984) and adult human hepatocytes (Rijntjes et al., 1986). Many of the biochemical activities that are possessed by fresh hepatocytes were retained following cryopreservation and thus stored cells could be used for studies in vitro of liver function.

Neural tissue

The clinical uses for neural tissue transplantation are discussed in Chapter 7. Fetal rat CNS neurons have been cryopreserved by Kawamoto & Barrett (1986) using dimethyl sulphoxide and slow cooling. Results appeared to be satisfactory but are difficult to assess in any quantitative manner with the tissue techniques involved in this study. Fetal rat cells (dopamine neurons of the substantia nigra pars compacta) as well as primate neurons of the African green monkey have been subjected to slow cooling in dimethyl sulphoxide, and rapid thawing (Collier et al., 1988). Both rat and primate neurons were affected by the freezing and thawing procedures but the surviving neurons (which excluded trypan blue) were functional as assessed by immunocytochemical tests on cells in tissue culture for tyrosine hydroxylase and neuron specific enolase. Functional monkey neuron grafts were obtained with cryopreserved material. Collier *et al.* (1987) have also looked at another source of dopaminergic neurons in the African green monkey, the ventral midbrain and olfactory bulb (crown–rump length 8–10 cm). Neurons were cooled slowly in dimethyl sulphoxide and thawed rapidly after storage in liquid nitrogen for a number of days. Immunocytochemical and tissue culture tests established the viability of the thawed nerons (9% survival). Grafts in suitably prepared recipients survived as judged by dopamine neuron specific tyrosine hydroxylase.

Human cortical cells in culture have been cryopreserved by Silani *et al.* (1988*a*); dimethyl sulphoxide in conjunction with slow cooling and rapid thawing gave survival rates of 62%. The cryopreservation of the different cellular phenotypes was demonstrated and there was no change in the cell ratio (45% neurons and 55% glial cells). Antineuron specific enolase serum was used for the detection of neurons and a monoclonal antibody to glial fibrillary acidic protein targeted glial cells. The synthesis of γ-aminobutyric acid by cryopreserved neuronal cells was also demonstrated.

Silani and his coworkers (1988*b*) also investigated the cryopreservation of human fetal adrenal medullary cells (14–18 weeks of gestation) for the possible treatment of parkinsonian patients. Chromaffin cells were isolated and cooled slowly in 10% dimethyl sulphoxide, stored for a short time in liquid nitrogen and thawed rapidly. More than 90% of the thawed cells were judged to be morphologically intact and excluded the dye, trypan blue. Stimulation of cryopreserved cells with neural growth factor caused the expected emission of cellular processes and they reacted normally to antityrosine hydroxlase antibodies. Silani *et al.* (1988*b*, p. 386) stated, 'In conclusion, to our knowledge, this report describes the first demonstration that human adrenal medullary cells can be frozen and thawed and exhibit a high percentage of viable cell recovery with morphological, immunocytochemical and functional characteristics similar to that observed in the fresh controls'.

Robbins *et al.* (1990) used propanediol to cryopreserve human ventral mesencephalic tissue obtained from aborted fetuses (9–12 weeks). Slow cooling and rapid warming were employed and the cryopreserved cells were assayed for their ability to grow in tissue culture. Normal neuron morphology was noted and immunocytochemical reactivity for tyrosine hydroxylase was maintained as well as the ability to synthesize dopamine. High levels of viability were seen in cells preserved with dimethyl sulphoxide. It was concluded that both cryoprotective agents were equally effective. This particular study was interesting because the fetal tissue was screened, before freezing, for the presence of infectious agents; three of the thirty two specimens were contaminated with microorganisms associated with the vagina. It should be emphasized that standard freezing and thawing procedures do not kill bacteria, fungi and viruses (Ashwood-Smith & Farrant, 1980).

The cryopreservation, culture, and transplantation of fetal human mesencephalic tissues into monkeys was reported by Redmond *et al.* (1988). Neural tissue was obtained from first-trimester abortions, cooled slowly in the presence of 7% dimethyl sulphoxide and stored in liquid nitrogen. The thawing rate was not mentioned but was probably rapid. After fourteen days in culture, cells that had been cryopreserved were positive for tyrosine hydroxylase and neuron specific enolase. Some of the thawed tissue was immediately implanted stereotaxically into the caudate nucleus of normal monkeys and each brain displayed the presence of functioning dopamine neurons, originating from the preserved graft. The authors concluded (Redmond *et al.*, 1988, p. 770) 'Further studies with human fetal neural tissue may also lead to the development of cultured cell lines that might have functional or immunological advantages over cadaver allographs'.

Such an objective has, in fact, been realized with the publication of two important papers on human brain cell culture. Haselbacher *et al.* (1989) have reported the long-term cultivation of human fetal brain cells in chemically defined media. Fetal brain stem fragments and tissue from the cerebral hemispheres obtained from legal abortions (tenth or fourteenth weeks) were cryopreserved with dimethyl sulphoxide according to the procedures described by Groscurth *et al.* (1986). Cultures were successfully established from cerebral hemisphere tissue only. The culture medium was defined chemically and augmented with insulin-like growth factor I and II. Primary cultures were kept for two weeks and secondary and tertiary cultures for three months; the cell cultures being characterized by morphology, electrophysiological and biochemical methods. Initially, glial cells were predominant, but neurons became more numerous with increasing time in culture. The cultured fetal brain cells produced somatostatin, substance P and neurokinin A. When insulin-like growth factor II or nerve growth factor was added to the medium an increase in acetyltransferase activity could be demonstrated. After six weeks in culture synaptic contacts between cells were seen. These results are illustrated in Figure 12.7.

Although the last paper to be reviewed in this section is concerned with cells that came from a very young child and not a fetus, it is sufficiently important and pivotal that it merits consideration. A continuous culture of a cell line derived from human cerebral neurons has been established for the first time (Ronnett *et al.*, 1990). The cells

Figure 12.7. Ultrastructure of secondary cultures of cryopreserved human fetal brain cells. (Reproduced from Haselbacher *et al.* (1989) with the permission of Elsevier Science Publishers, Amsterdam, Holland.) (A) Typical cell clusters found in prolonged (> 14 days) cultures. (B) Detail of a fibre bundle interconnecting adjacent aggregates; note the varicosities of the fibres. (C) Intricate network of cellular processes observed between the aggregates. (D) Bipolar neuronal cell surrounded by abundant processes. Inset – terminal bouton with clear vesicles.

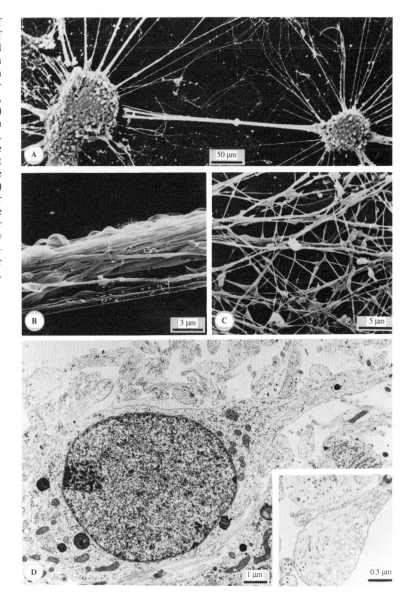

(designated HCN-1 and HCN-4) were derived from the cortical tissue of an 18-month-old female patient who had hemispherectomy performed for seizures. Cells were passaged twenty times over a period of nineteen months with no change in morphology or biochemical characteristics, and they have been cryopreserved by standard protocols involving dimethyl sulphoxide (G. Ronnett, personal communication, 1990). A number of cofactors were investigated for their effects on growth and differentiation, with nerve growth factor, 1-isobutyl-3-methylxanthine and dibutyryl adenosine 3′,5′-monophosphate (c-AMP) being necessary. A doubling time of 120 hours was consistent with the most mature growth; most mammalian cells in culture have a doubling time of about 24 hours.

Clone HCN-1 stained positively for neurofilament protein and neuron specific enolase, which are both selective markers for neurons. No staining for glial cell characteristics were observed (glial fibrillary acidic protein, S-100, and myelin basic protein markers). What is more, the HCN-1 cells gave positive staining reactions for a variety of neurotransmitter substances such as GABA, glutamate, somatostatin, cholecystokinin-8, and vasoactive intestinal polypeptide.

These cells were derived from a patient with an abnormal condition characterized by a continuous proliferation of immature neurons. Presumably they are genetically programmed and are not unlike tumour cells in some respects. The authors do make the point, however, that they do not display the primitive cell characteristics that are often seen with tissue culture cells obtained from tumours of the central nervous system. Ronnett *et al.* (1990) conclude 'As a continuous cell line, HCN-1A cells can be carried for numerous passages. They should be of use to investigators for study of biochemical, physiological, and pharmacological factors that regulate the function of human CNS neurones'.

Fetal pancreatic tissue

Considerable efforts have been made over the past decade in the experimental transplantation of pancreatic cells for the control of diabetes. Commensurate with these studies have been the many reports on the cryopreservation of insulin producing cells. The very necessary and fundamental animal models, mostly rat, that produced a firm foundation on which experiments with human tissues were built are summarized in Table 12.1. A number of important papers have shown convincingly that human fetal pancreatic tissues can be cryopreserved for extended periods of time and, therefore, can be used in clinical medicine (Kemp *et al.*, 1981). Brown *et al.* (1980) used a total of 33

Table 12.1. *Cryopreservation of animal pancreatic tissue*

Animal	Cryopreservation	Assay for viability	Comment	Reference
Rats (fetal 16.5–17.5 days) gestation	DMSO. Slow cooling rapid thawing.	Reversal of experimentally induced diabetes. In vitro stimulation by glucose	Apparent functional equivalence of cryopreserved to fresh pancreatic transplants	Kemp *et al.*, 1978
Rats (fetal 15–20 days) gestation	DMSO. Slow cooling	Transplantation response of fetal pancreas to glucose	Complete reversal of insulin-deficient diabetes	Brown *et al.*, 1978
Rats (fetal 17 day) gestation		Isotopic measurements of diffusion rates [^{14}C] glycerol and [^{14}C] DMSO	Permeability studies to glycerol and DMSO. Glycerol penetration very temperature dependent. (10 times more at 22°C than at 0°C)	Mazur & Rajotte, 1981
Rat (fetal 16.5–19 days) gestation	DMSO (2M) glycerol (2M) varying cooling and warming rates. Slow cooling (0.3°C/min). Thaw at 15°C/min	In vitro assay for ^{14}C-labelled amino acid incorporation into protein	No effect of warming & dilution rate. 100% survival with glycerol equally effective when equilibrated. (17 day +) tissues, poorly protected	Rajotte & Mazur, 1981
Mouse (fetal 17–18 days) gestation	DMSO. Slow cooling rapid thawing	Grafting in diabetic mice	Results with cryopreserved cells less good than with controls	Mendel & Carter, 1984
Mouse (fetal 17 days) gestation	DMSO. Slow cooling with seeding. Rapid thawing	Grafting. Histology & demonstration of viable alpha cells	A difficult study to quantify	Hegre *et al.*, 1984

fetuses obtained after prostaglandin-induced abortion with a mean gestational age of 100 days. The survival of pancreatic tissue after cryopreservation was assessed by measuring the synthesis of proteins using tritiated amino acids; this was identical to the methods used for the evaluation of fetal rat pancreases (Brown *et al.*, 1978). A slow cooling rate in dimethyl sulphoxide was used and the samples were thawed rapidly and a number of variables were studied including tissue culture prior to freezing. Survival rates after freezing and thawing varied between 70% and 10%.

Meunier *et al.* (1980) used pancreases from aborted fetuses (ninth to tenth week); cryopreservation involved glycerol as the cryoprotectant.

The cooling rate is difficult to determine from the information given in their paper; thawing was rapid, however. Fragments of fetal material were implanted into the pectoralis major muscle of a diabetic young man whose insulin requirements were considerably reduced following the graft, and injections of insulin were stopped after the tenth week. No glucosuria was seen 5 months postoperation. Sandler *et al.* (1982) successfully stored human fetal pancreas (obtained from prostaglandin induced abortions) for three to four months in liquid nitrogen using dimethyl sulphoxide in conjunction with slow cooling and rapid thawing. Viability was assessed by measuring insulin release when pancreatic fragments were challenged with glucose in the presence of theophylline and by the synthesis of (pro)insulin upon incubation of samples with ^{3}H-phenylalanine. It is difficult to make quantitative assessments of the results presented in this paper as adequate controls before cryopreservation were not done. However, in seven of the twelve cryopreserved pancreases, good morphology correlated with marked insulin responses.

Sandler *et al.* (1983) investigated the structure and function of fetal pancreas before and after cryopreservation with dimethyl sulphoxide in conjunction with slow cooling and rapid thawing. Again, prosta-glandin-induced abortions were used as a source of fetal material. Some deterioration in the responses of cryopreserved material to insulin release was noted and this correlated with observed morpholo-gical changes. The author concluded, however, that human fetal endocrine pancreas has functional B cell activity after cryopreservation.

An improved method for fetal pancreatic tissue cryopreservation involving a two-step method with dimethyl sulphoxide has been reported by Shiogama *et al.* (1987). In essence, tissue fragments from aborted fetuses at 14–23 weeks of gestation were cultured overnight before being exposed to increasing concentrations of dimethyl sul-phoxide (final concentration 2.1 M). A separate group was placed immediately in 2.1 M dimethyl sulphoxide. Both samples were cooled slowly, with several interruptions, and thawed at a moderate rate. The viability of the cryopreserved B cells was assessed by insulin release following a challenge with glucose and theophylline, incorporation of tritiated leucine into insulin and the content of insulin of the cryopreserved tissue grafted into athymic mice. One kidney received a frozen graft and the other the control unfrozen tissue. Results were better when pancreatic material had been frozen by the two-step method. However, even with the two-step method some cells were destroyed.

The evidence considered so far clearly supports the view that cryopreserved human fetal pancreatic tissue is functional. Two recent reports, although both demonstrating good in vitro survival, come to opposite conclusions in their in vivo results. Hullett et al., (1989) used dimethyl sulphoxide, which was added stepwise to fetal tissue that had been obtained from fetuses of 16–21 weeks of gestation. Slow cooling and rapid warming resulted in tissues, when cultured for a short time, responding normally to a standard challenge with glucose and theophylline. Diabetic mice that were given frozen grafts secreted insulin equally as well as those who received fresh tissue. The authors (Hullett et al., 1989, p. 452) state, 'The results described in this report are the first demonstration that cryopreserved human fetal pancreatic tissue maintains in in vivo capacity to differentiate and mature and the capacity to reverse diabetes in an animal system. Thus, cryopreservation is a suitable means for the accumulation and long-term storage of human fetal pancreas'.

However, Davidson et al. (1988) have considerable doubts about the ability of human fetal pancreas, following cryopreservation (slow cooling, in dimethyl sulphoxide and rapid thawing) to provide a long-term function graft in man. There was little doubt that the thawed tissue was viable as judged by standard in vitro tests for insulin release upon glucose and theophylline challenge. However, in six patients with insulin-dependent diabetes there was no evidence of the production, in vivo, of either insulin or C-peptide. The authors (Davidson et al., 1988, p. 83) concluded that, 'the usefulness of cryopreserved human fetal pancreata as a source of insulin-producing tissue for diabetic patients, therefore, remains to be demonstrated'. Failure could be attributed to a number of factors such as too little tissue surviving for the establishment of viable graft, graft rejection, and/or lack of vascularization.

Research by Warnock et al. (1991) at the University of Alberta indicates that adult human pancreatic cells, whether fresh or frozen, provided sustained function and reversed insulin dependence in an immunosuppressed patient who also received a kidney graft. It was felt by Warnock et al. that the success of this treatment, compared with previous attempts, was possibly related to the relatively large number of B cells that were transplanted. Sharp and coworkers (in a personal communication to R. Rajotte) has recently reported similar findings in patients transfused with fresh and cryopreserved isolated human islet cells.

The cryopreservation of functioning pancreatic cells from fetuses or adults is clearly well established. The preparation of the cells and the number of B cells necessary for a fully functioning graft are aspects still to be fully investigated, however.

316

Fetal organs

There is limited information on the cryostorage of fetal organs. Cacheiro *et al.* (1985) demonstrated the restoration of immune competence in immunodeficient mice by the transplantation of cryopreserved thymus material. Thymuses were obtained from 18 to 20-day-old fetal mice or from 1 to 2-day-old neonates and cryopreserved in 2 M DMSO added to RPMI tissue culture medium. The cooling procedures were very slow and, after seeding at $-60\,^{\circ}$C, involved cooling the samples at $0.6\,^{\circ}$C per minute to $-70\,^{\circ}$C prior to plunging in liquid nitrogen. A thawing rate of $15\,^{\circ}$C per minute in conjunction with this slow cooling rate yielded excellent results as measured by in vitro and in vivo tests. Frozen and thawed thymuses were grafted under the kidney capsule of athymic nude mice and apart from a slight retardation in the early growth of the cryopreserved material the results were judged to be as good as those obtained with fresh thymuses.

Conclusions

Fetal tissue behaves in a similar manner to adult tissue when subjected to the stresses associated with freezing and thawing. Banks of fetal tissue may be established at liquid nitrogen temperatures and cells can be expected, in general, to survive indefinitely. Between 80% and 90% survival should be obtainable with standard slow cooling and rapid thawing protocols in the presence of 10% dimethyl sulphoxide. The alternative approaches to cryopreservation involving either vitrification or desiccation are promising alternatives to the slow cooling procedures that involve expensive programmable freezing machines.

References

ASHORN, R., FOWLER, R. E. & ASHWOOD-SMITH, M. J. (1986) *Do cryoprotectants cause a risk of parthenogenetic activation when freezing unfertilized oocytes?* Second Annual Meeting of the European Society of Human Reproduction and Embryology, Brussels, Abstract no. 42, p. 13. IRL Press, Oxford.

ASHWOOD-SMITH, M. J. (1961) Preservation of mouse bone marrow at −79 °C with dimethyl sulphoxide. *Nature*, **190**, 1204–5.

ASHWOOD-SMITH, M. J. (1985) Genetic damage is not produced by normal cryopreservation procedures involving either glycerol or dimethyl sulfoxide: a cautionary note, however, on possible effects of dimethyl sulfoxide. *Cryobiology*, **22**, 427–33.

ASHWOOD-SMITH, M. J. (1986) The cryopreservation of human embryos. *Human Reproduction*, **1**, 319–32.

ASHWOOD-SMITH, M. J. & FARRANT, J. (eds.) (1980) *Low Temperature Preservation in Medicine and Biology*. Pitman Medical, Tunbridge Wells, UK.

ASHWOOD-SMITH, M. J. & GRANT, E. (1977) Genetic stability in cellular systems stored in the frozen state. In: *Freezing of Mammalian Embryos*, pp. 251–72. Elsevier, Amsterdam.

BARNES, D. W. H. & LOUTIT, J. F. (1955) The radiation recovery factor: preservation by the Polge–Smith–Parkes technique. *Journal of the National Cancer Institute*, **15**, 901–50.

BROWN, J., CLARK, W. R., RHODA, K., MAKOFF, R. K., WEISMAN, H., KEMP, B. A. & MULLENI, Y. (1978) Pancreas transplantation for diabetes mellitus. *Annals of Internal Medicine*, **89**, 951–65.

BROWN, J., KEMP, J. A., HURT, S. & CLARK, W. R. (1980) Cyropreservation of human fetal pancreas. *Diabetes*, **29**, Supplement 1, 70–3.

CACHEIRO, L. H., GLOVER, P. L. & PERKINS, E. H. (1985) Restoration of immune competence with cryopreserved thymus. *Transplantation*, **40**, 110–12.

CIBA FOUNDATION (1977) *The Freezing of Mammalian Embryos*. Elsevier, Amsterdam.

COHEN, J., SIMONS, R. F., FEHILLY, C. B., FISHEL, S. B., EDWARDS, R. G., HEWITT, J., ROWLAND, G. F., STEPTOE, P. C. & WEBSTER, J. M. (1985) Birth after replacement of hatching blastocyst cryopreserved at expanded blastocyst stage. *Lancet*, **i**, 647.

COLLIER, T. J., REDMON, D. E., Jr, SLADEK, C. D., GALLAGHER, M. J., ROTH, R. H. & SLADEK, J. R., Jr (1987) Intracerebral grafting and culture of cryopreserved primate dopamine neurons. *Brain Research*, **436**, 363–6.

COLLIER, T. J., SLADEK, C. D., GALLAGHER, M. J., BLANCHARD, B. C., DALEY, B. F., FOSTER, P. N., REDMON, D. E., Jr, ROTH, R. H. &

SLADEK, J. R., Jr (1988) Cryopreservation of fetal rat and non-human primate mesencephalic neurons: Viability in culture and neural transplantation. *Progress in Brain Research*, **78**, 631–6.

CROWDER, J. W., DUNN, C. D. R. & JONES, J. B. (1980) Cryopreservation of erythropoietin-responsive cells in murine hematopoietic tissue. *Cryobiology*, **17**, 18–24.

DAWIDSON, I., SIMONSEN, R., AGGARWAL, S., COORPENDER, L., DILLER, K., RAJOTTE, R., RASKIN, P., REDMAN, H. & ROSENSTOCK, J. (1988) Cryopreserved human fetal pancreas: A source of insulin-producing tissue? *Cryobiology*, **25**, 83–93.

DOWNING, B. G., MOHR, L. R., TROUNSON, A. O., FREEMAN, L. E. & WOOD, C. (1985) Birth after transfer of cryopreserved embryos. *Medical Journal of Australia*, **142**, 409–11.

EDWARDS, R. G. & STEPTOE, P. (1980) *A Matter of Life*, pp. 135–7. Hutchinson, London.

FAHY, G. M., MacFARLANE, D. R., ANGELL, C. A. & MERYMAN, H. T. (1984) Vitrification as an approach to cryopreservation. *Cryobiology*, **21**, 407–26.

FARRANT, J. (1965) Mechanisms of cell damage during freezing and thawing and its prevention. *Nature*, **205**, 1284–7.

GLENISTER, P. H., WOOD, M. J., KIRBY, C. & WHITTINGHAM, D. G. (1986) The incidence of chromosome anomalies in first-cleavage stage mouse embryos obtained from frozen-thawed oocytes fertilized *in vitro*. *Gamete Research*, **16**, 205–16.

GOMEZ-L, M., LOPES, P. & CASTELL, J. V. (1984) Biochemical functionality and recovery of hepatocytes after deep freezing. *In Vitro*, **20**, 826–32.

GROSCURTH, P., BALZER, M., JAKOB, H. P. & HASELBACHER, G. (1986) Cryopreservation of human fetal organs. *Anatomy & Embryology*, **174**, 105–13.

HARRISON, M. R., SLOTNICK, R. N., CROMBLEHOLME, T. M., GOLBUS, M. S., TARANTAL, A. F. & ZANJANI, E. D. (1989) In-utero transplantation of fetal haematopoietic liver cells in monkeys. *Lancet*, **ii**, 1425–7.

HASELBACHER, G., GROSCURTH, P., OTTEN, U., VEDDER, H., LUTZ, U., SONDEREGGER, P., BULATKO, A., GREEFF, N. & HUMBEL, R. (1989) Long term cultivation of cryopreserved human fetal brain cells in a chemically defined medium. *Journal of Neuroscience Methods*, **30**, 121–31.

HEGRE, O. D., SIMEONOVIC, C. J. & LAFFERTY, K. J. (1984) Syngeneic transplantation of cryopreserved fetal mouse proislets. *Diabetes*, **33**, 975–7.

HULLETT, D. A., BETHKE, K. P., LANDRY, A. S., LEONARD, D. K. & SOLLINGER, H. W. (1989) Successful long-term cryopreservation and transplantation of human fetal pancreas. *Diabetes*, **34**, 448–53.

JOHNSON, M. H. & PICKERING, S. J. (1987) The effect of dimethyl sulphoxide on the microtubular system of the mouse. *Development*, **100**, 313–24.

KAWAMOTO, J. C. & BARRETT, J. N. (1986) Cryopreservation of primary neurones for tissue culture. *Brain Research*, **384**, 84–93.

KEMP, J. A., HURT, S. N., BROWN, J. & CLARK, W. R. (1981) Recovery and function of human fetal pancreas frozen to −196 °C. *Transplantation*, **31**, 10–15.

KEMP, J. A., MULLEN, Y. & WEISSMAN, H. (1978) Reversal of diabetes in rats using fetal pancreases stored at -196 °C. *Transplantation*, **23**, 260–4.

KOHSAKI, M., YANES, B., UNGERLEIDER, J. S. & MURPHY, M. J., Jr (1981) Non-frozen preservation of committed hematopoietic stem cells from normal human bone marrow. *Stem Cells*, **1**, 111–23.

LASSALLE, B., TESTART, J. & RENARD, J.-P. (1985) Human embryo features that influence the success of cryopreservation with the use of 1,2 propanediol. *Fertility & Sterility*, **44**, 645–51.

LOVELOCK, J. E. (1953a) The haemolysis of human red blood cells by freezing and thawing. *Biochimica et Biophysica Acta*, **10**, 414–26.

LOVELOCK, J. E. (1953b) The mechanism of the protective action of glycerol against haemolysis by freezing and thawing. *Biochimica et Biophysica Acta*, **11**, 28–36.

MacFARLANE, D. R. & FORSYTH, M. (1990) Recent insights on the role of cryoprotective agents in vitrification. *Cryobiology*, **27**, 345–58.

MAZUR, P. & RAJOTTE, R. V. (1981) Permeability of the 17-day fetal rat pancreas to glycerol and dimethylsulfoxide. *Cryobiology*, **18**, 1–16.

MENDEL, T. E. & CARTER, W. M. (1984) Cryopreservation and transplantation of organ-cultured fetal islets. *Transplantation Proceedings*, **16**, 842–3.

MEUNIER, J. M., BERJON, J. J., CHASTAN, Ph. & GOMEZ, H. (1980) Homografts of fetal pancreas in adults; preparation by cryopreservation and organ culture. *Proc. Kon. Akad. Wet.*, **83**, 81–8.

ORLIC, D., PORCELLINI, A. & RIZZOLI, V. (1982) Electron microscopy of human fetal erythroid cells before and after cryopreservation. *Experimental Hematology*, **10**, 628–36.

PICKERING, S. J. & JOHNSON, M. H. (1987) The influence of cooling on the organizations of the meiotic spindle of the mouse oocyte. *Human Reproduction*, **2**, 207–16.

PICKERING, S. J., JOHNSON, M. H., BRAUDE, P. R. & HOULSON, E. (1988) Cytoskeletal organization in fresh and aged spontaneously activated human oocytes. *Human Reproduction*, **3**, 978–89

PRUMMER, O., RAGHAVACHAR, A., WERNER, C., *et al.* (1985) Fetal liver transplantation in the dog. I. Restoration hemopoiesis with cryopreserved fetal liver cells from DLA-identical siblings. *Transplantation*, **39**, 349–55.

RAJOTTE, R. V. & MAZUR, P. (1981) Survival of frozen-thawed fetal rat pancreases as functions of the permeation of dimethyl sulphoxide and glycerol, warming rate, and fetal age. *Cryobiology*, **18**, 17–31.

RALL, W. F. & FAHY, G. M. (1985) Ice free cryopreservation of mouse embryos at -196 °C by vitrification. *Nature*, **313**, 573–5.

REDMOND, D. E., Jr, NAFTOLIN, F., COLLIER, T. J., LERANTH, C., ROBBINS, R. J., SLADEK, C. D., ROTH, R. H. & SLADEK, J. R., Jr (1988) Cryopreservation, culture, and transplantation of human fetal mesencephalic tissue into monkeys. *Science*, **242**, 768–71.

RIJNTJES, P. J. M., MOSHAGE, H. J., VAN GEMERT, P. J. L., DeWAAL, R. & YAP, S. H. (1986) Cryopreservation of adult human heptocytes. The influence of deep freezing storage on the viability, cell seeding, survival, fine structures and albumin synthesis in primary cultures. *Journal of Hepatology*, **3**, 7–18.

ROBBINS, R. J., TORRES-ALEMAN, I., LERANTH, C., BRADBERRY, C. W., DEUTCH, A. Y., WELSH, S., ROGH, R. H., SPENCER, D. &

REDMOND, D. E., Jr (1990) Cryopreservation of human brain tissue. *Experimental Neurology*, **107**, 208–13.

RONNETT, G., HESTER, L. D., NYE, J. S., CONNORS, K. & SNYDER, S. H. (1990) Human cortical neuronal cell line: establishment from a patient with unilateral megalencephaly. *Science*, **248**, 603–5.

SANDLER, S., ANDERSSON, A., HELLERSTRÖM, B., PETERSSON, B., SWENNE, C., BJÖRKEN, C. & GROTH, C.-G. (1982) Preservation of morphology, insulin biosynthesis, and insulin release of cryopreserved human fetal pancreas. *Diabetes*, **31**, 238–41.

SANDLER, S., ANDERSSON, A., SWENNE, I., PETERSON, B., HELLERSTRÖM, C., BJÖRKEN, C., CHRISTENSEN, N. & GROTH, C. G. (1983) Structure and function of human fetal endocrine pancreas before and after cryopreservation. *Cryobiology*, **20**, 230–6.

SHIOGAMA, T., MULLEN, Y., KLANDORF, H., TERADA, M. & CLARK, W. R. (1987) An improved cryopreservation procedure for human fetal pancreas tissues. *Transplantation*, **44**, 602–7.

SILANI, V., PIZZUTI, A., STRADA, O., FALINI, A., BUSCAGLIA, M. & SCARLATO, G. (1988*a*) Human neuronal cell viability demonstrated in culture after cryopreservation. *Brain Research*, **473**, 169–74.

SILANI, V., PIZZUTI, A., STRADA, O., FALINI, A., PEZZOLI, G. & SCARLATO, G. (1988*b*) Cryopreservation of human fetal adrenal medullary cells. *Brain Research*, **454**, 383–6.

SMITH, A. U. (1952) Behaviour of fertilized rabbit eggs exposed to glycerol and to low temperatures. *Nature*, **170**, 374.

TROUNSON, A. & MOHR, L. (1983) Human pregnancy following cryopreservation, thawing and transfer of an eight-cell embryo. *Nature*, **305**, 707–9.

TROUNSON, A., PEURA, A. & KIRBY, C. (1987) Ultrarapid freezing: a new low-cost and effective method of embryo cryopreservation. *Fertility & Sterility*, **48**, 843–50.

WARNOCK, G. L., KNETEMAN, N. M., RYAN, E., SEELIS, R. E. A., RABINOVITCH, A. & RAJOTTE, R. V. (1990) Normal glycemia after transplantation of freshly isolated and cryopreserved pancreatic islets in type 1 diabetes. *Diabetologia*, **34**, 54–8.

WHITTINGHAM, D. G. (1971) Survival of mouse embryos after freezing and thawing. *Nature*, **233**, 125–6.

WHITTINGHAM, D. G., LEIBO, S. P. & MAZUR, P. (1972) Survival of mouse embryos frozen to −196 °C and −269 °C. *Science*, **178**, 414.

WILMUT, I. (1972) The effect of cooling rate, warming rate, cryoprotective agent and stage of development on survival of mouse embryos during freezing and thawing. *Life Science*, **11**, 1071–9.

ZEILMAKER, G. H., ALBERDA, A. Th., VAN GENT, I., RIJKMANS, C. M. P. M. & DROGEN-DIJK, A. C. (1984) Two pregnancies following transfer of intact frozen-thawed embryos. *Fertility & Sterility*, **2**, 293–6.

CHAPTER 13

Law and ethics of transplanting fetal tissue

J. C. POLKINGHORNE

IT IS IMPORTANT to recognize that the legal and the ethical are distinct, and only partially overlapping, categories. Lying is always ethically dubious but it becomes illegal only in certain circumstances, such as when one is under oath. Moral theory holds that in certain situations there can be an ethical obligation to break unjust laws. The mechanism of written statutes and the decisions of the courts is designed to provide ascertainable answers to legal problems. Ethical judgements, on the other hand, call for acts of discernment on which there may well not be universal agreement. Not only may the principles be in dispute but also many moral decisions involve the weighing of conflicting claims (the welfare of the mother against the welfare of the fetus, for example), which different people may assess in different ways. Consensus is sometimes difficult to achieve in the moral realm. Because of this, it should not be assumed that all adherents of a particular religious tradition hold exactly similar views on all moral issues.

While there are inescapable acts of individual judgement involved in ethical decisions, nevertheless, it is desirable that conclusions should be reached in ways that result in as consistent a practice as possible. A way of achieving this in a given area of activity is to formulate a code of practice, providing general guidelines within which individual decisions are to be made. In the area of the transplantation of fetal tissue, the Code of Practice currently operative in Britain is that recommended by the Government-appointed Committee to Review the Guidance on the Research Use of Fetuses and Fetal Material (FFMC), which reported in July 1989 (FFMC, 1989). Its Code of Practice is reproduced in the Appendix.

In English law, the fetus, while in the uterus, is not a legal person. A fetus which is born and lives *ex utero*, even if only briefly, becomes a legal person and acquires all the rights and status thereto attached.

A fetus which dies *in utero*, either naturally or as the result of a therapeutic abortion, has not been a legal person and, in consequence, the provisions of the Human Tissue Act (1961) do not apply to it. There is some uncertainty about what, if any, legal requirements there are in relation to consent for the use of material derived from such a fetus. In practice, this does not give rise to perplexity because there are ethical requirements for such consent (see below), which are incorporated in the Code.

There is also legal uncertainty about what property rights, if any, exist in the fetal material and derivatives from it (such as cell lines). A related case has arisen in the United States but the matter has not been tested in the English courts.

Fetal material in the embryological state arising from fertilization *in vitro* is governed by the Human Fertilization and Embryology Act (1990). It may be brought into existence and used only under licence from the Authority that was established by that Act, and it is restricted to embryos not older than fourteen days, in whom the primitive streak has not yet appeared.

The fundamental ethical question, in relation to the use of fetal material, concerns the status of the fetus. Is it at any stage to be regarded ethically as a person? There is considerable difference of opinion among responsible people about what the answer to that question ought to be. Some believe that, from the moment of fertilization, the embryo possesses full personal status, and the consequent ethical rights of a human being (concerning whose rights there is little dissent). Others would defer that status until the fourteen day period has elapsed, signifying the beginning of cell differentiation with the appearance of the primitive streak and the end of the possibility of development into more than one person through uniovular twinning. Others would place the onset of personality yet later in fetal development; or wish to speak of the gradual development of personhood between conception and delivery.

The debate has a long history. Christian writers of the patristic period frequently differentiated the ensouled from the unensouled fetus, and Augustine set the division at forty six days. In the Middle Ages, Thomas Aquinas, following Aristotelian notions of fetal development, placed ensoulment at forty days for male fetuses and ninety days for female.

The matter cannot be settled by simple appeal to the vastly improved modern knowledge of embryology, for the difficulty arises from uncertainty about what criteria to apply in the definition of a person. Some have argued that in that case, a policy of caution should be followed, usually concluding that it would be best to accord human status to all embryos and fetuses. It is difficult, however, to think that caution should be made so absolute a principle, not least because there seems to be a need to balance the possibility of desirable gains, such as the cure of disease, against this ethical uncertainty.

An alternative approach, suggested in the Report of the Warnock

Committee (1984) inquiring into Human Fertilisation and Embryology is to bypass the question of status and proceed directly to the question of praxis:

> 'Although the questions of when life and personhood begin appear to be questions of fact susceptible of straightforward answers, we hold that the answers to such questions in fact are complex amalgams of factual and moral judgements. Instead of trying to answer these questions directly we have therefore gone straight to the question of *how it is right to treat the human embryo*.' (Warnock, paragraph 11.9).

This approach was also adopted by FFMC, which concluded that 'On the basis of its potential to develop into a human being, a fetus is entitled to respect, according it a status broadly comparable to that of a living person' (paragraph 9.1). (The Committee defined a fetus as relating to the state 'from implantation in the womb until the time gestation ends, whether alive or dead, and whether inside or outside the womb' (paragraph 1.5). It did not address the question of embryos produced *in vitro*.) On this understanding, the indisputable fact that a fetus is capable of developing into a human person is sufficient of itself to grant high ethical status, independently of whether or not the fetus can be said already to have attained personhood. A consequence is that the only ethically relevant categories of fetus are 'alive' or 'dead'. An earlier code of practice, produced by the Peel Committee in 1974, had introduced the category of 'pre-viable fetus' but FFMC rejected this as being of no ethical relevance. No enhanced ethical status attaches to the other uterine contents, such as the placenta, which do not have the potentiality to develop into a human being.

A living fetus should be treated on principles broadly comparable to those applicable to children and adults: no intervention above minimal risk except on balance for the benefit of the fetus. The only exception relates to termination of pregnancy under the Abortion Act (1967), in which case ethical considerations relating to the welfare of the mother come into play.

There are, of course, difficult ethical questions relating to trial procedures (e.g. trials of diagnostic techniques for conditions that may cause serious handicap) which may be of considerable benefit to the group to which the subject belongs. Decisions in such cases call for the same delicacy of moral judgement in relation to the fetus that must be exercised in similar trials relating to children.

Material from a dead fetus only is ethically available for use in research or therapy. Where abortion techniques (such as the use of RU486 with prostaglandins) may result in the delivery of a live fetus, tissue is not ethically available from that fetus while it lives, whatever its stage of development. The Code states that care is needed in framing a definition of fetal death (see article 1 of the Code).

A consequence of the high ethical status accorded to the fetus is that a living fetus is never to be treated instrumentally, merely as a means to an end that is unrelated to itself. This status is not abrogated by severe handicap. It would, for instance, be wrong to allow an anencephalic fetus, which it had been decided to abort, to go to term simply to provide tissue that was better developed. A fetus cannot properly be a source of monetary gain, so that payment for fetal material (other than necessary handling costs) is ethically unacceptable. It would be wholly wrong to conceive a fetus with the intention of producing fetal material for subsequent use. [This raises ethical questions about the production of embryos *in vitro* with the sole intention of using them in research, as opposed to the use of 'spare' embryos resulting secondarily from activity primarily aimed at solving fertility problems. The present writer believes that it is not ethically acceptable to create embryos for research purposes only, although this has now been allowed by Parliament under licence. The practical argument about availability of material for research should not be allowed to over-ride ethical considerations.] A dead fetus is to be treated with the respect comparable to that accorded to a human cadaver.

A further set of ethical problems arise for the use of fetal tissue because most of the tissue made available will result from therapeutic abortions. Almost all people recognize that the decision to terminate a pregnancy by abortion is a grave moral decision. Major differences of opinion arise over whether there are circumstances in which this is justified ethically. Few would see abortion as an intrinsically desirable – or even morally neutral – action, but many ethical dilemmas are concerned with the attempt to choose the lesser evil in an inescapably imperfect situation. In the case of abortion (at least in the circumstances as laid down by the 1967 Act) there is the balancing consideration of the mental and physical welfare of the mother and her existing family.

There are basically two types of contending moral theory. One is called the deontological approach and relies on the existence of what it believes are absolute moral laws. The other approach is the teleological, which seeks to evaluate action in terms of its expected consequences. A version of this approach is so-called 'situation ethics', which emphasizes the unique character of each occasion of moral choice. The two approaches can be contrasted by the advice they might offer to someone faced with a would-be murderer and asked whether his intended victim was hiding in their house. If the victim is, in fact, known to be inside, is a lie about his whereabouts permitted in this desperate circumstance? A deontologist might say no; a teleologist would say yes.

Those who take a deontological view of ethics have often thought that the prohibition on taking (potential) human life is over-riding to an extent that makes abortion impermissible on all occasions. Those who take a teleological view of ethics have been inclined to permit abortion in some circumscribed set of circumstances. In considering the ethics of transplanting fetal tissue, it is not necessary to settle the moral problem of abortion in precisely such terms. Instead, one can address the problem of whether the act of abortion (even if it were ethically dubious in itself) produces such a moral taint that any subsequent beneficial use of material resulting from it would be ethically unacceptable. There are clearly situations in which such moral taint exists: most would consider that the use of organs derived from those who had died under torture would be unacceptable. There are clearly cases where it does not: organs may be used from those who have died as a consequence of a culpably careless accident. Those who take a deontological view of the wrongness of abortion have frequently felt a moral prohibition on using the resulting fetal tissue. Those who take a teleological view are inclined to feel that the act of abortion, even in circumstances where there may be room for doubt whether the moral balance has been weighed sufficiently carefully, is not so heinous an act as to incur an ineluctable moral taint, so that the resulting fetal material is ethically available for beneficial use in certain circumstances. This was the view taken by FFMC, provided that two important conditions are satisfied.

The first is that there is a clear separation between decisions and actions relating to the abortion, and decisions and actions relating to the use of the material. It is ethically imperative that no considerations resulting from the possible beneficial use of consequent fetal material should be allowed to influence the mother in her decision about whether to have the pregnancy terminated or to influence the timing and management of the termination. The Code of Practice lays down stringent regulations to that end (article 3) and FFMC recommended that the best way of implementing this requirement was by means of a Government-funded Intermediary (Tissue Bank), acting as a buffer between the sources of supply of the fetal material and the places of its use. This recommendation has been accepted by the Department of Health.

Only the most general information should be transmitted across the barrier of the Intermediary. It is ethically acceptable for a user to ask the Tissue Bank for material with certain characteristics (first trimester fetus, or a mother who had been smoking, for instance) and for the

Tissue Bank to supply this material *if it is available*. It would not be ethically correct to ask the sources of supply, either directly or indirectly, to provide material of specified type, lest this should lead to unacceptable influence on mothers in the appropriate category to have their pregnancies terminated. Thus, it would be permissible for the Tissue Bank to ask suppliers to record the trimester of the fetuses, but not to express preference or need for material from a specific trimester.

Another consequence of the impenetrability of the barrier between source and user is that it is not permissible for mothers to know for what purpose the tissue will be used or even if it will be used at all. Consent, therefore, is given for the general possibility of use, not for specific applications. Although this will deprive mothers of a certain satisfaction which might result from the knowledge of specific beneficial use, FFMC regards this provision as essential, not least to prevent the possibility of the ethically improper practice of 'targeting', i.e. deliberately generating fetuses to provide material for some particular purpose or even individual need.

A particular problem arises from the possible use of fetal ovarian tissue to enable women who have no ovaries to conceive. In this case the fetus would be the genetic mother of the resulting child, and the mother providing the tissue would be its genetic grandmother. It seems clear to this writer that it would be ethically wrong to allow the creation of a human person linked in this way with a family without the *explicit* consent of the mother involved. Such consent could not, in fact, be given under the condition of an impenetrable barrier. It follows that, while material might be made available in ethically acceptable ways for preliminary experimentation, it would not be possible ethically to proceed to implantation and pregnancy using this procedure. (There are also grave ethical problems about parents who might wish to propagate a further generation from a prematurely dead child.)

A second important requirement for the ethical availability of fetal tissue is that the informed consent of the mother has been obtained for its use (article 4 of the Code). The necessity for this arises from the close bond between the mother and the fetus she has been carrying. Some people have suggested that this bond is broken by the mother's decision to have her pregnancy terminated. FFMC were of the opinion that this was too dismissive a judgement, in view of the moral complexities that are involved in reaching the decision to have an abortion. 'Because abortion is a decision of moral ambiguity and perplexity for many, reached only through a conflict of considerations, it seems too harsh a judgement of the mother's relation to her fetus to suppose that she is no longer in a special position with regard to it, following an abortion' (paragraph 2.8 of the Report). They also considered that the father's consent, though desirable, was not indispensable. (His consent has been held not to be legally necessary for the termination itself.) Since the use of fetal material will involve its being subjected to certain tests (such as those for HIV and hepatitis B), whose results could have grave implications for the mother, it is a necessary part of her informed consent that she should be counselled in this respect, according to the best currently operative guidelines. The seeking of consent for the use of fetal tissue must be separate from, and subsequent to, the decision to have an abortion. It should precede the actual act of termination, as the effects of anaesthesia and possible distress make the postoperative period unsuitable.

The use of fetal material raises delicate ethical questions, about which there is considerable public concern and whose answers do not attain universal agreement. As a consequence of the degree of public concern, FFMC recommended that 'All research or therapy of an innovative character should be described in a protocol and be examined by an ethics committee'. This is required in article 6 of the Code, despite ethics committees normally being concerned only with research on living subjects.

As a consequence of the fact that responsible people will not all agree on the ethical propriety of using fetal material at all, the Code (article 5) includes a conscience clause that allows medical and nursing staff the right to decline to participate in the actual use of fetal material, but not, for instance, to decline to care for someone who has received a fetal transplantation.

Another conscience problem arises in connection with potential recipients of fetal transplants. There are some people who, for ethical reasons, would be prepared to accept suitable material only if it had arisen from a spontaneous, rather than therapeutically induced, abortion. FFMC concluded that 'the potential recipient of a fetal tissue transplant does not have the right *to insist* on knowing whether the tissue originates from a spontaneous abortion or from a termination' (paragraph 2.9 of the Report, my italics). The Committee referred here to its rejection of the moral taint argument, but a similar conclusion would follow from the general principles of separation which, for example, do not permit a researcher to be able to insist on knowing whether the material provided originates from a woman who has been a smoker. However, just as the Intermediary may be able to make the latter type of material available with propriety, so it might also be able to make spontaneously aborted material available in an ethically acceptable way without breaking the necessary condition of separating supply from use, if such material does indeed prove suitable for use in transplantation. An essential condition would be that no specific request for such material was passed on to the source of supply by the Intermediary, for otherwise mothers having undergone a spontaneous abortion might be under ethically unacceptable pressure to make tissue from their fetuses available for use.

The consistent thread in this complicated web of ethical considerations has been the high respect due to the human fetus, at the very least because of its potentiality to develop into a human being. A necessary ethical corollary of that status, is that material derived from the fetus should be used only for beneficial purposes and with serious intent, and never for trivial or merely speculative purposes.

Appendix: Code of practice on the use of fetuses and fetal material in research and treatment*

In this Code *fetus* means the embryo or fetus from implantation until gestation ends and, unless qualified by the words *in utero*, includes the fetus outside the womb.

1. Treatment of the fetus

1.1.   Two categories of fetus are recognised:

(a) The *live* fetus, whether *in utero* or *ex utero*, which should be treated on principles broadly similar to those which apply to treatment and research conducted with children and adults.

(b) The *dead* fetus. The determination of death shall be by reference to the absence of vital functions, as indicated by the absence of spontaneous respiration and heartbeat after consideration of possibly reversible factors, such as the effects of hypothermia in the fetus, or of drugs or metabolic disorders in the mother. This determination shall be made or confirmed by a doctor responsible for the clinical management of the mother and the fetus and not involved with the subsequent unconnected use of fetal tissue.

Only tissue from the dead fetus is ethically available for use in therapy.

1.2.   It is unethical to administer drugs or carry out any procedures during pregnancy with the intent of ascertaining whether or not they might harm the fetus.

1.3.   In the case of nervous tissue only isolated neurones or fragments of tissue may be used for transplantation.

2. Contents of the uterus other than the fetus

The contents of the uterus resulting from pregnancy other than the fetus (ie the placenta, fluid and membranes) may be used for research or

*FFMC (1989) Reproduced with the permission of the Controller by Her Majesty's Stationery Office.

therapeutic purposes subject to the conditions relating to screening at section 4.5 of this Code and those relating to finance at section 7.

3. Separation of the supply of fetal tissue from the practice of research and therapy

3.1.   The decision to carry out an abortion must be reached without consideration of the benefits of subsequent use. The generation or termination of pregnancy to produce suitable material is unethical.

3.2.   The management of the pregnancy of any mother should not be influenced by use of the fetus in research or therapy. In this context, management of the pregnancy should be taken to include:

   (a) the method and timing of an abortion;

   (b) the clinical management of a mother whose fetus dies *in utero* or who has a spontaneous abortion.

3.3.   No inducements, financial or otherwise, should be put to the mother or to those who are in a position to influence her decision to have her pregnancy terminated, or to allow fetal tissue to be used.

3.4.   The mother should not be informed of the specific use which may be made of fetal tissue, or whether it is to be used at all.

3.5.   Those involved in the process of abortion and responsible for the clinical care of the mother should not knowingly be involved in research on the fetus or fetal tissue collected. Dissection of the dead fetus, research on it, or transplantation of fetal tissue should, when practicable, be on separate premises and certainly not in the same room. However, ethically acceptable exceptions to this degree of separation occur when research is concerned with the investigation of cases of fetal death *in utero* or spontaneous abortion, or analogous post-mortem concerns arising from previous medical history.

3.6.   *The source* must keep records indicating the next destination of any fetal tissue which is released for purposes of research or therapy, and it should have a means of satisfying itself that anyone to whom tissue is sent has satisfied the requirements of this Code. The mother's identity should not be revealed when fetal tissue is released, although some coding will be necessary which will enable her to be traced by those responsible for her clinical management, should relevant information come to light through examination of the fetal tissue.

3.7.   Any *intermediary* or tissue bank which receives or passes on fetal tissue must keep a record of the destination and origin of all tissue and not reveal details of the identity of the source to the user and *vice versa*.

3.8.   On the same principle the *user* should be able to satisfy itself that any material it receives has been procured in accordance with the requirements of this Code. It must keep records indicating the proximate source of any fetal tissue and the use to which it is put, but should not reveal details of the use to the source.

3.9.   Details about a fetus (eg gestational age) which might be of significance for research but could not be used for identification may be released by the source, but it is not acceptable for the source to be approached with requests for fetuses with particular characteristics.

4. Consent

4.1.   The written consent of the mother must be obtained before any research or therapy involving the fetus or fetal tissue takes place. Sufficient explanation should be offered to make the act of consent valid.

4.2.   Consent to the termination of pregnancy must be reached before consent is sought to the use of fetal tissue, and without reference to the possibility of that use. Provided the question of use is not introduced until consent to the termination of pregnancy has been obtained, it is permissible to deal with the two issues on the same occasion.

4.3.   It may be desirable to consult the father since, for example, tests on fetal tissue may reveal a finding of potential significance to him, and because he may have knowledge of a transmissible or hereditary disease, but his consent shall not be a requirement nor should he have the power to forbid research or therapy making use of fetal tissue.

4.4.   In the case of spontaneous abortions (or where death of the fetus has occurred *in utero*) consent to use fetal tissue should preferably be sought only after the fetus has died.

4.5.   Consent should be obtained from the mother to tests if any screening is to take place for transmissible disease or if any procedure is contemplated which could have similar consequences for the mother and affect her clinical management. Any such tests, and the counselling to accompany them, should be conducted according to the best current practice and guidance, in a manner which ensures that the principles of separation are maintained.

5. Conscientious objection

No member of the medical or nursing staff should be under any duty to participate in research or therapy involving the fetus or fetal tissue if he or she has conscientious objection. This right of non-participation does not extend to the prior or subsequent care of a patient thus treated.

6. Ethics committees

All research or therapy of an innovative character involving the fetus or fetal tissue should be described in a protocol and be examined by an ethics committee. Projects should be subject to review until the validity of the procedure has been recognised by the committee as part of routine medical practice. The ethics committee has a duty to examine the progress of the research or innovative therapy (eg by receiving reports). It should have access to records and be able to confirm that the material is in fact being used for the purpose set out in the protocol. It should also be able to examine the record of any financial transactions involving fetal tissue. Before permitting research the ethics committee must satisfy itself:

(a) of the validity of the research or use proposed;
(b) that the objectives of the proposed use cannot be achieved in any other way;
(c) that the researchers or clinicians have the necessary facilities and skill.

7. Finance

There should be no monetary exchange for fetuses or fetal tissue. Profit from any dealing in fetal tissue or the other contents of the uterus is unethical.

References

FFMC (1989) *Code of Practice on the Use of Fetuses and Fetal Material in Research and Treatment* – Sections 1–7, CM 762. HMSO, London.

WARNOCK COMMITTEE (1984) *Report*, Cmnd 9314. HMSO, London.

Brief bibliography on various aspects of transplanting fetal tissue

The following bibliography offers a group of references on various topics that are covered only briefly in the other chapters of this book. It is meant to complement the contributions of the various authors, and is by no means intended as a comprehensive reference list on the use of fetal tissues in medicine. It is intended as a source of reading, offering recent references to those who may wish to follow up work or concepts that are not fully dealt with elsewhere. In general, the references that are given relate to authors who have not contributed to the present book.

The references were culled from various literature searches, and from general reading in libraries. The list presents work that is connected only with the grafting of fetal tissues for clinical purposes, or studies that are judged to be of significant value in improving the understanding and application of clinical work. Research on animals, or on the differentiation of fetal tissue, has not been included. The reference list is divided into seven sections, as follows: general reading; ethics; haemopoietic tissue; fetal liver (some of these references are relevant to haemopoietic tissue); brain tissue; pancreatic tissue; and other tissues.

General articles

DRUGAN, A., EVANS, W. J. & EVANS, M. I. (1989) Fetal organ and xenograft transplantation. *American Journal of Obstetrics & Gynecology*, **160**, 289–93.

(EDITORIAL) (1988) Fetuses and parkinsonism. *Nature*, **332**, 667.

(EDITORIAL) (1989) Using fetal tissue. *Nature*, **340**, 327–8.

(EDITORIAL) (1990) Tolerance and the fetal graft. *Lancet*, **336**, 538–9.

INNES, A., CUNNINGHAM, C., POWER, D. & CATTO, G. (1990) Tolerance and the fetal graft. *Lancet*, **336**, 1133.

JOHNSON, J. M. & ELIAS, S. (1988) Prenatal treatment: medical and gene therapy in the fetus. *Clinical Obstetrics & Gynecology*, **31**, 2, 390–407.

MARZUSCH, K., DIETL, J., HORNY, H. P., RUCK, P., KAISERLING, E., GRIESSER, H. & KABELITZ, D. (1991) Tolerance and the fetal graft. *Lancet*, **337**, 52.

NADLER, H. L. (1989) Fetal tissue transplantation (editorial). *American Journal of the Diseases of Childhood*, **143**, 149.

NOLAN, K. (1990) The use of embryo or fetus in transplantation: what there is to lose. *Transplantation Proceedings*, **22**, 1028–9.

TULIPAN, N. (1988) Brain transplants. A new approach to the therapy of neurodegenerative disease. *Clinics in Neurology*, **6**, 405–20.

Ethics

ANNAS, G. J. & ELIAS, S. (1989) The politics of human fetal tissue. *New England Journal of Medicine*, **320**, 1079–82.

CLARK, R. D., FLETCHER, J. & PETERSEN, G. (1989) Conceiving a fetus for bone marrow donation: an ethical problem in prenatal diagnosis. *Prenatal Diagnosis*, **9**, 329–34.

COUNCIL ON SCIENTIFIC AFFAIRS AND COUNCIL ON ETHICAL AND JUDICIAL AFFAIRS. (1990) Medical applications of fetal tissue transplantation. *Journal of the American Medical Association*, **263**, 565–70.

CULLITON, B. J. (1988) Panel backs fetal tissue research (news). *Science*, **242**, 1625–6.

DAFLER, C. E. (1989) Transplanting fetal tissue: how ethics and emotions interact. *Colorado Journal of Medicine*, **86**, 264.

DICKSON, D. (1989) Fetal tissue transplants win U.K. approval (news). *Science*, **245**, 464.

DOSSETOR, J. B. & STILLER, C. R. (1990) Ethics, justice, and commerce in transplantation. *Transplantation Proceedings*, **22**, 892–5.

EDER-RIEDER, M. A. (1990) Effects of 'the embryo protection law' on 'encapsulated' organ transplantation. *Beitrage zur Gerichtlichen Medizin*, **48**, 643–8.

EMBRYOS AND PARKINSON'S DISEASE (Ed.) (1988) *Lancet*, **i**, 1087.

FINE, A. (1988) The ethics of fetal tissue transplants. *Hastings Center Report*, **18**, 5–8.

FREEDMAN, B. (1989) Fetal tissue transplantation: politics, not policy. *Journal of the Canadian Medical Association*, **141**, 1230–2.

GILLON, R. (1988) Ethics of fetal brain cell transplants (editorial). *British Medical Journal*, **296**, 1212–13.

HU, Y. F., GU, Z. F., ZHANG, H. D. & YE, R. S. (1989) Fetal islet cell transplantation in China. *Transplantation Proceedings*, **21**, 2605–7.

JONSEN, A. R. (1988) Transplantation of fetal tissue: an ethicist's viewpoint. *Clinical Research*, **36**, 5–9.

KING, P. & AREEN, J. (1988) Legal regulation of fetal tissue transplantation. *Clinical Research*, **36**, 205–8.

LOWY, F. H. (1989) Fetal tissue transplantation: time for a Canadian policy. *Journal of the Canadian Medical Association*, **141**, 1227–9.

MAHOWALD, M. B. (1988) Placing wedges along a slippery slope: use of fetal neural tissue for transplantation. *Clinical Research*, **36**, 220–2.

MAHOWALD, M. B. (1989) Neural fetal tissue transplantation. Should we do what we can do? *Clinics in Neurology*, **7**, 754–7.

MAHOWALD, M. B., SILVER, J. & RATCHESON, R. A. (1987) The ethical options in transplanting fetal tissue. *Hastings Center Report*, **17**, 9–15.

MARWICK, C. (1988) Committee to be named to advise government about fetal tissue transplantation experiments (news). *Journal of the American Medical Association*, **239**, 3099.

NELSON, R. M. (1990) A policy concerning the therapeutic use of human fetal tissue in transplantation. *Western Journal of Medicine*, **132**, 447–8.

NOLAN, K. (1988) Genug ist genug: a fetus is not a kidney. *Hastings Center Report*, **18**, 13–19.

PALCA, J. (1989) Fetal tissue transplants remain off limits (news). *Science*, **246**, 752.

338

ROBERTSON, J. A. (1988) Rights, symbolism, and public policy in fetal tissue transplants. *Hastings Center Report*, **18**, 5–12.

ROBERTSON, J. A. (1990) The ethical acceptability of fetal tissue transplants. *Transplantation Proceedings*, **22**, 1025–7.

ROSNER, F., BENNETT, A. J., CASSELL, E. J., FARNSWORTH, P. B., LANDOLT, A. B., LOEB, L. NUMANN, P. J., ONA, F. V., RISEMBERG, H. M., SECHZER, P. H., *et al.* (1989) Fetal therapy and surgery. Fetal rights versus maternal obligations. *New York State Journal of Medicine*, **89**, 80–4.

SEIGER, A. (1988) Collection and use of aborted central nervous system material. Commendation and controversy. *Fetal Therapy*, **3**, 8–13.

THORNE, E. D. & MICHEJDA, M. (1989) Fetal tissue from spontaneous abortions; a new alternative for transplantation research? *Fetal Therapy*, **4**, 37–42.

TOURAINE, J. L. & TOURAINE, F. (1986) Fetal tissue transplantation: medical and ethical aspects. *Agressologie*, **27**, 771.

TUCH, B. E., DUNN, S. M. & DE VAHL-DAVIS, V. (1990) The effect on researchers of handling human fetal tissue. *Transplantation Proceedings*, **22**, 2109–10.

WALTERS, L. (1988) Ethical issues in fetal research: a look back and look forward. *Clinical Research*, **36**, 209–14.

Haemopoietic tissue

ALMAZOV, V. A., AFANAS-EV, B. V., SHATROV, V. A., ZUBAROVS-KAIA, L. S., EFIMOV. K. V., ZARITSKII, AIU & SIMBIRTSEVA, NIU. (1990) Effects of embryonal bone tissue on hemopoiesis. *Vestnik Akademii Meditsinskikh Nauk, USSR*, **930**, 37–41.

BHARGAVA, M., KARAK, A. K., SHARMA, S. & KOCHUPILLAI, V. (1987) Bone marrow recovery following fetal liver infusion (FLI) in aplastic anaemia: morphological studies. *Thymus*, **10**, 103–8.

BROXMEYER, H. E., DOUGLAS, G. W., HANGOC, G., COOPER, S., BARD, J., ENGLISH, D., ARNY, M., THOMAS, L. & BOYSE, E. A. (1989) Human umbilical cord blood as a potential source of transplantable hematopoietic stem/progenitor cells. *Proceedings of the National Academy of Sciences, USA*, **86**, 3828–33.

ENDE, N., RAMESHWAR, P. & ENDE, M. (1989) Fetal cord blood's potential for bone marrow transplantation. *Life Sciences*, **44**, 1987–90.

FETAL LIVER TRANSPLANTATION (1987) Developments in hematology and immunology. *Thymus*, **10**, 1–158.

GALE, R. P. (1987) Fetal liver transplantation in aplastic anemia and leukemia. *Thymus*, **10**, 89–94.

JEDRZEJCZAK, W. W. & POJDA, Z. (1987) Technique of preparation of hemopoietic cells of human fetal liver for transplantation. *Archives of Immunological and Experimental Therapy*, **35**, 71–8.

KELEMEN, E., JANOSSA, M., CALVO, W., FLIEDNER, T. M., BOFILL, M. & JANOSSY, G. (1987) What kind of morphologically recognizable haemopoietic cells do we inject when doing foetal liver infusion in man? *Thymus*, **10**, 33–44.

KOCHUPILLAI, V., SHARMA, S., FRANCIS, S., NANU, A., MATHEW, S., BHATIA, P., DUA, H., KUMAR, L., AGGARWAL, S., SINGH, S. *et al.* (1987) Fetal liver infusion in aplastic anaemia. *Thymus*, **10**, 95–102.

KOCHUPILLAI, V., SHARMA, S., FRANCIS, S., NANU, A., VERMA, I.

C., DUA, H., KUMAR, L., AGGARWAL, S. & SINGH, S. (1987) Fetal liver infusion in acute myelogenous leukaemia. *Thymus*, **10**, 117–24.

LINCH, D. C. & BRENT, L. (1989) Marrow transplantation. Can cord blood be used? (news). *Nature*, **340**, 676.

MEHRA, N. K., TANEJA, V., JHINGHON, B., CHAUDHURI, T., SHARMA, S. & KOCHUPILLAI, V. (1987) HLA status following fetal liver transplantation in aplastic anaemia and acute myeloid leukaemia. *Thymus*, **10**, 131–6.

NATHAN, D. G. (1989) The beneficence of neonatal hematopoiesis (editorial). *New England Journal of Medicine*, **321**, 1190–1.

PHAN, D. T., MIHALIK, R., BENCZUR, M., PALOCZI, K., GIDALI, J., FEHER, I., DOMOTORI, J., KISS, C., PETRANYI, G. G., NATONEK, K. *et al.* (1989) Human fetal liver as a valuable source of haemopoietic stem cells for allogeneic bone marrow transplantation. *Haematologia*, **22**, 25–35.

TOURAINE, J. L. (1983) European experience with fetal tissue transplantation in severe combined immunodeficiency (SCID). *Birth Defects*, **19**, 139–42.

TOURAINE, J. L., RAUDRANT, D., ROYO, C., REBAUD, A., BARBIER, F., RONCAROLO, M. G., TOURAINE, F., LAPLACE, S., GEBUHRER, L., BETUEL, H., *et al.* (1991) In utero transplantation of hemopoietic stem cells in humans. *Transplantation Proceedings*, **23**, 1706.

TOURAINE, J. L., RONCAROLO, M. G., ROYO, C. & TOURAINE, F. (1987) Fetal tissue transplantation, bone marrow transplantation and prospective gene therapy in severe immunodeficiencies and enzyme deficiencies. *Thymus*, **10**, 75–87.

TOURAINE, J. L., ROYO, C., RONCAROLO, M. B., MURRAY, K. & DE BOUTEILLER, O. (1989) Unmatched stem cell transplantation as a possible alternative to bone marrow transplantation. *Transplantation Proceedings*, **21**, 3112–13.

Fetal liver
(See also Haemopoietic tissue)

BHATIA, P., KOCHUPILLAI, V., MATHEW, S., MEHRA, N. K., NANU, A., JAYASURYAN, N., SHARMA, S., FRANCIS, S. & MENON, P. S. (1987) Studies on engraftment following fetal liver infusion. *Thymus*, **10**, 125–130.

GALE, R. P., TOURAINE, J. L. & KOCHUPILLAI, V. (1987) Synopsis and prospectives on fetal liver transplantation. *Thymus*, **10**, 1–4.

ROYO, C., TOURAINE, J. L., VEYRON, P. & AITOUCHE, A. (1987) Survey of experimental data on fetal liver transplantation. *Thymus*, **10**, 5–12.

TAFRA, L., BEREZNIAK, R. & DAFOE, D. C. (1990) Beneficial effects of fetal liver tissue on fetal pancreatic transplantation. *Surgery*, **108**, 734–40.

TOURAINE, J. L. (1983) Bone-marrow and fetal-liver transplantation in immunodeficiencies and inborn errors of metabolism: lack of significant restriction of T-cell function in long-term chimeras despite HLA-mismatch. *Immunological Reviews*, **71**, 103–21.

TOURAINE, J. L., GRISCELLI, C., BETUEL, H., DURANDY, A., BETEND, B. & SOUILLET, G. (1983) Chimerism following fetal liver transplantation: cell cooperation despite HLA mismatch. *Birth Defects*, **19**, 143–5.

WU, C. T. & YE, G. Y. (1987) Advances in experimental studies and clinical application of fetal liver cells. *Thymus*, **10**, 109–16.

Brain tissue

ABROUS, D. N., STINUS, L., LE MOAL, M. & HERMAN, J. P. (1990) Intra-accumbens implants of embryonic dopaminergic neurons reverse the behavioral supersensitivity to opiates evoked by lesion of the mesolimbic dopaminergic pathway. *Brain Research*, **525**, 155–9.

BLUNT, S. B. (1989) Fetal brain tissue and Parkinson's disease (letter). *Lancet*, **i**, 1021.

BREDESEN, D. E., HISANAGA, K. & SHARP, F. R. (1990) Neural transplantation using temperature-sensitive immortalized neural cells: a preliminary report. *Annals of Neurology*, **27**, 205–7.

BREEZE, R. E. (1990) Implanting fetal tissue to treat Parkinson's disease. *Western Journal of Medicine*, **153**, 543–4.

BRUNDIN, P., STRECKER, R. E., CLARKE, D. J., WIDNER, H., NILSSON, O. G., ASTEDT, B., LINDVALL, O. & BJORKLUND, A. (1988) Can human fetal dopamine neuron grafts provide a therapy for Parkinson's disease? *Progress in Brain Research*, **78**, 441–8.

DECKEL, A. W. & ROBINSON, R. G. (1986) Status marmoratus in fetal cortical transplants. *Experimental Neurology*, **91**, 212–8.

FETAL BRAIN GRAFTS AND PARKINSON'S DISEASE (Ed.) (1990) *Science*, **250**, 1434–5.

FREED, C. R., BREEZE, R. E., ROSENBERG, N. L., SCHNECK, S. A., WELLS, T. H., BARRETT, J. N., GRAFTON, S. T., HUANG, S. C., EIDELBERG, D. & ROTTENBERG, D. A. (1990) Transplantation of human fetal dopamine cells for Parkinson's disease. Results at 1 year. *Archives of Neurology*, **47**, 505–12.

GUSTAVII, B. (1989) Fetal brain transplantation for Parkinson's disease: technique for obtaining donor tissue (letter). *Lancet*, **i**, 565.

HITCHCOCK, E. R., CLOUGH, C., HUGHES, R. & KENNY, B. (1988) Embryos and Parkinson's disease (letter). *Lancet*, **i**, 1274.

HITCHCOCK, E. R. R., CLOUGH, C. G., HUGHES, R. C. & KENNY, B. (1989) Fetal brain tissue (letter). *Lancet*, **i**, 839.

LEES, A. J. (1989) Transplantation in Parkinson's disease (editorial). *British Journal of Hospital Medicine*, **42**, 261.

LIEBERMAN, A. N. (1988) The use of adrenal medullary and fetal grafts as treatment for Parkinson disease. *New York State Journal of Medicine*, **88**, 287–9.

LINDVALL, O. (1989) Transplantation into the human brain: present status and future possibilities. *Journal of Neurology, Neurosurgery & Psychiatry*, Supplement, 39–54.

LINDVALL, O., REHNCRONA, S., GUSTAVII, B., BRUNDIN, P., ASTEDT, B., WIDNER, H., LINDHOLM, T., BJORKLUND, A., LEENDERS, K. L., ROTHWELL, J. C., et al. (1988) Fetal dopamine-rich mesencephalic grafts in Parkinson's disease (letter). *Lancet*, **ii**, 1483–4.

LOPEZ-GARCIA, J. C., FERNANDEZ RUIZ, J., BERMUDEZ-RATTONI, F. & TAPIA, R. (1990) Correlation between acetylcholine release and recovery of conditioned taste aversion induced by fetal neocortex grafts. *Brain Research*, **523**, 105–10.

MacDONALD, A. S. (1990) Foetal neuroendocrine tissue transplantation for Parkinson's disease: an institutional review board faces the ethical dilemma. *Transplantation Proceedings*, **22**, 1030–2.

MADRAZO, I., FRANCO-BOURLAND, R., OSTROSKY-SOLIS, F., AGUILERA, M., CUEVAS, C., ZAMORANO, C., MORELOS, A., MAGALLON, E. & GUIZAR-SAHAGUN, G. (1990) Fetal homotransplants (ventral mesencephalon and adrenal tissue) to the striatum of parkinsonian subjects. *Archives of Neurology*, **47**, 1281–5.

MADRAZO, I., LEON, V., TORRES, C., AGUILERA, M. C., VARELA, G., ALVAREZ, F., FRAGA, A., DRUCKER-COLIN, R., OSTROSKY, F., SKUROVICH, M., *et al.* (1988) Transplantation of fetal substantia nigra and adrenal medulla to the caudate nucleus in two patients with Parkinson's disease (letter). *New England Journal of Medicine*, **318**, 51.

MAHOWALD, M. B., AREEN, J., HOFFER, B. J., JONSEN, A. R., KING, P., SILVER, J. SLADEK, J. R., Jr & WALTERS, L. (1987) Transplantation of neural tissue from fetuses (letter). *Science*, **235**, 1037–8.

MELAMED, E. (1988) Brain grafting may reverse loss of responsiveness to levodopa therapy in Parkinson's disease. *Clinical Neuropharmacology*, **11**, 77–82.

MELONI, R. & GALE, K. (1990) Pharmacological evidence for feedback regulation of dopamine metabolism in solid fetal substantia nigra transplants. *Journal of Pharmacology and Experimental Therapy*, **253**, 1259–64.

MICHEJDA, M. (1987) Treatment of Parkinson's disease in adult patients by transplantation of human fetal brain tissue obtained from elective abortions. *Fetal Therapy*, **2**, 129–34.

PEARCE, J. M. (1988) Adrenal and nigral transplants for Parkinson's disease. *British Medical Journal*, **296**, 1211–12.

PERLOW, M. J. (1987) Brain grafting as a treatment for Parkinson's disease. *Neurosurgery*, **20**, 335–42.

SILANI, V., PEZZOLI, G., MOTTI, E., FERRANTE, C., FALINI, A., PIZZUTI, A., ZECCHINELLI, A., MOGGIO, M., BUSCAGLIA, M. & SCARLATO, G. (1988) Characterization of purified populations of human fetal chromaffin cells: considerations for grafting in parkinsonian patients. *Progress in Brain Research*, **78**, 551–7.

TEMLETT, J. A. (1990) Transplantation, fetuses and Parkinson's disease (editorial). *South African Medical Journal*, **78**, 710–71.

WIDNER, H., BRUNDIN, P., REHNCRONA, S., GUSTAVII, B., FRACKOWIAK, R., LEENDERS, K. L., SAWLE, G., ROTHWELL, J. C., MARSDEN, C. D., BJORKLUND, A., *et al.* (1991) Transplanted allogeneic fetal dopamine neurons survive and improve motor function in idiopathic Parkinson's disease. *Transplantation Proceedings*, **23**, 793–5.

Pancreatic tissue

FARKAS, G. & KARACSONYI, S. (1985) Clinical transplantation of fetal human pancreatic islets. *Biomedica Biochimica Acta*, **44**, 155–9.

FARKAS, G., KARACSONYI, S., SZABO, M. & KAISER, G. (1987) Results of cultured fetal pancreatic islet transplantation in juvenile diabetic patients. *Transplantation Proceedings*, **19**, 2352–3.

FORMBY, B., WALKER, L. & PETERSON, C. M. (1986) Rapid selection of viable transplantable human fetal pancreatic islets by trypan blue exclusion. *Proceedings of the Society for Experimental Biology & Medicine*, **182**, 245–7.

GRAY, D. W. & MORRIS, P. J. (1987) Developments in isolated pancreatic islet transplantation. *Transplantation*, **43**, 321–31.

HELLERSTROM, C., ANDERSSON, A., KORSGREN, O., JANSSON, L. & SANDLER, S. (1989) Aspects of pancreatic islet transplantation in diabetes mellitus. *Baillieres Clinical Gastroenterology*, **3**, 851–63.

HU, Y. F., CHENG, R. L., SHAO, A. H., YE, R. S., GU, Z. F., ZHANG. H. D., ZHANG, Z. G., HEN, L. R., BI, H. F. & SHI, G. F. (1989) The influences of islet transplantation on metabolic abnormalities and diabetic complications. *Hormone and Metabolic Research*, **21**, 198–202.

HU, Y. F., ZHANG, H., ZHANG, H. D., SHAO, A. H., LI, L. X., ZHOU, H. Q., ZHAO, B. H. & ZHOU, Y. G. (1985) Culture of human fetal pancreas and islet transplantation in 24 patients with type 1 diabetes mellitus. *Chinese Medical Journal*, **98**, 236–43.

HULLETT, D. A., BETHKE, K. P., LANDRY, A. S., LEONARD, D. K. & SOLLINGER, H. W. (1989) Successful long-term cryopreservation and transplantation of human fetal pancreas. *Diabetes*, **38**, 448–53.

HULLETT, D. A., FALANY, J. L., LOVE, R. B., BURLINGHAM, W. J., PAN, M. & SOLLINGER, H. W. (1987) Human fetal pancreas – a potential source for transplantation. *Transplantation*, **43**, 18–22.

HULLETT, D. A., FALANY, J. L., LOVE, R. B., BUTLER, J. A. & SOLLINGER, H. W. (1987) Human fetal pancreas: potential for transplantation. *Transplantation Proceedings*, **19**, 909–10.

JOVANOVIC-PETERSON, L., WILLIAMS, K., BRENNAN, M., RASH-BAUM, W. & PETERSON, C. M. (1989) Studies of human fetal pancreatic allografts in diabetic recipients without immunosuppression. *Journal of Diabetic Complications*, **3**, 107–12.

KONDRATIEV, Y. Y., SADOVNIKOVA, N. V., PETROVA, G. N., FEDOTOV, V. P., BLJUMKIN, V. N., IGNATENKO, S. N. & PANKOV, Y. A. (1989) Islet cell transplantation in type I diabetes mellitus: evaluation of humoral immune response. *Experimental and Chemical Endocrinology*, **93**, 147–50.

KHUN, F., WACHS, J. H., RUCKERT, J., SETTMACHER, U., SCHULZ, H. J., MATTHES, G., BOLLMANN, R., HAHN, H. J., RATZMANN, K. P. & WOLFF, H. (1990) Tissue bank of human fetal pancreas. *Transplantation Proceedings*, **22**, 683–4.

LACY, P. E. & SCHARP, D. W. (1986) Islet transplantation in treating diabetes. *Annual Review of Medicine*, **37**, 33–40.

LAFFERTY, K. J., HAO, L., BABCOCK, S. K. & SPEES, E. (1989) Is there a future for fetal pancreas transplantation? *Transplantation Proceedings*, **21**, 2611–13.

LISSING, J. R., TUCH, B. E. & SURANYI, M. G. (1988) The use of gliotoxin in human fetal pancreas transplantation. *Transplantation Proceedings*, **20**, 76–8.

MORRIS, P. J., GRAY, D. W. & SUTTON, R. (1989) Pancreatic islet transplantation. *British Medical Bulletin*, **45**, 224–41.

MULLEN, Y., CLARE-SALZLER, M., STEIN, E. & CLARK, W. (1989) Islet transplantation for the cure of diabetes. *Pancreas*, **4**, 123–35.

PETERSON, C. M., JOVANOVIC-PETERSON, L., FORMBY, B., GON-

DOS, B., MONDA, L. M., WALKER, L., RASHBAUM, W. & WIL-
LIAMS, K. (1989) Human fetal pancreas transplants. *Journal of Diabetic Complications*, **3**, 27–34.

ROBERTSON, R. P., LAFFERTY, K. J. HAUG, C. E. & WEIL, R., 3rd (1987) Effect of human fetal pancreas transplantation on secretion of C-peptide and glucose tolerance in type I diabetics. *Transplantation Proceedings*, **19**, 2354–6.

SHIOGAMA, T., MULLEN, Y., KLANDORF, H., TERADA, M. & CLARK, W. R. (1987) An improved cryopreservation procedure for human fetal pancreas tissues. *Transplantation*, **44**, 602–7.

SHUMAKOV, V. I., BLJUMKIN, V. N., IGNATENKO, S. N., SKA-LETSKY, N. N., SLOVESNOVA, T. A. & BABIKOVA, R. A. (1987) The principal results of pancreatic islet cell culture transplantation in diabetes mellitus patients. *Transplantation Proceedings*, **19**, 2372.

SIMONSEN, R., DAWIDSON, I., AGGARWAL, S., DILLER, K. R., RAJOTTE, R., COORPENDER, L. & ABSHIER, D. (1987) Intraportal transplantation of cryopreserved human fetal pancreata. *Transplantation Proceedings*, **19**, 2365–7.

TUCH, B. E., GRIGORIOU, S. & TURTLE, J. R. (1988) Long-term passage of human fetal pancreas in non-diabetic nude mice fails to allow maturation of the response to glucose. *Transplantation Proceedings*, **20**, 64–7.

TUCH, B. E. & LENORD, K. A. (1989) Time required for grafted human fetal pancreas to reverse diabetes is dependent on the amount of tissue implanted. *Transplantation Proceedings*, **21**, 3801–2.

TUCH, B. E. & LENORD, K. A. (1989) Insulin is advantageous to the growth of human fetal pancreas after its implantation. *Transplantation Proceedings*, **21**, 3803–4.

TUCH, B. E., SHEIL, A. G., NG, A. B. & TURTLE, J. R. (1986) Long-term survival of human fetal pancreatic tissue transplanted into an insulin dependent diabetic patient. *Diabetic Medicine*, **3**, 24–8.

TUCH, B. E., SHEIL, A. G., NG, A. B. & TURTLE, J. R. (1986) Transplantation of cultured human fetal pancreas into insulin-dependent diabetic humans. *Transplantation Proceedings*, **18**, 260–3.

TUCH, B. E., SHEIL, A. R., NG, A. B. & TURTLE, J. R. (1987) Experience with human fetal pancreatic allografts over a three-year period. *Transplantation Proceedings*, **19**, 2357.

YDERSTROEDE, K. B. (1987) Pancreatic islet transplantation. Experimental and clinical aspects. *Danish Medical Bulletin*, **34**, 323–9.

Other tissues

ASPENBERG, P. & ANDOLF, E. (1989) Bone induction by fetal and adult human bone matrix in athymic rats. *Acta Orthopaedica Scandinavica*, **60**, 195–9.

HAN, J. Q. & LIANG, R. X. (1987) Fetal cartilage graft in periodontal disease. *Chinese Medical Journal*, **100**, 429–30.

HINDERER, U. T. & ESCALONA, J. (1990) Dermal and subdermal tissue filling with fetal connective tissue and cartilage, collagen, and silicone: experimental study in the pig compared with clinical results. A new technique of dermis mini-autograft injections. *Aesthetic Plastic Surgery*, **14**, 239–48.

MAYUMI, M., KIMATA, H., SUEHIRO, Y., HOSOI, S., ITO, S., KUGE, Y., SHINOMIYA, K. & MIKAWA, H. (1989) DiGeorge syndrome with hypogammaglobulinaemia: a patient with excess suppressor T cell activity treated with fetal thymus transplantation. *European Journal of Pediatrics*, **148**, 518–22.

YAN, Z. B., BING, Z. X., YANG, W. R. & LONG, W. L. (1990) A study of cadaveric fetal adrenal used for adrenal transplantation to treat Addison's disease: thirteen cases reported. *Transplantation Proceedings*, **22**, 280–2.

Index

DATE DUE

L-2971 due 3/27/96		
OC 9 '97		
APR 0 5 1999		
MAR 2 9 2000		
APR 0 2 2001		